P9-CQC-553

FEELING STRONG

ETHEL S. PERSON, M.D.

FEELING

The Achievement of
Authentic Power

STRONG

WILLIAM MORROW An *Imprint of* HarperCollins*Publishers*

HarperCollins books may be purchased for educational, business,
or sales promotional use. For information please write:
Special Markets Department, HarperCollins Publishers Inc.,
10 East 53rd Street, New York, NY 10022.

FIRST EDITION

Designed by Kate Nichols

Printed on acid-free paper

Library of Congress Cataloging-in-Publication Data
Person, Ethel Spector.
Feeling strong : the achievement of authentic power /
Ethel S. Person.—1st ed.
p.   cm.
ISBN 0-688-17577-5 (alk. paper)
1. Control (Psychology) 2. Interpersonal relations.
3. Meaning (Psychology) I. Title.
BF611 .P47 2002
158—dc21   2002023893

02   03   04   05   06   WBC/BVG   10   9   8   7   6   5   4   3   2   1

In loving memory of my parents,

Anna Zimmerman Spector and Louis Spector,

who gave me the freedom to pursue

love and power

Contents

Introduction

Who has power and how best to achieve and wield it have long been questions about which most of us display a healthy interest. Look on any bestseller list and there you will likely find one or more books on the subject of power. Most of them focus on how to achieve worldly power, giving us detailed instructions in the neo-Machiavellian techniques of dreaming and scheming our way up the corporate or entrepreneurial ladder. *The 48 Laws of Power*, published in 1998 and reviewed as "rules for suits," is a good example of this venerable tradition—a collection of prescriptions for attaining and wielding power, as exemplified by some of its most noted practitioners, from Sun Tzu and von Clausewitz to Swifty Lazar and Henry Kissinger.

Then there are the multitudes of books that depict the powerful while not explicitly telling us how to join their ranks—the biographies of great men (and occasional women) of destiny, the stories of extreme ambition brought to success or ruin, pop novels with titles like *Total Power* and *Absolute Control*, all the Mafia "godfather" sagas. Many of these books are nothing more than a kind of dreamy pornography of power, showing it at its most glamorous and dangerous, luring us in.

Not that we need to be lured. Our fascination with power goes back to the ancient myths depicting humankind's struggle to take on the powers, prerogatives, and perks of the gods—Prometheus stealing fire from heaven, Hercules performing his twelve labors, Eve persuading Adam to eat from the Tree of Knowledge. Indeed, the longing for power—whether it is acquiring secret knowledge, wresting magical control over our fate, or even securing immortality—is so ancient in our history that it's easy to conclude that the longing for power is hot wired into our psyches.

Despite the depth and duration of our interest in power, many of us feel ambivalent if not downright uncomfortable about its pursuit. The whiff of evil we catch when the subject of power is in the air comes from one particular conception of power—as the drive for dominance over other people or, in its most extreme form, as an overriding, often ruthless lust for total command and control. And it is true that this lust for interpersonal power may be extreme and its possession abused. However, dominance over others is not all there is to power. We misunderstand its true nature if we see it only as the assertion of blunt force operative in the lives of others—the politicians and business leaders who seem to be in charge or the rich and famous who monopolize the headlines—while failing to acknowledge the central role it plays in everyone's life. In the most general way, power can be defined as our ability to produce an effect, to make something that we want to happen actually take place.

Power issues are a part of all of life's activities and are key to our inner lives as well. As the psychoanalyst Rollo May observed, ". . . power is not a theory but an ever-present reality which we must confront, use, enjoy, and struggle with a hundred times a day."[1] Even those who are not gripped by any desire to command or control must, nonetheless, deal with power issues from infancy to old age. We all have a stake in possessing power, using it, understanding it, and negotiating it. This holds true not just in managing or mediating our sex and love lives, our family lives and friendships, and our work relationships with our peers, subordinates, and superiors, but also in seeking to realize our dreams, whether in the pursuit of our ambitions (many of which are solitary rather than joint endeavors), in the expression of our creative impulses, or in our need to identify with or participate in something that takes us beyond our daily lives. The true heart of power is two-chambered; it comprises both our ability to negotiate relationships and our ability to initiate independent goal-oriented

interpersonal power → ability to negotiate relationships
personal power → ability to initiate independent goal-oriented activities .

INTRODUCTION \ xi

activities—two different, complementary capacities that I call, respectively, interpersonal power and personal power.

We can see these two aspects of power in even the youngest children. The little boy wants to control his mother; he wants her *now*, wants her to play with him, to stroke him, to take him out to the park. And to get what he wants, he uses all the ploys at his disposal to persuade her, cajole her, and plead with her. But he also wants to prove to himself and others that he can build a big sand castle without help and climb up the highest sliding board all by himself. In other words, he wants to test and to assert his mastery of his own little world. This latter effort is what I call *personal power*, distinguishing it from the boy's wish to exert *interpersonal power*, to persuade, influence, or force someone else to bend to his will.

Describing interpersonal power is easier than describing personal power. We are born into a power grid called a family, and it is in that intimate context that we first learn about the power differentials among people. All power relationships, all desires either to dominate or submit, have their psychological roots in the fact that we were once little children with big parents, and their existential roots in our feeling of being small people in an out-of-control big world that we need to be able to tame. Our response to these issues is to want either to be like our parent figures or to charm and disarm them—and this is true not just in the intimate realm but also in our work and social lives.

We have all thought about what we need to do in our relationships in order to get our way, and we know what it feels like to submit to someone else's will. We know, too, about power struggles. Minor disagreements can erupt into fierce battles, whether among schoolchildren, in an academic faculty, or in a political party. And we know that when there is a contest for dominance, the outcome depends in some measure on how assertive and aggressive the players are and sometimes on how cunning they are.

We are so accustomed to using power to mean dominance, that depending on who we are and who we are judging, we have a ready-made evaluation which we describe as "powerful." Most of us can intuit who holds the power in any given situation. When we make the judgment that someone is powerful, we are generally referring to the strength or clout a person wields in a particular situation—clout being the capacity to pull strings, to make things happen. We appear to have software that preconsciously categorizes people as "powerful" if they are both strong and active. And, depending on who is judging, that designation is either very good or very bad.

There are powerful people and not so powerful people, and given a list, say, of a hundred names, we could probably select the twenty most powerful, the twenty least powerful, and the great middle with some reliability from one rater to the next. In this context, power is inevitably hierarchical. But—and this is the important point—the list is always subject to change. Some such lists actually exist—for example, the yearly list of the most important people in the entertainment industry or the list of the best dressed women. When someone is added to the list, another person is dropped. So, too, in the political world. Bush won his fight to be President—now he's in and Gore is out. And so forth.

The same kind of evaluation can be made among friends and associates. If we know the same people, we would probably come up with lists of the most powerful and least powerful that would not vary much. But this list, too, would be subject to change. Larry has just lost his job, Betty just married a Broadway producer, and Ralph has finally finished his residency at Mount Sinai—changes, changes, changes. If someone in the group wants tickets to a hot new show, Betty suddenly becomes a powerful friend; Ralph can be tapped for medical advice; and Larry—well, perhaps we never thought too much of Larry to begin with. The point, of course, is twofold: power is context-related and we're very sensitive to shifts in the winds of power.

We live in several different power grids simultaneously, and we exert different kinds of power depending on which one we're in. Children are dependent on adults, and this dictates the inevitability of the family structure, which is, in significant ways, the model for the hierarchical structure of larger organizations that distinguish between leaders and followers, dominants and submissives.

Even when power is intensely personal—as it is in a family—it may be intensely political. For example, a younger son's goal may be to best or unseat his older brother. A beautiful daughter knows how to melt her father's opposition on cue. Family power is also tacitly ideological; the child's obedience to his or her parents is ratified by the biblical injunction to "honor thy father and thy mother that thy days may be long" upon this earth. And until the 1960s, the husband's traditional dominance over his wife seemed to be sanctioned by the belief that woman was the weaker vessel. Similarly, social power and organizational and political power get connected to a system of ideas or philosophy. The political theorist Adolph Berle emphasizes that "Absent such a system or philosophy, the institutions essential to power cease to be reliable, power ceases to be effective, and the power holder is eventually displaced."[2] While some form of control and command is necessary to the stability of social organizations, including families, what gives groups their staying power is some kind of shared belief system that legitimates them.

As for personal power, or agency, it is enacted when the little boy wants to build his sand castle, the young woman seeks to scale a mountain, or the old man is set on mastering a third language. This is the power of self-expression and mastery. It does not necessitate mediating power with others; rather, it is an expression of personal will.

Agency encompasses self-assertion, the ability to choose the direction that our lives take, to control our time and how we use our minds and bodies. The desire for this kind of self-determination is apparent very early in life, and it generally stays with us till the end of life. It takes form in the most basic of ways—for example, it is expressed when we decide what and when to eat—as well as the most complex ways, such as seeking control over the degree and kind of life-prolonging medical care we are willing to accept.

In addition, agency encompasses our control over animals and inanimate matter. This kind of personal power may seem insignificant at first glance, compared with other kinds of personal power—that is, until we remember that our species' development as social beings was jump started by the taming and domestication of wild animals and that our control of the physical world could not have developed without our intimate knowledge of inanimate matter and physical forces.

In our exercise of personal agency, however, an interpersonal component is almost always at play. Positive identification with someone who is himself or herself independent—whether a beloved parent, someone we know, someone we observe from afar, or someone we have merely read about or seen in a movie, for example—can facilitate our achievement of a sustained sense of self-control and mastery. At the same time, we may be discouraged if our efforts are depreciated by a naysayer. Sometimes we assert pseudo autonomy early in life as a response to an absent or undependable parent. In other cases, we may be robbed of our chance to achieve authentic personal power gradually if we are prematurely forced to take on an adult role that leaves us with an underlying sense of weakness or resentment.

Individual acts of personal power well up from the unconscious as often as they are deliberately enacted. In 1928, at a time of mounting crisis in Europe, the essayist and critic Walter Benjamin observed: "These are days when no one should rely unduly on his 'competence.' Strength lies in improvisation. All the decisive blows are struck left-handed."[3] For Sigmund Freud, the individual possesses "a scrap of independence and originality" only to the degree that he can escape from what we would now call groupthink or conformity.[4] That is, personal power is contingent on our ability to trust to our instincts and hunches and so doing to express our deepest selves.

will?

We might think of personal power as akin to willpower. Willpower is to self-control, self-determination, and agency what the will to power is to the control of other people. Yet the term *will* is not altogether applicable in either instance. While we sometimes assert our power with conscious intent, more often our intent first reveals itself to us in our actions. Taken together, personal and interpersonal power constitute the sometimes elusive capacity to write our own life stories.

AS A PSYCHIATRIST AND PSYCHOANALYST, I am frequently forced to think about power explicitly, although it is seldom discussed in any course work nor is it a major topic in mental health journals. Yet every conversation I have with patients touches on their feelings of powerlessness or of power run amok—even if they do not explicitly identify those feelings as such. They complain of their failure to act, to apply themselves to a project, to get a promotion; of their inability to control their weight, their calendar, or their children; of their fear of being unable to fall in love or their fear of being swept away; of their hesitancy in confronting disagreements or of hastiness in acting out angry impulses. These problems, among others, are intimately tied to issues of power and powerlessness.

I remember vividly two psychotherapy patients who gave me a crash course in power. The year I finished my psychiatric training, instead of taking August as the standard therapist's holiday, I stayed in the city so that I could pick up a little extra income by covering some senior psychiatrists' practices. A few of the patients who call in while their regular therapist is away want only to have prescriptions refilled or other minor help, but most are in great distress.

My first call was from Eve, who was in a suicidal depression. I began seeing her every day and also talked to her regularly between sessions. A mental health professional herself, Eve knew all the buttons to push to alarm me, and she pushed them so skillfully that I felt compelled to answer her middle-of-the-night calls, sometimes several times a night. She also used an emergency telephone signal, intended only for acute crises, to alert me to an emergency during my therapeutic hours with other patients.

One of my ongoing patients, Mark, whose sessions she broke into several times, had been diagnosed as what was then called a psychopath. A young man of great charm and slickness, Mark had made stacks of money by renting apartments in very elegant buildings and then illegally subletting them at inflated prices to pimps, who otherwise would not have been able to operate in such tony neighborhoods. But he was in a panic because his lavish spending had prevented him from paying some of the rent bills, and the landlords were harassing the pimps, disrupting business at the apartments, and causing the pimps to threaten his life if he didn't pay up. To find a safe haven, he wanted to be hospitalized. I shared the same goal, but for different reasons, my naive hope was that forced inactivity might help him identify some of his underlying problems. While I waited for him to be admitted, he came in regularly, only to have his sessions broken into by Eve, whose calls he greatly resented. Finally Mark cheerfully explained to me that she was not in real danger but was simply manipulating me, probably hoping that I would call her regular psychiatrist, interrupting his vacation. Not convinced, I challenged him: "How do you know she's not in danger?" He replied, "Because if she was really going to kill herself she wouldn't call so frequently." An expert at manipulation, Mark knew it when he saw it. And how was I to handle this situation? "Well," Mark told me, "you had better set limits and refuse to see her until she stops calling."

Having delivered this invaluable advice, which I subsequently took and which proved entirely successful, he promptly went into the bathroom, threw up, and then left for home. I was left to clean up the mess, as I pondered some of the complexities of power and powerlessness. One small mystery is why Mark needed to throw up. Having empowered me to deal with my suicidal patient, he apparently needed to disempower me vis-à-vis himself, casting me as the mommy who had to clean up after her bad little boy. He could never give without taking away, perhaps replicating some interaction from his early life or redressing some injustice he felt he had experienced then.

Eve and I survived the summer, as did Mark, whose intervention was helpful not only to me but also to its target. Years later I learned from her regular psychiatrist that Eve went on to have a successful career and a relatively happy marriage to a man who didn't mind being controlled by her periodic bouts of manipulation. And I eventually managed to get Mark admitted to a hospital, where he promptly organized a patient government, which survived long often his stay, tyrannizing the staff for years to come. Alas for Mark, despite his great insight into interpersonal processes and manipulation, he had virtually no self-knowledge. He was unable to give up the rush of adrenaline and excitement his scams brought him. He lost his wife, and when last heard from was still living in the havoc that invariably followed in his wake.

Of course, what transpired during that long hot month had to do with my inexperience and my never having adequately contemplated the mechanics of interpersonal processes. It was also the last August I ever spent in New York City.

But I did learn several things about power. From Eve I learned how manipulation propelled by weakness distances others and depletes the self. As for Mark, despite his shrewd insights into people and how to play them, his life drifted irretrievably downhill, a common fate for those with his kind of problem. He had mastered certain power gambits—how to read other people, how to bend them to his way of thinking, how to prosper financially—but ultimately what he lacked was any sense of internal coherence, self-control, or conscious awareness of the long-term consequences of his destructive and self-destructive behavior (for example, spending the pimps' money instead of paying the rent). He was comfortable only "in action," whether a particular action served him well or ill. Doomed to live only in the moment, he never calculated the consequences of his behavior. Though a veritable master of interpersonal power plays, he lacked authentic power—a sense of being comfortable and content within himself. Like all of us, he was motivated by forces of which he was unaware: in his case, by destructiveness and self-destructiveness.

OUR PUSH TO EXERT POWER is wired in, instinctual. But as we become more and more self-aware, power enters into our mental lives as part of our motivational system, whether conscious or preconscious. Our longing, our need for power, is nourished, paradoxically, by the weakness that is our common lot. While feelings of weakness and helplessness can be intensified by unfortunate circumstances or by neurotic conflict, they are also an ineluctable part of the human condition, based on the total dependency we experience in infancy and the terrible knowledge of mortality we acquire in adolescence if not before. Just as gnawing are our fears and the day-to-day frustrations of our intimate lives and our work lives. We worry about financial security and health. We fret about small inconveniences and mishaps—missing the bus, burning the dinner, wondering why our adolescent son forgot to check in when he was supposed to. To deal with the inevitable setbacks of daily life, we must have inner resources that can counter negative events and preserve our sense that life is worthwhile. Such inner resources constitute one or another form of interpersonal or personal power. Without these resources we come to feel anxious, cheated, angry, or depressed. ← symptoms of lack of authentic power

Although it's a much visited (if sometimes inadequately theorized) subject in philosophy, political science, and sociology, power has been largely neglected by psychology and psychoanalysis—with the exception of a few psychoanalysts, foremost among them Alfred Adler, Erich Fromm, and Rollo May.

Far from being esoteric, power is the stuff of everyday life. Yet with all the pop-psychological talk of "personal empowerment," we have yet to fully address the issue of experiencing ourselves as authentically powerful and of realizing genuine self-worth. Psychoanalysts do talk about omnipotence, but generally in terms that depict its expression in adulthood as a pathological regression to the infant's fantasy of omnipotence. Yet they fail to theorize the concept of authentic power.

Authentic power encompasses the ability to face adversity, to overcome fear and inhibitions, to be sufficiently in touch with our inner lives that we are able to genuinely express ourselves and chart our life's direction, to be open to a range of interpersonal relationships, to be assertive without being confrontational, and to create meaning in our lives.

To understand ourselves, we must come to know just what kind of power we personally aspire to—competence as lover, parent, or friend; command of a kitchen, a lectern, or a business; mastery of a skill; or possession of convictions or religious beliefs that provide meaning in our lives. Whatever it is, we can generally achieve it only through a process of psychological development, often involving a power struggle. Those power struggles we engage in may be wholly internal (for example, a psychological conflict between our wish to be assertive and our fear of being punished for assertiveness) or may be played out with adversaries who are sometimes our nearest and dearest.

When we think about power and its distortions, it is impossible to ignore ethical considerations. There is an inherent conflict—some have called it an unbridgeable gulf—between the demands of most Western religions and the natural impulse to act in one's own interest. As the political scientist Hans Morgenthau put it: "Christian ethics demand love, humility, the abnegation of self; Man as a natural creature seeks the aggrandizement of the self through pride and power."[5] The best one can do is to try to narrow the gap between ethical injunctions and one's own conduct. Self-abnegation is not the solution. Ethicists argue that we must regard ourselves as equal in value but not superior to any other individual. While the rewards that come from behaving ethically may be less clear-cut than those of pragmatic politics or psychological insights, the power of taking a moral stance may allow us to enjoy our real achievements. Taking shortcuts on the road to power can often leave us feeling, if not guilty, then less than true to ourselves and thus less deserving of our achievements than we would otherwise feel.

Many of us, including some psychoanalysts, view anger as primarily maladaptive or destructive, not accounting for the downside should we fail to experience or express it. In the same way, we sometimes view the exercise of power as nothing more than a dangerous contaminant in our lives. Often, the use of power *is* corrupt—whites against blacks, men against women, rich against poor, the ruling class against the proletariat, imperial powers against colonies. But apart from its corrupt forms, power is as essential to the stability of personal relationships and family structure as it is to the body politic. In fact, the precise disposition of power in a given family inevitably shapes a child's emerging personality and leaves an indelible stamp on how he or she views power as an adult. Intimate relationships cannot endure without a workable balance of power.

Power, like anger, has many constructive, adaptive dimensions. In fact, I would suggest that weakness is more likely than power to be bad, because the inability to exert power—as a result of psychological or external factors—can become the most corrosive force in our lives. Many abuses of power—for example, acts of untriggered violence—are perpetrated not only by those who are disenfranchised but also by those who may appear powerful but experience themselves as weak, vulnerable, and isolated.

Political scientists, ethologists, sociologists, and organizational psychologists are all theoreticians of power, but their focus on hierarchies often restricts their analyses to issues of domination and submission. Some argue that extending the definition of power beyond such considerations would make power a concept so general as to be meaningless. However, my observations about the reasons patients seek therapy lead me to disagree. *← argument from personal experience* ,

In our personal lives, many of us feel ensnared, unable to change or improve our relationships or initiate new ones because we fear confrontation or confuse assertion with aggression. In our work or professional lives, we may feel stuck, unable to act, trapped, paralyzed, or inhibited by fear, depression, or a depreciated sense of our capacities. We often describe ourselves as impotent, and not just in the sexual sphere. Resolving these problems ultimately entails issues of power, whether in our ability to effect the changes we seek or to open new avenues to self-governance.

Bertrand Russell wrote an entire book "to prove that the fundamental concept in social science is Power in the same sense in which Energy is the fundamental concept in physics."[6] I make the more modest claim that power is a central concept in self-understanding and that it needs to be integrated into our theories of the mind. This book is about how power, in its various forms and disguises, permeates our lives. It is about power's uses and abuses, its illusions and realities, its fragility despite its appearance of immutability. The fundamental power motives that drive us are often veiled, remote from our consciousness, even while they are central to our daily lives. I will redefine and elaborate what constitutes individual power in a way that illuminates its positive effects on our lives, focusing not only on the power strategies and tactics we bring to bear in our personal relationships but also on self-governance—self-control, mastery, creativity, and agency—and on our need for transcendental pursuits.

I will use power as a prism through which to view aspects of human relationships and aspirations, and vice versa. The first section addresses the anatomy of power, what it is and the sources from which it flows. The second and third sections, respectively, treat interpersonal power and personal power as separate domains that meet different fundamental needs, although, as will become abundantly clear, they intersect all the time. The reason this is so resides in our earliest lives: we learn about intimacy with our mother and father at the same time that we are seeking independence—learning to feed ourselves, to walk, to escape control or turn our back in anger. How we fare in either domain ultimately impacts the other. I will conclude with our need to seek meaning in our lives, whether through transcendence or some other modality, as key to what I view as authentic power.

To find something that matters; to live at a higher pitch; to feel inner certainty; to find a personality of one's own and effectively plot one's own life story—these are the forms of power I will explore. These aspects will become visible through stories, vignettes, and observations drawn from life, literature, clinical practice, and research findings, and in the process will point the way to a self-empowerment that is broader and more deeply fulfilling than what is so often touted in pop psychology. To achieve and maintain such empowerment always entails struggle. Power is never achieved once and for all, never possessed with any degree of finality. The possession of authentic power is an ongoing process.

PART

Power and
Powerlessness

ONE

I

Seeking Authentic Power

"We are lived by powers we pretend
to understand"

—W. H. AUDEN, "In Memory of Ernst Toller"

What constitutes power, who has it, where it comes from, and how it is played out in the real world are much more complicated matters than we generally think. Our desire for power is often far from transparent, our longing for it deeply rooted in the mysteries of our existence such as Auden captures in his remarkable phrase, "We are lived by powers we pretend to understand." Power originates from a deep psychological source, from the very center of the self.

But what exactly is power? The word derives from the Latin *posse*, "to be able." As the dictionary defines it, power is the ability to mobilize, "the strength and potency to accomplish something . . . the vital energy to make choices and decisions."[1] While some people restrict the meaning of power to dominance, the ability to compel the obedience of others, power is more fundamentally the ability to act, to effect whatever goal we have in mind. It is the vehicle through which we exert some measure of control over the course of our own lives, but the way we express it takes many forms.

The essence of power is found in the phrase the *power to* do something not—as commonly thought—in the phrase the *power over* someone else. John O. Whitney, a management consultant, catches its protean character: "Power is a freighted idea, filled with shifting cargo: power to build, power to tear down; power to hasten, power to delay; power to inspire, power to frighten; power to give, power to withhold; power to love, power to hurt; power to do good, power to do evil."[2] It is the ability to say "yes" or "no," to act or refuse to act, to make things happen or to keep something from happening.

Power is the ability to exert command over the self. Self-control encompasses control of our voluntary actions, but it also entails self-regulation over what are sometimes thought of as our vegetative functions—our appetite and sleep patterns—and over the maintenance of our health. Moreover, self-control encompasses the ability to manage our time, to do our chores, to fulfill our obligations, to order our lives based on the paths we choose and the demands we face. Taken together, self-regulation, self-care, and self-determination constitute agency. And agency is the prerequisite to freedom.

Power is also the ability to maintain relationships, the capacity to mediate the inevitable power clashes that arise in our personal and professional relationships, and to exert influence on others. It is the ability to forgive, to work at our relationships, and to accept the fact that our self-interest may sometimes conflict with that of our loved ones. Overbearing behavior, excessive compliance, and unnecessary defiance are all distortions of interpersonal power.

Power in and of itself is neutral, neither good nor bad, nothing more or less than a force or an energy. While the power of electricity lights up our lives, a tornado has immense destructive power. Ideas have the power to change the world for good or evil. Similarly, the power we exert individually may be constructive or destructive.

In contrast, weakness—the inability or failure to exert power in any significant way whatsoever—can be a major corrosive force in our lives. Not surprisingly, our longing for power is sometimes driven by the powerlessness all of us experience. Feelings of weakness and helplessness can be intensified by neuroses and mental maladies (inhibitions, phobias, major anxiety, or depression) or by limitations in our life circumstances (poverty, poor health, low status), but they are also intrinsic to our experience—our helplessness as infants and our knowledge of death. Unless we have developed some capacity for control over our day-to-day lives, we feel inert, at the mercy of external forces. Seen this way, our impulse to exert power or to form alliances with people who are more powerful than we are is an attempt to combat our feelings not just of personal weakness and vulnerability but also of existential fragility. Seeking power, then, is an antidote for vulnerability. But it is also something more.

The impulse to power is a kind of life force that propels us into the world to sing our song. To experience ourselves as the author of our own actions, based on our own desires, expands our sense of self-identity and self-worth. Power is made up of acts that enable us to feel that we are the creators of our own experience. Almost from birth, we seek power as a way of defining ourselves and our needs in a world that seems bent on shaping us to respond to its demands. As the author and editor Michael Korda has written: "Without power, we might as well be trees, rocks, oysters, whatever you like, estimable objects in the sight of God, useful even, obeying the complex laws of nature but without the capacity to alter the world, *to control our own lives.*"[3] Although Korda's book *Power* dispenses plenty of power-mongering advice (for example, positioning your desk at a slight elevation so that people literally have to look up to you), here he is depicting power in a more general, philosophical way, proposing that it enables us to define ourselves and our needs, to shape our own destiny.

Our desire to direct our day-to-day experiences is evident in early life. Years ago, the psychologist Robert Whyte identified this desire in what he calls the "battle of the spoon." A tiny child, still in a high chair, insists on feeding himself even though the baby food ends up everywhere but in his mouth. But power in the form of agency extends beyond day-to-day choices. Ultimately, it entails being independent enough to frame our own ambitions *and* to take the responsibility for seeing them through to the finish line. It encompasses our ability to act independently *and* to appraise our chances of success in our undertakings.

Childhood teaches us a range of different power ploys. We begin to develop a repertoire of interpersonal maneuvers not only to control, influence, or cooperate with others but also to establish a sense of agency, the capacity to nudge destiny instead of simply responding to it. These two, sometimes intersecting, paths of power constitute *interpersonal power* and *personal power*.

AUTHENTIC POWER, power that we can own, derives more from a strong sense of self than from any position we might hold. What we want is not simply to be in command; we also want to feel in command. This occurs only when our power, over ourselves or over others, comes from within and is experienced as an integral part of our self. To be sure, how successfully we exert power depends on what sources of power we command. Many young boys may want to grow up to play professional basketball, but they must have the height, the talent, and the opportunity, not just the wish. The wish without the physical gifts is virtually useless, as are the physical gifts absent the drive. The phrase *power to* describes the thrust of power; the phrase *power of* describes the sources of power. Whatever our gifts may be, we always need enough self-knowledge to grasp the true range of our potential and enough drive to exercise it. Ethel Merman, we can all agree, had a powerful, commanding voice. But she also had a commanding presence, a powerful theatrical sense. Her very presence on the stage was as brassy, as loud, and as satisfying as that magnificent voice. And she really felt that way, felt that she belonged right there onstage. Asked once if she ever got stage fright, "No," she replied, "I never thought about it." Well, then, did she ever get even a little nervous before an audience? "No," she said. "If they could sing as good as I can, they would be up here and I would be down there watching them." She owned her gift. This is authentic power.

There are many potential sources of power. One of the most important is self-understanding, because it gives us the capacity to change and grow. We also derive power from intelligence, resourcefulness, likeability, and from an inner sense of strength engendered early in life. There are many intangibles that add to power: visibility, availability, self-confidence, and, when necessary, combativeness. We benefit, too, if we possess concentration and staying power. Other personal sources include physical qualities: brawn, vigor, high reserves of energy, youth in some cultures and age in others. Power can coalesce around some natural gift—creativity or a talent for music, mathematics, or language.

Many important sources of power are innate. This is particularly true when it comes to being assertive and dominant. Here, our similarity to other animals is evident. Whenever horses are "let out," one of them automatically comes to the gate first. It doesn't seem to matter if the horse is male or female, large or small, a gelding or not; it has something to do with the horse's innate spirit. Even if a rider comes to fetch his or her horse and calls for it, the dominant horse comes first.

Some of us possess a natural aptitude for leadership. With my Uncle

Phil, it was his charisma—the power of his personality that let him hold sway over people. All his nieces and nephews were in thrall to this idealistic bachelor who always took time to play with us. He challenged us to find a rhyme for the word "orange," and promised us a million dollars if we could. He was virtually penniless so he must have been sure that no such rhyme existed, though he took the reason for his certainty to the grave with him. Ultimately, it was his communal vision of the world that we bought into, not the entrepreneurial glory propounded by our Uncle Abe. But our allegiance to Phil surely had as much to do with the emotional connection he created as with the strength of his ideas.

Our sources of power are intimately connected to our emotional profiles. Some people, like Uncle Phil, are naturally empathic and nurturant, sensitive to the needs of others without relinquishing a healthy self-interest. This is a kind of power. Indeed, in the emotional realm, it's hard to overestimate the constructive power of love, compassion, forgiveness, and mercy. Positive feelings confirm our sense of self and add to our sense of intrinsic value, promoting our experience of ourselves as strong and effective. Joy, gladness, ecstasy, and love make us feel expansive, worthy, and important. These feelings, too, are empowering; they enhance our ability to reach out, to form bonds with others, to enter into new activities. Even in bad times, the feeling of hope keeps alive the possibility that we can reorder our lives in such a way that the future will be brighter.

By contrast, certain feelings are connected to a sense of powerlessness. Generally speaking, anxiety, fear and terror, and shame are connected to a sense of depletion and may inhibit our ability to act. Depression, whether its genesis is biological or situational, renders the afflicted person weak and helpless, sometimes even paralyzed.[4] Because depression is so often associated with a sense of powerlessness, a pharmaceutical house promotes its antidepressant drug Zoloft as "the power that speaks softly."

There are many other sources of power: access to a good education and, if we are lucky, to mentors. Traditional sources of power reside in our position in life, one to which we may be born or which we may achieve. They include wealth, social access, professional achievement, and relationships with people who are powerful or potentially useful. As Mark Twain once remarked: "In Boston they ask, how much does he know? In New York, how much is he worth? In Philadelphia, who were his parents?"

People sometimes strive for social status or some other kind of power by positioning themselves close to those who have it, sometimes shame-

anxiety, fear
terror, shame } inhibit power
depression

lessly so. The writer Sally Quinn tells a funny and perhaps apocryphal story about the Washington hostess Gwen Cafritz and her clumsy but apparently successful campaign to achieve proximity to the powerful: "Years ago, Mrs. Cafritz called the wife of Congressman Joe Casey to invite the couple over for drinks one evening. After Mrs. Casey replied that they would love to come, the conversation continued: 'I understand your husband has just been nominated to be Secretary of Labor,' said Mrs. Cafritz. 'That's right,' replied Mrs. Casey. 'Well,' continued Mrs. Cafritz, 'if he gets confirmed, we would love to have you stay for dinner.'"[5] Social life in this context, as in many others, is not so much about pleasure as it is about positioning ourselves so that other people's power will rub off on us.

But being powerful in the social world is not a static condition. As Edith Wharton once advised, you should always be nice to young girls; you can never tell whom they will marry. Or, in our time, become.

Power is often role-related, as with parent and child, teacher and student, employer and employee; power is also age-related, the power gradient operating against both the very young and the very old. It may be affected by social, physical, or financial factors, by class, race, and sex. Formal factors can confer power in intimate relationships—the authority of parents vis-à-vis their children, the greater prestige often accorded to a husband vis-à-vis his wife.

The Italian film *Swept Away* shows how social convention shapes the power gradient. A wealthy socialite and her manservant are shipwrecked on a deserted island. Because of his superior physical strength and basic survival skills, he gains power, and she, who previously scorned him, comes to idealize him. The change in their balance of power is a prelude to a torrid affair in which he proves an ardent and commanding lover; she is emotionally swept away. But the minute they are rescued, social convention takes over, and the socialite barely acknowledges her lover. Yet personal psychology sometimes upends the status conferred on us by role, resulting in unexpected reversals: a self-doubting father leans on his pubescent son to make decisions for him; the king's wife or mistress is the power behind the throne.

Our sources of power do not reside exclusively in our own abilities and gifts, in our status, or in our emotional strength. Some of our greatest deeds and misdeeds are inspired by the power of conviction, whether religious or political; consider, for example, the acts of heroism and the acts of barbarity so often observed in war. When we add conviction to the list of factors that already includes natural talent, social role, and emotional profile, among other variables, we begin to see how truly complicated the sources of power are.

THE LATE SENATOR THOMAS PRYOR GORE once wrote to his grandson Gore Vidal, "The power to excel is not the same thing as the desire to excel."[6] Where does the desire or the drive to assert oneself come from? The origins of power are complicated even when we're talking about the quintessentially macho version of a character like Don Corleone in *The Godfather*.[7] Head of a Mafia family, Don Corleone ruthlessly wields his power over a vast and vicious crime empire. In an interview with the critic Camille Paglia, the Godfather's creator, Mario Puzo, explained, not so surprisingly, that he loved writing scenes that depict the operation of power, especially those that allowed him to explore the subtle manipulations through which a strong-willed person manifests his power over others.[8]

To read Puzo is to assume that he had intimate knowledge of Mafia leadership. How else would he have acquired such an intimate understanding of the brutal workings of power? From quite a different source, it turns out. In the preface to his reissued novel *The Fortunate Pilgrim*, Puzo revealed the true inspiration for the Godfather: "Whenever the Godfather opened his mouth, in my own mind I heard the voice of my mother. . . . I heard her wisdom, her ruthlessness, and her unconquerable love for her family and for life itself. . . . without [her], I could not have written *The Godfather*."[9] His *mother*! But why should I be surprised, given that the advancement of "family," in both senses of the word, is Don Corleone's central passion? In fact, we think of him as being as much paterfamilias as crime lord, a man who values his power most for enabling him to shore up the wealth, safety, and security of his blood family as well as his crime family.

For those who believe that will and dominance are fueled strictly by testosterone, the origins of the fictitious Don Corleone's personal power should give them pause. All of us, not just Mario Puzo, acquired our basic ideas about power and powerlessness in intimate relationships, first at our mother's breast and then at her knee. The writer and feminist June Jordan describes childhood as "the first inescapable political situation each of us has to negotiate. . . . You are powerless. You are on the wrong side in every respect. Besides that there's the size thing."[10] Yes and no.

Who has power and how it is exerted are complicated questions even when we're talking about a mother and child. Totally weak and dependent at the beginning of life, the infant dramatically shows us the spectacle of power being exerted without conscious will. For playwright Thornton Wilder, the baby is Nero in the bassinette. The psychologists Erik and Joan Erikson describe the baby's power in terms of how he affects others: "The baby's genuine weakness exerts a spiritual power over those around him. . . . Our newborns . . . are able to move us with mere whimpers and ever-so-faint smiles and even to cause crises among the strongest of us, forcing us to be for a little while more helpfully human."[11] The baby's inborn but limited repertoire of strategies to enthrall its caregivers include cuteness, helplessness, and cries of distress, what the Eriksons call the baby's "native powers of seduction." These powers will become progressively elaborated upon—smiles and tears used ever more consciously—as the baby learns what kind of response they get. However, the baby's inborn power and his ability to build on that power depends equally on the parents' capacity for appreciation—what Rollo May called nutrient (or nurturant) power. If the parents do not respond, or worse, if they are abusive, the baby's power is negated.

Just because the baby's power depends on the parents granting it a kind of permission to exercise it does not mean that the power is not real. Paradoxically, the baby's powerlessness evokes its parents' protectiveness. Clearly, powerlessness and not just power shapes our private and communal lives.

We arrive at our earliest forms of self-determination—personal power— when we learn to hold a biscuit between thumb and forefinger. Once we can feed ourselves, we are on the road to dispensing with mother. However, we begin to experience personal power as such only when we *intend to assert it*. Early in our lives, the push for autonomy and independence is instinctual. But as we become increasingly self-aware, power enters into our mental lives as part of our motivational system, whether in or out of our awareness. Learning to sit up, toddle, walk, and run are all steps in learning to separate, and our longing for separation is so strong that we become very protective of whatever independence we have gained.

The psychoanalyst Althea Horner relates the key event in the development of autonomy: "If one is to become a grown-up in a world of grown-ups, sooner or later there must be an 'overthrow' of parental authority, with a resultant change in the locus of security, direction, decision-making and the taking of responsibility."[12] What she is saying is that our independence can only be won as the result of a power struggle with our parents, and one in which we are ultimately successful to some degree.

Self-will is evident from infancy on. The baby's desire to have his own way inevitably meets opposition from his parents, resulting in a clash of wills. Beginning toward the end of the first year and accelerating during the second year, the toddler is developing a new set of skills and abilities that often brings his noisy self assertion—"I can do it for myself"—into immediate clashes with his parents. The terrible twos are good evidence of our natural resistance to power as we strive for self-expression. Many a parent has seen a little child tottering at the top of a steep flight of stairs after an unsupervised—and explicitly forbidden—climb, and fearing for his safety, runs to offer the child assistance. "No! Do it myself!" the child cries when the parent offers a helping hand (or worse a controlling one). Though most parents view the terrible twos as a disagreeable period of negativity, the child's ebullience of will evident in his insistence on "no" or "yes" is actually a crystallization of himself as an autonomous being.[13] The toddler's mastery of these two words and his eagerness to stand by his judgments are major leaps toward forming an independent sense of self—and often enough the beginning of an overt power struggle with his parents. Here we see that, from the beginning, interpersonal power and personal power develop in tandem.

The toddler's struggle is not just an external struggle with his parents. Toddlers are also struggling to exert control and constraint over their own impulses, a prerequisite for the acquisition of personal power. The writer and psychoanalyst Judith Viorst describes how you sometimes hear a child mumbling about whether or not to do something forbidden: "I will take the cookie. No, I shouldn't." Not only "no and yes" but also "should and shouldn't." Language is a brand new tool for the toddler, not only for controlling others but also for self-control.[14]

Describing the child's acquisition of self-control, Viorst cautions that it is not an easy lesson: "It takes a while to accept the on-the-face-of-it preposterous point of view that self-control may be the royal road to freedom . . . allowing us to master ourselves—and the world." The paradox Viorst emphasizes is that each of us must struggle "to manage, master, dominate, regulate, influence, curb, or restrain [our own] impulses."[15] We must curb gratification in order to take control. On the face of it, this is an improbable lesson: self-limits as a positive good, not as an imposition!

Power is a desire and a drive; it is a motivational force as basic as sex, bonding, and aggression. The impulse propelling us to exercise power is both innate and shaped by learning and experience. As infants, we act instinctively rather than volitionally—we suck a nipple, grasp a bottle, cry in discomfort—and it is the same with our impulse to exert power. Among psychoanalysts and psychologists this instinct goes by many names—among them, life force and élan vital. Althea Horner calls it "intrinsic power," the power of the self.[16] For the former monk and writer Thomas Moore, "personal power is almost indistinguishable from the life that is in us."[17] The London pediatrician turned psychoanalyst D. W. Winnicott calls it, with a very un-British directness, "aggression," but what he actually describes is more like self-assertion, not destructiveness. In fact, aggression is generally the default position, mobilized only when self-assertion is thwarted.[18]

The psychoanalyst Michael Schulman distinguishes between the infant's preintentional force (when the infant does not yet possess a conscious awareness of himself as an active agent) and the later appearance of will, in which his awareness of his own agency is paramount.[19] Like Schulman, I believe that the power "drive" is initially hardwired and spontaneous, and only later becomes intentional. Yet our earliest instinctual form of self-assertion, of "aggression" in Winnicott's terms, is the kernel of the power drive or power motive.

As we leave infancy, and enter babyhood, our instinctive drive to power gets elaborated into an ever more conscious and deliberate exercise of power. Viorst describes the growth of autonomy as "hatching out of dependency" and "taking possession of ourselves."[20] The developmental psychologist Robert White calls it the development of a feeling of "efficacy," which encompasses a theme of "mastery, power, and control."[21] Of course, "intention" is itself complicated, a mixture of conscious elements fueled by unconscious ones.

Granted that there must be an instinctive kernel in the expression of power, competing theories assign different priorities to the ways we develop our personal patterns of power—whether we grow into independence or dependency, strength or weakness. Behavioral geneticists believe that temperament and biological predisposition have more impact on behavior and personality than experience does, while psychoanalysts believe that experience, particularly the events of early life, have the most effect on our patterns of power. Viorst comments, perhaps ironically, that just as "biological determinists . . . see us as the prisoners of our genes, environmental determinists see us as the prisoners of our childhood."[22]

The nature side of the debate draws credibility from ethologists and their studies of animal behavior, particularly the study of dominance in primates. Dominance, in a nutshell, entails who can beat up whom, whether we are talking about flying squirrels or marmosets or chimpanzees or men. Dominance entails aggression, the beating up occasionally being quite real, but it is clearly more than that. Indeed, an evolutionary advantage for species capable of forming dominance hierarchies is that they no longer have to waste time and energy or risk life and limb engaging in aggression against one another, since, except when the hierarchy is in flux, everyone knows who is top dog or top marmoset and no fighting occurs. Indeed, an animal making a submissive display is basically immune to aggressive assault. If you don't believe me, take a look at two dogs going at it, or rather not going at it, the next time you check out the local dog run. If things get heated, one dog will first run and then, if the other catches up, will offer its neck; this causes the more aggressive dog not to bite it. But from then on, the two are not necessarily friends. If you look carefully, you can see that the more aggressive dog is still furious and will start in again the moment the other stops making submissive gestures. If we could read the stronger dog's thoughts, he would probably be thinking something like, "Dammit, fight like a man," or a dog, that is. But this way of *not* fighting is predominant among dogs, with the exception of just a few breeds; there is nothing the dominant dog can do about it, not while the underdog is behaving like the underdog. So not only is aggression involved in dominance, but also the inhibition of aggression. This inhibition of aggression, moreover, is communicative; that is, it is something the submissive animal evokes in the dominant one. Once you are familiar with a pack or two of animals you realize that dominance is power in the sense that every animal knows who has it and who doesn't. Of course, the dominance hierarchy changes as young animals mature and mature ones age.

All this is worth noting because with a moment's thought it becomes clear that such communicability is taking us, and the dog, in the direction of social organization. Is power then the equivalent of dominance? Yes and no. Yes, it is, in the sense that humans clearly use the same sort of

dominance hierarchy ——> Social organization

expressions and body attitudes that higher primates (especially the great apes) do in threatening and appeasing aggression. You can see comparable expressions, postures, and actions in small children. If you sent ethologists into a nursery for toddlers, they could quickly rattle off the organization chart for the dominance hierarchy. This dominance hierarchy in the nursery is, in fact, the first time children become part of a stable social organization beyond their families—the first time they begin to form relationships on their own.

But the applicability of the dominance model has its limitations. As children begin to develop, dominance does not remain the only means of social organization, and power does not remain limited to dominance. Other attributes come into play in social organization, such as sheer likability and ingenuity in fashioning play. By high school, athletic prowess, good looks and academic competence all play a role. Moreover, humans live in multiple power hierarchies concurrently. Bertrand Russell, writing in 1938, made this point brilliantly: "A woman who enjoys power in the management of her house is likely to shrink from the sort of power enjoyed by a prime minister; Abraham Lincoln, on the contrary, while not afraid to govern the United States, could not face civil war in the home."[23]

The idea that the impulse to express power is at least in part hard-wired draws additional support from studies which found temperamental similarities in identical twins separated at birth and raised in separate households. It is bolstered, too, by long-term studies that track the stability of infants' temperament throughout childhood and into adulthood. The psychiatrists Stella Chess and Alexander Thomas, two pioneers in this field with whom I was privileged to work when I was a medical student, observed children at regular intervals from early infancy until their teens and were able to demonstrate the stability of temperament.[24] Tracking several characteristics—fussiness, ease of feeding, regularity of sleep, fearfulness, and reciprocity with others—they put children into three categories: "easy to handle," "difficult to manage," and "slow to warm up to other people." Certainly, parents observe similar differences in newborns. Like Chess and Thomas, the developmental psychologist Jerome Kagan has observed what appear to be inborn differences that persist over time. He concluded: "Of all the temperamental qualities that had been studied—activity, irritability, and fearfulness are the most popular—an initial display of inhibition to the unfamiliar [what parents call 'shyness,' 'cau-

Temperament

tion,' or 'timidity,'] and its opposite [what they call 'sociability,' 'boldness,' or 'fearlessness'] are two qualities that seem to persist from the first birthday to late childhood."[25] (Boldness and fearlessness are of course traits customarily linked to dominance, timidity and caution to powerlessness.) But, as Kagan points out, parents can change the behavioral surface of the inhibited child insofar as they "encourage a less fearful approach to unfamiliar people and situations."[26] What this means is that while innate differences in natural assertiveness are important, they are not decisive.

The major limitation of applying the biological model to humans is that among humans, power is not synonymous with dominance. While dominance is one facet of interpersonal power, power has a much broader meaning—the ability to produce a desired effect. Many factors—some known, some that we can only guess at—combine to make our acquisition of self-determination and interpersonal competence relatively easy or difficult.

What psychologists and psychoanalysts add to our understanding of power is how our pursuit of it is shaped by experience. Initially we adopt power strategies in identification with our parents and others we admire. A great deal depends on our family dynamics during childhood, the identifications we form, the unresolved conflicts that may burden us, and the circumstances of our lives. While the powers we live by are innate, they are also evidently molded by experience and our knowledge of our own limitations.

Neither the geneticists nor the environmentalists give much room to (free) will. But we experience ourselves as controlling our behaviors and choices either through our will or through our failure to exert it. We also observe that our ability or inability to assert our will is connected to feeling strong or feeling weak. Those of us who feel able to control ourselves and our relationships feel powerful, whereas those of us who are beset by demoralizing feelings like fear, depression, or shame feel relatively powerless.

Gill is a brilliant young man whose parents had every reason to expect that he would become a prominent mathematician or physicist, given his natural intellectual gifts. But also evident from early childhood was an almost paralyzing passivity. As a toddler, Gill never tried to climb out of his crib. Some babies attempt this before they can walk, and some who toddle early not only make it out of the crib but also get all the way to the door, ready to explore the outside world if only their arms were long enough to reach the doorknob. But Gill remained in his crib, contentedly waiting to be lifted out, even at the relatively advanced age of two.

This quality, which I would call passivity, made him easy to care for in late infancy and early toddlerhood. But his passivity was not restricted to staying put. He never became a self-starter. His persistent lack of initiative appeared so early in his life that it appeared to be part of his nature rather than engendered in psychological interaction with his parents.

As a result, despite his intellectual brilliance, Gill ended up in adulthood in a low-level computing position, though he is able to help his senior colleagues solve difficult problems. He has married a similarly passive woman, and he appears perfectly happy, though his situation saddens his parents. In their value system, his life trajectory is a tragic case of unfulfilled potential.

The fact is that the inborn life force that propels us to assert our will is not distributed equally. You only have to contrast Gill with Nat to see the extremes. The youngest of six children, Nat lost his beloved mother when he was five years old. He remembers the funeral, remembers looking at the gaping hole in the ground, remembers his sense of devastation, and remembers the exact moment when he affirmed himself as his own source of strength. As he stood by the grave, someone told him to say the Kaddish, the Jewish prayer for the dead. He knew how to do this, and, focusing all his energy on remembering the words and not giving way to tears, he got through it successfully. When he was done he heard all the women crying and praising him. What he remembers most vividly was the exhilaration of knowing he had the power to perform a grown-up act and through it to touch and control the emotions of those around him. For many years, the memory of that exhilaration helped him modulate the grief he felt. He had discovered something valuable about the rewards that accrue to self-generated actions—that is, to agency. He later was able to transform his own loss into compassion for others and grew up to become an eminent psychoanalyst.

POWER IS a universal obsession; power issues are ubiquitous in all our activities and in our internal psychic lives as well. But power is not expressed in only one way, nor is a manifestly powerful act always consciously experienced as power. Over the course of our lives, each of us comes to develop conscious but also subliminal (or preconscious) ideas about power—what it is, in what domains it exists, who has it, what forms are available to us, and what forms are precious to us. Gradually, each of us arrives at different concepts of power as well as different preferences— what I call *fantasies* or *dreams*—about how we personally hope to exert power.[27] Our dreams are shaped by the factors I've already discussed in connection with power: our level of drive, our temperament, our experiences, our personal gifts, the values we incorporate from our parents and families, our emotional life in general, and, most of all, what we judge to be not only desirable but also plausible for us. Our dreams are influenced, too, by the network of relationships in which we grew up and by the values that obtain in our culture. To put it another way: Though we may be consciously aware of an intense desire for one or another kind of power, our preferences are profoundly shaped by factors we only "pretend to understand."

Although we may never be able to fully realize all our dreams of power, many of us can manage to exert control and command over a large swath of life. The power adaptation we achieve in our interpersonal lives is not the same in every situation. We position ourselves on different rungs on the ladder of various power hierarchies: our families, our peer group, the workplace, and the clubs, religious organizations, and other groups to which we belong. A few of us crave extremes—either striving for control over the destinies and welfare of those we command in the role of employer, military officer, Mafia don, or local political boss; or seeking the hoped-for safety of depending on someone else, even resorting to extreme submissiveness. Our dreams of personal power can be recruited to long-term or short-term goals. They may be invoked in the pursuit of grand ambitions (for example, plotting a corporate takeover or running for political office) or simply in establishing a sphere of autonomy (for example, establishing financial security by accumulating a personal nest egg). We call upon a variety of power ploys to deal with the daily grind of competition and jealousy at work and to establish our place in the pecking order. Some among us have plotted how to keep a rival and sometimes even a friend out of a club we belong to or off a board of directors on which we sit.

Power is not only a matter of seeking positions of command and control; it is also a matter of the mastery of specific skills: owning the knuckleball; speaking up in a classroom; lovingly tending a baby; proudly organizing one's first dinner party. Being a beauty and being a belle. Being the life of the party. Commanding a playing field or an orchestra. Organizing shelters for the homeless. Leading a rent strike. Writing a poem. Learning to ride a motorcycle. Growing a perfect tomato.

No one can with impunity ignore power (manifest or wished for) or powerlessness (experienced or dreaded) as a theme in the narrative of our lives. Some exercise of power is a prerequisite for full humanity. The main obstacle to pursuing our goals, to exerting our power, is fear. But the danger of failing is nothing compared with the danger of feeling that we have never lived, never taken the risk of feeling wholly vulnerable and alive.

It is the theme of the unlived life that Henry James so tellingly portrays in his story "The Beast in the Jungle."[28] John Marcher, who believes he has been chosen for a special destiny, lets life pass him by while he waits for the defining moment—for the great thing to happen. Only after May Bartram, who has loved him, dies, and Marcher, at her grave, hears the true grief of a mourner at the next grave, does he understand the emptiness of his life: "The escape would have been to love her; then, *then* he would have lived." Marcher let what *was* possible slip by, waiting instead for the great thing that failed to materialize. That James himself may have felt life was passing him by is suggested in the reminiscences of two of his friends. Hugh Walpole described James as lonely, perhaps because he was an American abroad, but more likely because he was "a spectator of life." He believed that James, with his Puritanical temperament, had probably suffered some sexual frustration: "What that frustration was I never knew but I remember him telling me how once in his youth in a foreign town he watched a whole night in pouring rain for the appearance of a figure at a window. 'That was the end . . .' he said, and broke off."[29] James made the same confession to Edmund Gosse, who understood him much as Walpole did: "So discreet was [James], and so like a fountain sealed that many of those who were well acquainted with him have supposed that he was mainly a creature of observation and fancy, and that life stirred his intellect while leaving his senses untouched."[30] Only seldom did James give Gosse a "flash or glimmer of deeper things." Gosse then relates the identical story of the figure in the window and James's feeling of tearful disconnection.[31] While James was brilliant and socially engaged, he appears to have lacked the capacity for any deep romantic (and perhaps sexual) attachment. And yet it may be that some kind of emotional engagement is integral to the subjective sense of authentic power.

WE OFTEN ASSUME that worldly power confers inner strength. Yet the feeling of authentic power, of inner strength, is not necessarily, and perhaps only rarely, associated with power in the external world. To establish a *raison d'être* whether in work or love or religious devotion, to commit to activities that one chooses, to be able to live in the moment without abandoning either the past or the future; to have a life relatively free of fear, anger, or envy and filled with love and concern for at least a few others—these are all facets of authentic power. Authentic power is the ability to live fully, with few regrets and fewer recriminations. When we are internally free to pursue our goals, we experience neither excessive apathy nor doubt, and we remain untroubled by fear of failure or of success.

Authentic power is not the same thing as worldly power. Like the proverbial needle in the haystack, it is often difficult to find those among us who experience themselves as authentically powerful, who feel anything like inner strength or a sense of being in command of themselves. Some of us are denied the realization of authentic power because of the demands our current life places on us, demands that sometimes preclude our being in touch with our innermost selves. The high school student is cramming for the SATs, the mother is devoting all her time and energy to her young brood, the new father is plagued by escalating expenses and can see no clear way to increase his income. (In this frantic age, it is perhaps appropriate that the last refuge for many is the gym. Some of us go to a gym out of duty or fear, but others go because it's one of the few places where we can escape interminable demands from the world, a place where no one can metaphorically put a hand on our neck and tell us what urgent task we must immediately attend to—a place where we can let our psychic center of gravity come to the fore.)

It's perhaps even harder to identify people who experience themselves as genuinely powerful among those apparently powerful people who inhabit the headlines. In part this is because there are so few absolute rulers today and so few solo buccaneers. Many who command worldly power experience themselves as lacking in strength because of the constant effort they expend to hold on to their power, what with competitors and challengers nipping at their heels. The CEO is worried about profits, the loyalty of the staff, and the tension among the board of directors, not to mention the economy.

There is, however, a more fundamental factor that severely limits the satisfaction of being top dog in any field. So many major players feel as if they're trapped on a hamster wheel. Some are so consumed by the frustration of trying to fulfill their ever-escalating ambitions that they cannot contemplate personal time or downtime. Their well-being and sense of security depend on perpetual striving. Simply to look at the schedule of some manifestly powerful people—often beginning with a business breakfast at 6 A.M. and ending with a business dinner at 10 P.M.—is to understand the cost of their achievements.

Indeed, those who hold the most exalted posts often lack the kind of personal freedom many of us take for granted. Paradoxically, those "in power" may in some ways be the least powerful because they must be on call night and day to handle crises, demands, requests, and challenges, while at the same time needing to negotiate with political power blocs. The perpetual plaint of those "in power"—at least in the psychiatrist's office—is a lack of time to cultivate an inner life or a personal relationship. The urge to gain power in the "world" is almost antithetical to being able to enjoy stretches of time with few external demands. Freedom may be harder to acquire than either position or money. The frenzied life of today's "powerful" represents a shift from earlier generations, when social class and inherited money defined power, enabling people to lead pampered and leisurely lives. The powerful of that earlier era looked down on those who were forced to work. And if they were tempted by public office, they certainly did not feel it had to be a round-the-clock job.

Still others fail to experience themselves as powerful because power in the boardroom does not translate into power in the bedroom. Or it may be because of a failure to maintain a permanent relationship or because the sometimes neglected or resentful children of the powerful arrange for payback time. Some of these problems stem from the fact that powerful people often prioritize worldly power over their personal lives.

The popular HBO television series *The Sopranos* is both a story of power and a telling riff, a send-up of it. The mob boss Tony Soprano, despite his powerful position, is subject to anxiety attacks and intermittent sexual impotence. He is unable to handle his mother or discipline his children. And, wouldn't you know it, he has a full-blown erotic transference to his female psychiatrist. In *Analyze This*, Robert De Niro is another Mafia boss suffering from anxiety to the point of a nervous breakdown who lassoes, almost literally, a terrified psychiatrist, played by Billy Crystal, to minister to his overwhelming anxiety.

Neuroses can get in the way of any sense of fulfillment and pleasure we might otherwise enjoy as the fruit of our labor and success. Mr. Jackson, for instance, was referred for treatment only because his internist thought some personal problems might be contributing to an ongoing medical problem that is generally thought to have a psychosomatic component. He was happily married and had two successful adult sons. Acknowledged by his friends as a powerful man and among the leaders in a high-profile profession, he was frequently written up in magazines and quoted in newspapers. Yet he had long been aware that he relished his competitors' setbacks, particularly as these were publicly recounted in the *New York Times* or the *Wall Street Journal*. But he failed to connect his extreme competitiveness to his favorite reverie: he soothed himself to sleep delivering a brilliant eulogy at the funeral of one or another of his cronies, all of whom happened to be alive and well. In addition, he scrutinized the *New York Times* daily, looking for the obituary of one of these successful "friends." What had never occurred to him was that his fantasies might involve a death wish or that he was selectively fantasizing about the funerals of the competitors whom he most envied for their seemingly authentic power. Only slowly could he acknowledge how much he hated, feared, and envied his rivals. His pride had stood in the way of acknowledging how small they made him feel and how his fantasies about their obituaries reflected his wish that his rivals would die. Because they were powerful, he had no way of humiliating them in real life, so he cast them as dead men in his fantasies.

Toward his employees Mr. Jackson was critical, stingy with praise, and controlling, insisting that they work long and sometimes unremunerated hours. This aggressiveness appeared to be the way he protected himself from experiencing any conscious sense of weakness. Under the guise of upgrading her, he sent his wife to a speech therapist to "remediate" her accent, and he made innumerable other assaults on her self-image and self-esteem. What he was doing was projecting onto her the loathing he felt for himself—a projection he was aware of only sometimes, and then just barely. While his worldly power was real, it was not internalized in a way that permitted him to be proud of his many authentic achievements.

His inauthentic power—acts of dominating and humiliating others—was mobilized to counteract sudden dips in his sense of well-being, as were his reveries when he was going to sleep.

As he gradually gained insight, he came to understand that his core problem was related to his father's having made him feel inadequate when he was growing up—a feeling he was now inflicting on those near and dear to him, his wife and two sons. Mr. Jackson's mother had been sickly and "inadequate," so he grew up more or less at the mercy of his overcontrolling though not particularly successful father, who pushed him to excel even while ceaselessly criticizing and nagging him. Although Mr. Jackson internalized his father's values and ultimately achieved success, his father's power to demean him trumped any sense of authenticity and pride he might have had in his accomplishments. Though they maintained a superficially cordial relationship, his father was preserved in his psyche as his tormentor. He identified with his father and criticized, humiliated, and controlled others in the way his father treated him. Only when he gained insight into his inner feelings of weakness was he able to make the first step toward change.

Death fantasies like Mr. Jackson's are more common than some of us might imagine and are generally a product of feelings of weakness or competitive disadvantage. They occur fairly frequently among children who are angry at their parents with no mode of redress, and sometimes among patients in relationship to their psychotherapists. One of my patients checked the obituaries in the New York Times every morning to see if I had died. But while some death fantasies are indeed death wishes, motivated by a desire to be rid of a heavy hand or overt disapproval, other such fantasies may be fearful fantasies encapsulating the dread of losing a necessary support system. And some fantasies are both.

Authentic power—though sometimes in short supply among those publically proclaimed as powerful—certainly exists. Most of us have been privileged to know people who experience themselves as fulfilled and strong while actually possessing few of the external trappings of power. For me, one of these people was my grandfather.

I was born and raised in Louisville, Kentucky, sometimes described as the most northern of the great southern cities. Mine was a family of eccentrics, with strong and diverging interests and beliefs—capitalists and communists, believers and atheists, the learned and the barely literate— so I was presented with a dramatic diversity of perspectives. But I don't think my fundamental experiences of learning about power were different from anyone else's. Like most people, I knew unquestioningly who among my relatives possessed the greatest inner strength: it was my maternal grandfather, Abraham Zimmerman, our personal patriarch, our *Zayde*. His ability to live in and possess the moment always seemed like a rare gift, the outward manifestation of a deep-seated core of contentment and centeredness, the hallmark of authentic power. Whatever he happened to be doing felt to him—and to those around him—like the best thing possible to do it that moment, whether it was wandering around a dusty construction site to stay abreast of the changing contours of Louisville; reading the Russian classics in Russian; betting on the horses like a proper Kentuckian; playing pinochle once a week with his brother-in-law (my Great-Uncle Philip), my father, and the local tailor; or strolling the aisles of his beloved bookstore. He remained enthralled with the external world and had great acumen about it throughout his life. When he was in his late nineties, still a keen observer of the political scene, he authoritatively told me that President Nixon would be forced out of the presidency one way or another, long before this even remotely seemed to be a possibility. Not even my closest friends, several of whom were political scientists, got there before *Zayde* did.

Starting out as a peddler, my immigrant grandfather sold everything that came his way *except* books—these, at the insistence of his first wife (my grandmother), he saved until he had collected enough to open the secondhand bookstore she wanted. It was she who finally made him a businessman. Over the years the store became a legend among the locals of Louisville, in part because *Zayde* lived so long and was such a presence there, in part because his bookstore, recently written up in a journal of Kentucky history, had become a meeting place for the local intelligentsia.[32] *Zayde* worked in his store until he was a hundred years old, when he fell off a ladder and broke his hip while packing up to move to a new store, a necessity because the city had bought the building where the store was situated and evicted him. He died one week short of his 101st birthday.

Whatever gave *Zayde* his remarkable durability, both physically and emotionally, it was not apparent in his early years, when he seemed rather sickly, especially in comparison with a younger brother, who was viewed as the strong, powerful one in the family. From the time I was a little girl, I remember that every Passover *Zayde* would announce that this one might be his last and would then thank God for letting him live so long. As the years accumulated, however, and *Zayde* approached extreme old age, outliving not only the younger brother he had seen as his rival but most of his contemporaries, he became very proud of his longevity. There's no doubt that my grandfather relished the power of having turned out to be the long-distance runner compared with his brother, whom he regarded retrospectively as a sprinter. Thus, in his own imagination, at least, he was the victor in an ancient power struggle. His underlying strength, however, was also derived from the unconditional love his mother had for him, as her oldest son and the one who needed her protection because of his sickliness. Then, too, it must have had something to do with his deep religious commitment. Even in his nineties he walked to *shul*, never traveling by car on the Sabbath, despite a dispensation his rabbi had urged upon him.

By the time I was old enough to understand my grandfather, he was in his late sixties. Having reached a stage in life where he had to navigate several enormous personal crises, which he did without flinching, he appeared to me as a man whose power seemed to well up naturally from sources deep within him. As far as I could see, that strength continued to sustain him in the years that followed through all the crises inevitable for those who live long lives. When my grandmother died, he mourned her fully and then promptly remarried, falling passionately in love for what was perhaps the first time in his life. When he was told, in his early nineties, that he had colon cancer and would probably not live through an operation, he considered his options carefully. His near and dear were too upset to help him with the decision, so he made it by himself and took his chances with surgery. Under minimal anesthetic, he survived, and indeed thrived for nearly another decade. When his business nearly failed because his most reliable source of income, the sale of textbooks, eroded after the state legislature voted to provide free books for all public schools, my religious and traditional grandfather began to sell pornography under the counter—though nothing hotter than magazines featuring naked women—in order to save his bookstore and keep his independence. This was illegal at the time, and he was soon arrested and convicted. He would have gone to jail, too, but the judge, fearing that a man in his late nineties might die in prison, commuted his sentence.

What made my grandfather so powerful was the inner sense of serenity he had first developed only in middle life. It has always seemed to me to be a mark of serenity that one is comfortable enough in one's own skin that there is no nagging doubt about the road not taken, the opportunities missed, the shortness of the road remaining. My grandfather had this gift. Among other things, he taught me through example that authentic power develops over the years and is seldom a gift of youth.

The inner strength my grandfather acquired through the decades was not transmitted to any of his five children, except perhaps one. While we may benefit from our parents' inner strength, authentic power seems to be something we must struggle to reach on our own. My grandfather was perhaps too much of a patriarch and too orthodox in his faith to guide his children in a changing world. Also, the very strength of his will may have cowed his children. Though I adored my grandfather, I always suspected that his strength and inner certainty might have made him overwhelming as a father.

WHILE POWER IS an inborn drive—the ubiquitous human impulse to self-assertion—it is nourished by parental support and encouragement. And our own vulnerability and negative experiences can also goad us to build on whatever kernel of power we already possess. For the political scientist Hans Morgenthau, the *experiential* roots of the power drive are to be found not only in our search for an antidote to our weakness but also in the human need to overcome existential loneliness. We may assuage our loneliness, he said, through either power or love. "Through love, man seeks another human being like himself, the Platonic other half of his soul, to form a union which will make him whole. Through power, man seeks to impose his will upon another man, so that the will of the object of his power mirrors his own."[33] Another way a man responds to the terrible feeling of isolation, Morgenthau said, is "to seek the extension of his self in offspring—the work of his body; in the manufacture of material things—the work of his hands; in philosophy and scholarship—the work of his mind; in art and literature—the work of his imagination; in religion—the work of his pure longing for transcendence."[34] Although Morgenthau was a political theorist, he located the source of our yearning for power within the psyche, not in the political world, grasping intuitively that "the powers we are lived by" arise in large measure from our deepest psychological longings.

Morgenthau saw power as simply one of a number of strategies we use to assuage our human condition, but from my perspective power is an important ingredient in all the strategies he describes. These encompass interpersonal power, the ability to mediate power vis-à-vis another person, so as to maintain a core of vigorous relationships; personal power, the ability to direct our own life trajectories and have an impact on the external world beyond the interpersonal domain, such mastery to include the work of the hands and the work of the mind; creative activity; and transcendence, achieved through identification with a cause larger than the individual self.[35]

Those power strategies we come to favor may act in unison or may be antagonistic, one to the other. To the degree that we are consumed by the pursuit of one kind of power, we may well neglect others. When Gustave Flaubert was writing *Madame Bovary*, he wrote to his long-suffering and complaining mistress, Louise Colet, excusing himself for the extended "paralysis" that kept him from visiting her: "If I haven't written sooner in reply to your sad, discouraged letter, it's because I have been in a great fit of work. . . . I am leading an austere life, stripped of all external pleasure, and am sustained only by a kind of permanent frenzy which sometimes makes me weep tears of impotence but never abates. I love my work with a love that is frantic and perverted as an ascetic loves the hair shirt that scratches his belly."[36] Here Flaubert chooses personal power in the form of creativity over the power implicit in love. But in truth he was also expressing a kind of interpersonal power, dominating and dangling Louise, keeping her on call as muse to his genius, as an "outlet—for chronicle, ideas, protests, and her brand of affection."[37] He would give her up altogether within a few years.

Most of us are neither totally powerless nor totally powerful but have some combination of weaknesses and strengths. Dominance is not the same thing as authentic power; in fact, those who rely on dominating others in order to establish their own self-esteem are often papering over an underlying sense of weakness and often doubt whether they are authentically loved or even liked. Nor should we view vulnerability as synonymous with weakness. To develop real empathy, we must at one time or another have permitted ourselves to feel frightened, overwhelmed, or helpless. Indeed, a certain amount of strength is required for us to open ourselves up and express vulnerability. Authentic power wells up from within, and as the story of my grandfather suggests, it seldom appears full-blown early in life. Rather, it is an outcome of our ability to integrate our experiences in such a way that even adversity is ultimately incorporated into the process of growth. Authentic power is gained through vigorous participation in life, coupled with an openness to new experiences, emotional sure-footedness, strong ties to other people, the ability to find interest and pleasure in whatever we encounter, and, most of all, the ability to construct meaning in our lives.

2

Feelings of Powerlessness

"He who desires but acts not breeds pestilence."
—WILLIAM BLAKE,
from *The Marriage of Heaven and Hell*

Not many people would describe themselves as powerless. Yet as the psychoanalyst Rollo May observed, when "powerlessness is referred to by its more personal name, helplessness or weakness, many people will sense that they are heavily burdened by it."[1] By acknowledging feelings of helplessness or weakness as the result of powerlessness, and not something else, we are better able to look for its underlying causes and can begin to figure out how we might achieve authentic power.

While we loathe our powerlessness, we intermittently yearn for its close cousin, passivity. Allowing ourselves to experience moments of passivity is not always bad or undesirable. Not only are such moments inevitable; they are also necessary and can be the source of a particular kind of pleasure. Letting go serves as a periodic release from the all-too-pressing demands of preserving a strong, self-reliant self-image. And some kinds of passivity have nothing to do with powerlessness; they are an appealing, delicious release—for example, sighing with relief when we put an obligation behind us or letting go in sex, both of which may enhance our sense of self.

The security of being taken care of, letting someone else be the decision maker, permitting that person to be the power in our life, can mirror the warm safe cocooning some of us happily experienced in childhood. This can be deeply seductive, pleasurable, and, again, sometimes completely necessary. The joy of being looked after and provided for may continue unabated into adulthood, and it sometimes intensifies in old age. (It's hard to say who gets the most gratification from intermittent dependency—someone who had too much of it in childhood or someone who had too little.) In our everyday lives, some of us relax only when we can admit to ourselves that a problem is no longer in our hands, if ever it was. We rejoice when we are able to leave it to someone else or to fate, happy to be done with it, win, lose, or draw. Dropping the reins, even if only occasionally, gives us a chance to breathe fresh air.

We sometimes feel powerful when we finesse responsibility—that is, it can be empowering to pass our problems and the responsibility for finding solutions on to someone else. What we want most in such situations is to free ourselves of making daily but inconsequential decisions. This is why some adoring mothers can't wait for their children to go to sleepaway camp, and why a father may be happy when his wife and children spend the week at a summer house and he needs to appear only on weekends. Sometimes in pursuit of our desire to temporarily halt the demands on us, we may even welcome the dentist's chair, where all that is required of us is to open the mouth.

There are few things more deeply if oddly pleasurable than intermittently giving up the reins. This is often mirrored in the sheer glee we take in vicarious identification with comic moments. Our laughter in response to low comedy shows our pleasure in helplessness. For low comedy, in the theater, in movies, or on television, puts physical ineptitude at center stage. Slapstick plays on the absurdity of our bodies and our physical limitations, acted out in pratfalls, slips on banana peels, fat men stuck in doorways. No one has expressed the psychology of low comedy better than the drama critic Walter Kerr:

> Low comedy is a birth experience, and for a time traumatic. It consists in the discovery that we have a backside and that it is going to be slapped. Total humiliation comes with our first breath of air, is a condition of our breathing. We are embarrassed to have a body that can be subjected to such treatment, and whenever it is

subjected to such treatment again—in a first slap from a mother, in a misstep that leaves us astonished on our noses in the playpen—we are freshly outraged.[2]

Laughing at humiliating and ridiculous aspects of the flesh gives us relief. Kerr asks why it is that "With so much dust in mind . . . we continue to regard comedy as a warm house?" His answer is that although we may deplore our limitations, we're also deeply enamored of them:

> Each of the nuisances that retards man's free movement, that calls him back imperiously to attend to an around-the-clock need, repays him somewhat for his trouble. . . . Physical necessity summons him, deflecting him from his free course; it then hands out cookies. A filled gullet and an empty bladder are equally rewarding; and when the body becomes so demanding that all free activity must stop, sleep is as pleasant as can be.[3]

For Kerr, the truth is that "in one part of his mind man likes being helpless. It is his only form of hooky, the only holiday he gets. . . . Food and sex and sleep and a warm bath have all been imposed upon [men]. And they look at their helplessness in the matter and laugh. They laugh because the imposition is ridiculous. And they laugh because they like it."[4] The body betrays us, but the body is where the pleasure is.

As adults, we often cordon off the pleasures of passivity into circumscribed arenas. We work hard at our jobs and wait until we go on vacation to abandon our responsibilities. During this time, we rationalize our passive longings as recharging. Before the advent of instantaneous communication, many people liked to go on long flights so they could be shielded from the incessant demands of the telephone. The yearning for passivity often emerges in our sexual preferences, too—for example, in being made love to instead of making love. Such longing is transparent in the wish to be tied up, symbolically rendered helpless. Freud might describe these pleasures as regressive, but as he knew full well, regression has its uses.

Passivity is a problem only if we give away freedom in return for full-time protectors, propelled by a strong urge to lean on those who are more powerful. Then we are flirting with true powerlessness. Obsequious spouses, submissive employees, and acolytes, desirous of the gratification of dependency, sometimes discover to their chagrin just how high the dues may be. Part of the bargain with people who are controlling partners is that while they take responsibility for most organizational tasks, we necessarily relinquish our role in decision making.

Occasionally, powerlessness can confer real power, or at least permit one to get one's way. A Spanish woman I once knew married a Puerto Rican man and did not have the will to resist his demands that they relocate to his homeland. Then her body intervened. Either her unconscious spoke or she actually developed an allergic reaction in Puerto Rico, but in either case she became so asthmatic that they had no alternative but to move back to New York and ultimately to Spain.

Yet powerlessness generally fails when it becomes the main course rather than the spice. Powerlessness and pervasive passivity, if unmodulated, lead to grief. The reason many people seek psychotherapy is that they are feeling weak or powerless, sometimes to the point of being inhibited or even paralyzed in their attempts to initiate change. They may be unable to form a permanent relationship or they may be stuck in an unsatisfactory one, confused about why their love life always tanks. They may be unmotivated or inhibited at work, troubled by their lack of direction and purpose or defeated by every power struggle. Sometimes they recognize that they must be repeating the same mistake over and over again, but they cannot put their finger on what it is. For example, a creative furniture designer is always in a breakout mode, gets shown in one or another prestigious outlet every year, but fails to turn any of his opportunities into ongoing success. He does not see that his problem lies in his choice of business partners to whom he cedes authority.

People come into treatment, too, because they are swamped by feelings—shame, fear, anxiety, depression, uncontrollable anger—that drain away their sense of power. A sense of powerlessness can be short-lived, a result of some transient event or circumstance that we can often identify. We may be intermittently frightened about not having enough money, having missed a stock market boom or fearing a plunge; anxious or depressed about the inevitable ups and downs in emotional relationships; concerned that our sexual desire is diminishing; worried about the adequacy of our children's social life and grades and, later, about their marital prospects; or we may suffer the sadness of an empty nest. Then, too, there are many ongoing threats to our security and well-being that are more fundamentally threatening—helplessness in the face of a loved one's chronic illness, the failure to get a job we desperately need, or the aftermath of natural disasters or political upheavals that can uproot us from our home and even our homeland. Our sense of whether we are weak and powerless or competent and powerful is not static but is closely connected to what we are experiencing at any particular time.

All of us know what it feels like to be weak. Certain universal aspects of the human condition teach us about powerlessness—the dependency of childhood, imbalances of power in relationships, the experience of being mistreated with no opportunity for redress, a lack of control in determining the circumstances and outcome of our lives, bouts with illness, the knowledge of death, and a sense, throughout our days, of the existential loneliness that intermittently afflicts us all. Some of us really are born disadvantaged: our parents are abusive, we have physical or mental disabilities, our family is impoverished and marginalized, or we are members of a powerless group, political, racial, economic, or sexual.

Often, though, our sense of powerlessness is rooted in our psyches. It is a component of the way we feel about ourselves, not a result of current events or cataclysmic challenges to our personal ecosystems. For example, Beatrice, a married woman in her early thirties, entered therapy to explore her inhibitions in her professional life and the low self-esteem that resulted. What proved pivotal was a fantasy she had in response to a newspaper article describing a woman who had been raped in Central Park and the loving attention this woman had received from her family: "I found myself wishing that I could be her. I was envious of all the attention she was getting and of her spirit to be able to fight back. Her mother and both her sisters gave up everything and sat at her bedside around the clock. Each of them slept just two hours at a time. And then I just put myself in her place, with my parents and sisters by my side. I know it's sick how I felt."

Although she was ashamed of her fantasy, Beatrice realized that was gravitating toward a scenario of victimhood, of feeling "special," a default kind of power, because other possibilities seemed blocked. Her fantasy covered over a previously unexplored catacomb of similar masochistic fantasies and self-defeating behaviors, the product of her dependency on and psychological submission to her authoritarian parents. Her mother and father had undermined her attempts to achieve independence by disparaging her creative impulses and criticizing her friends, undercutting any sense of healthy pride, based on self-confidence and self-esteem, except for pride in being a dutiful daughter. Beatrice wanted to be an energy source like the sun, not a reflective moon, but deep down, crippled by her parents' systematic disparagement and her learned passivity, she feared that she could best get attention as a victim. Such a fantasized mode of garnering attention, even in a demeaned role, provides a kind of recognition, an ersatz form of power that substitutes for authentic personal power.

The journalist Marie Brenner, writing of her mother Thelma Brenner, catches the subtle off-centeredness of those who feel vaguely apprehensive and somehow insufficient:

> The largeness of [my father's] personality diffused her anxiety that they would be shunned; in fact, she never was. . . . But sometimes I would find her wandering the hallway in the middle of the night, distracted and melancholy. "What is it, Mother?" I would ask. "Oh, nothing. Everything is fine," she would say, unconvincingly. . . . I understand now that she was adrift in a marriage which had given her security and fidelity, but that wasn't enough. . . . Sensitive to slights of all kinds, she would puzzle over ambiguous remarks. What did this mean? . . . Why did someone say this to her? . . . Oddities of behavior would play out as hypochondria— she kept files of clippings on nitrates in processed meats, carcinogenic substances, contagions found on toilet seats. It feels to me now that she was looking for a catch-all for her anxieties, but her coping mechanism was motion, a trait she has passed on to me. . . . It could not be coincidence that she became obsessed with the rights of victims of all kind. . . . The shelves in the game room filled with new books, Elie Wiesel and William Shirer, memoirs of survivors.[5]

Just like Beatrice and Thelma Brenner, many of us readily identify with victims. In the same way that so many of us are fascinated by tales of power, we are also drawn to stories of long-suffering powerlessness. We are especially empathic toward artists and celebrities who publicly display despair—Judy Garland, Marilyn Monroe, Princess Diana. At Diana's funeral Elton John sang a revised version of his song "Candle in the Wind," which was originally written for Marilyn Monroe. Some details were changed, but the refrain remained the same, likening Diana's frail life to a flickering candle.

Our preoccupation with the meteoric rise and fall of celebrities and public figures can come close to a cult of victimhood and martyrdom. Sometimes we are defending ourselves against an envy of celebrities, thinking that so-and-so got his comeuppance, but more often an element of identification is at play.

At an extreme, powerlessness carries moral authority. Of Sonia, the beloved of Raskolnikov in *Crime and Punishment*, the critic Philip Rahv wrote that she is one in whom "the incapacity for resistance becomes morality," who experiences "any resistance, even any compulsion to resist, as unendurable *displeasure* . . . and finds blessedness (pleasure) only in no longer offering any resistance to anybody, neither to evil nor to him who is evil—love as the only, as the *last* possible way of life."[6] Her religious faith, which protects her, rationalizes what we might otherwise view as a pure culture of submissiveness verging on masochism.

Some of us, like Dostoyevsky's Sonia, believe that suffering confers a special goodness, a sense of self-abnegation that is wholesome or even saintly, and so we elevate powerlessness to a virtue, a sign of sensitivity. Some religious poor proclaim with Jesus that it is easier for a camel to get through the eye of a needle than for a rich man to enter the kingdom of heaven. In some eras, there is even a vogue for specific kinds of suffering. Many Christian saints were canonized because of their suffering. In the 1950s and 1960s, the suffering artist, linked in the imagination to tortured geniuses like Dostoyevsky, could still achieve cult status, the degree of psychic pain believed to be correlated with the greatness of the masterpiece-to-be, even though that work as yet existed solely in his imagination.

Over the past decade or so, victimhood has provided, if not cachet, then a kind of honorable self-identity, particularly if one has been awarded survivor status. After World War II, the word *survivor* was appropriated to refer specifically to those who survived the Nazi extermination camps. Today the term refers to self-designated survivors of broken homes, divorce, personal tragedies, afflictions, and sexual abuse. And the word *holocaust*, which mainly referred to Hitler's systematic eradication of Jews, has been usurped to describe everything from the plight of various ethnic minorities to all the devastations of personal life.

Such rampant fascination with and reverence for survivors may sometimes stem from genuine empathy for victims, but our co-opting the term to apply to a spectrum of greater or lesser problems of our own suggests that many of us share an underlying sense of frailty that we try to mythicize and transmute into heroism. The survivor script gives dignity to the suffering we have invited through our own bad choices. It offers us the opportunity to soar, powered by the hope of redemption to traverse the arc from victim to survivor, and sometimes even to guru. Whatever its source, this script can help us heal, provided that we use it to rewrite our own lives, not simply to attach ourselves to a generic identity. Becoming a professional victim is itself a kind of victimization.

Many contemporary films and novels center on powerlessness that is confronted and surmounted, or on adversity and handicaps that are overcome by ordinary people who rise to heroism. They play on our vulnerability and nourish our hopes for recovery from confusion, paralysis, a sense of insecurity or inferiority, hard times, or bad situations. Such themes are found in movies such as *Field of Dreams, Forrest Gump,* and the now classic *It's a Wonderful Life.* Sometimes, though, the outcome for a despairing hero or heroine is death. Consider Judith Rossner's novel *Looking for Mr. Goodbar* (and the movie based on it), in which we find ourselves morbidly fascinated with the desperation and loneliness of a young woman who looks for love in all the wrong places and makes a fatal pickup.

Popular interest in vulnerability is evident in Oprah Winfrey's television show and in her successful magazine, *O.* The writer Alex Kuczinski of the *New York Times* sums up *O*'s appeal: "The editorial mix is unlike that of most women's magazines. . . . There are articles about how to recover after your husband walks out, how to diagnose your own depression, and how a homeless women became a chief executive, and interviews with celebrities such as Sidney Poitier, Martha Stewart and Jane Fonda—each revealing some vulnerable part of themselves to Ms. Winfrey. (Ms. Stewart admitted that she cries every day.)"[7] The novels selected for Oprah's book club often have similar themes.

A fascination with vulnerability, particularly when vulnerability is overcome, may be particularly prominent today but is by no means of recent origin. A 1910 novel for adolescents, *A Girl of the Limberlost,* tells the story of Elnora, a country girl who lives with her mother and struggles against poverty and her mother's disparagement of and opposition to her wish to go to high school. Overcoming her mother's negativity is not Elnora's only hurdle. On the first day of school, "in one burning flash

[Elnora] came [to] the full realization of her scanty dress, her pitiful little hat and ribbon, her big, heavy shoes, her ignorance of where to go or what to do; and from a sickening wave which crept over her, she felt she was going to become very ill."[8] Here the author catches the way we often feel when our clothing and our lack of money and sophistication cause us to be excluded. Elnora must overcome her poverty and her ignorance of city ways as well as her mother's scorn. Yet through true grit, knowledge of the natural world, an ability to collect and sell butterflies, and the help of loving neighbors and a few classmates, Elnora prevails.

Whatever the source of our feelings of weakness and powerlessness, our sense of insufficiency waxes and wanes with our circumstances. We never achieve complete command of our lives. Yet, our feelings of weakness may intensify our longing for self-determination, our desire for power, and our drive to achieve it.

Before our feelings of powerlessness can prompt us to change, we must first allow ourselves to experience them. Many people are sensitive to powerlessness; they register it quickly and pertinently both in themselves and, through identification, in others. This natural sensitivity needs to be accounted for. Our easy identification with feelings of powerlessness has many sources, the most profound of which is the residue of our total dependency as children. Completely helpless at birth, we are totally at the mercy of a caregiver. Infancy gives us our first encounter with our inadequate control of our bodies, which much later elicits our laughter when it becomes the subject of low comedy. But the other side of humor is anxiety. We come to feel more or less secure, or more or less vulnerable, depending on the quality and the consistency of the parental care we receive in early life. Even the best parent sometimes fails to minister to our needs, and this demonstrates to us the limits of our self-sufficiency. Cherished though we may be, lapses in our care will give rise to periodic eruptions of anxiety.

The process of socialization places many demands on children. If all goes well, we grow out of our dependency, but this process requires "an overthrow of parental authority," resulting in a shift of power.[9] The child gradually assumes responsibility for her own care and begins to shape the direction her life takes, replacing total dependency with some degree of mastery. Parents can discourage or inhibit this process not only by overprotection and overcontrol but also by their attitude about the child's strengths. One pair of parents whose first child had died in infancy treated their daughter as someone who could be lost, and through their oversolicitousness evoked in her both hypochondriasis and a fear of the physical world.

While the child's overthrow of her parents' authority can be rebellious, it does not have to be. Part of a child's growth into autonomy draws on her internalization of parental strategies and values that become part of her essential being. The child takes on the parents' strength. As children relinquish dependency in favor of exercising their own powers, they gradually create for themselves a world they can manage. They do this by virtue of what has been called an innate healthy-mindedness, which expresses itself in the pleasures of the senses, in a feeling of expansiveness as the children get behind their particular skills and gifts, and in a sense of the newness and seeming limitlessness of life and its experiences.[10]

Children's weakness motivates them to cope independently, to learn self-reliance, to relinquish their wish for a parent's divine intervention, and to problem-solve for themselves. When parents stop dealing with all their children's small and large emergencies, children became aware that helping themselves may be essential. However, surmounting weakness and dependency is rarely a smooth process and is always incomplete.

Unfolding oneself into the world is often discouragingly difficult and frightening. The social theorist Ernest Becker beautifully describes how children experience a broad spectrum of anxieties in response to the demands of socialization:

> We . . . understand . . . why children have their recurrent nightmares, their universal phobias of insects and mean dogs. In their tortured interiors radiate complex symbols of many inadmissible realities—terror of the world, the horror of one's own wishes, the fear of vengeance by the parents, the disappearance of things, one's lack of control over anything, really. It is too much for any animal to take, but the child has to take it, and so he wakes up screaming with almost punctual regularity during the period when his weak ego is in the process of consolidating things.[11]

Feelings of weakness also arise from specific traumas—childhood illnesses, separation from parents, natural disasters—and our fears of them constitute an essential part of the human condition. How else might we explain the universality of children's terrors and nightmares?[12]

Children who are ill cared for, excessively punished, or abused experience an intensified feeling of powerlessness and realistic fear because they lack the means to protect themselves. They eventually come to resent their parents, sometimes even wishing them dead. Their hatred may allow them to feel more powerful, at least temporarily. But there may be another outcome. An undercurrent of their resentment and their wish for revenge may stay with them throughout their lives. By virtue of the talion principle (an eye for an eye, a tooth for a tooth), as adults, they often become fearful of retaliation and feel increasingly anxious.

Sometimes we opt for guilt over anxiety. If parents are overly strict, and their requirements are hard to meet, a child may experience anxiety based on a need to be watchful, alert to her parents' wishes. To the degree that a child holds her tongue, swallows her anger, shoulders the blame, she may come to experience her compliance as weakness. This sense of weakness, in turn, may inspire rebellion. Feeling guilty is often preferable to feeling weak. Some excessively compliant people feel guilty if they diverge even fractionally from their parents' or partner's guidelines, in part to create the illusion that they maintain some independence. Mobilizing guilt this way, they disguise from themselves their real problem— excessive compliance, motivated by anxiety and fear of abandonment.

No matter how ideal our childhood, we invariably experience a sense of weakness that stays with us in adulthood. Even when we are unaware that we feel powerless, our unconscious still periodically erupts to reveal an underlying fragility, in the form of anxious dreams or nightmares, in flash fantasies of danger or impoverishment. When we dream of being chased by menacing animals and monsters, of falling, of running from a fire that is licking at our heels, the symbolic language of dreams is allowing us to express feelings of weakness that may be inaccessible in our waking hours. One patient has recurrent dreams of herself producing unending bowel movements while sitting in an overflowing public toilet where the door won't stay shut. By now she knows that the dream is her unconscious alerting her to a humiliation in her waking life which she is blocking out, failing to identify—probably having to do with her abject submission to her parents' dictates. Something similar is happening when we experience spontaneous outbreaks of fear, often in the form of vivid images of disaster—getting fired, a spouse leaving, a child dying, the doctor telling us we have cancer, the car we are driving crashing.[13]

WHAT MOVES US—sometimes into action, reaction or assertion, sometimes into withdrawal and even apathy—is the power of our feelings. Feelings tell us different things about ourselves. They help us scan the inner and outer worlds, prodding both self-knowledge and knowledge of the outside world. Being in touch with our feelings is one of the primary ways we can navigate through our lives.[14] Just as important, feelings are instruments of our global self-evaluations, telling us how we're doing, mediating our sense of power or powerlessness, our experience of ourselves as weak or strong.[15] Alerted to feelings of weakness, we are sometimes able to change course and avoid a downward spiral. But sometimes we can be so overwhelmed by almost exactly the same feelings that we become paralyzed—incapacitated and powerless.

Shame and bodily vulnerability are often turned into comedy in TV sitcoms, and it is true, as Walter Kerr noted, that we like to laugh at other people's fleshly frailty. Yet shameful memories or events can be of such magnitude that they become a major part of our self-identity and can threaten our sense of wholeness and healthy narcissism. Some adults, still ashamed of their parents or their early lives, conceal some of the events in their lives, even from their spouses, and as a result feel unknown, unknowable, and isolated. Closely guarded secrets include illegitimacy, pregnancy out of wedlock, giving a child up for adoption, "passing," victimization by battering or sexual abuse, and skeletons in the family closet. The price we pay is that no one can really know us unless they know where we come from, what bumps and wounds we experienced in early life, and how we reacted to them emotionally. This is perhaps why friendships of youth and early adulthood are often among our strongest bonds. Our lifelong friends have known our hurts and secrets from the get-go.

Not all negative feelings diminish our sense of power. Rage, resentment, anger, fury, jealousy, and envy are feelings often connected with action, assertion, and the exertion of one or another kind of power. They propel us to right the wrongs we have suffered and to fight on our own behalf. As a result, they often lift our spirits. Sometimes we misuse the high that recriminations and anger can provide us by transposing these emotions from their real object to a loved one or even to an innocent bystander. In other words, we mobilize anger—even if it is unjustified—to get over any narcissistic injury that leaves us feeling diminished. A teenager, fearful that he has failed an exam, may explode in anger when asked by his parents about how he thinks he did on a test. As a consequence, he may feel relief. A lawyer who loses a client may displace his sense of inadequacy by betraying an associate. Although a blowup may cost us dearly in the long run, in the short run it acts to heal our wounded sense of self.

Many of us express hostility in the form of subtle put-downs or stinging questions in order to allay our own feelings of insecurity and inadequacy. In social situations, people who are feeling at a disadvantage often ask seemingly concerned questions as a way of making others feel bad. At a lavish party, an overweight woman whose dress has a high neck and long sleeves asks a newcomer, a glamorous woman in a strapless dress, if she isn't cold. The question is meant to make the newcomer feel uncomfortable—a kind of indirect put-down. Or one dinner guest will ask a divorced woman how she feels about her ex-husband's notorious exploits. I categorize this kind of remark as a "concerned" put-down. There are other, more shattering self-preserving gambits that we sometimes resort to in response to our negative feelings.

While we sometimes use guilt to squelch our anxiety and our feeling of powerlessness, guilt may itself become unbearable. In *The Iceman Cometh*, Eugene O'Neill gives a stunning demonstration of how self-depleting guilt can morph into rage. Sitting in Harry Hope's bar, Hickey tells his drinking buddies that his wife, Evelyn, is dead. He counters their various hypotheses about how she died—that she killed herself, that someone else killed her, or that he killed her because she was sleeping with "the Iceman." Then Hickey tells them what really happened. For years, he has guiltily agonized over being an alcoholic, a periodic binger, who betrayed Evelyn time and again:

> . . . I hated myself more and more, thinking of all the wrong I'd done to the sweetest woman in the world who loved me so much. I got so I'd curse myself for a lousy bastard every time I saw myself in the mirror. I felt such pity for her it drove me crazy. . . . It got so every night I'd wind up hiding my face in her lap, bawling and begging her forgiveness. And, of course, she'd always comfort me and say 'Never mind, Teddy, I know you won't ever again.' Christ I loved her so, but I began to hate that pipe dream! . . . I couldn't forgive her for forgiving me. I even caught myself hating her for making me hate myself so much. There's a limit to the guilt you

can feel and the forgiveness and the pity you can take! You have to begin blaming someone else, too. I got so sometimes when she'd kiss me it was like she did it on purpose to humiliate me, as if she'd spit in my face! . . . You'd never believe I could hate so much, a good-natured, happy-go-lucky slob like me. . . . I went in the bedroom. I was going to tell her it was the end. But I couldn't do that to her. She was sound asleep. I thought, God, if she'd only never wake up, she'd never know! And then it came to me—the only possible way out, for her sake. I remembered I'd given her a gun for protection while I was away and it was in the bureau drawer. She'd never feel any pain, never wake up from her dream. So I . . . [16]

Disillusioned with himself and his deception and enraged that his wife could not accept the truth, Hickey kills her. In so doing, he asserts a kind of power and takes revenge on the pity she feels for him, something he saw as a product of her feeling superior to him. (Here, O'Neill gives us an important insight. Being pitied is not ultimately comforting.) Hickey then takes it on himself to disabuse his drinking cronies of their pipe dreams, to put them down under the guise of setting them straight. For Hickey there are no longer any dreams, just pipe dreams, a condition he finds unbearable. And although what he does, and did, is thoroughly illogical, the audience accepts it because the sudden metamorphosis of intense negative feelings is all too familiar.

Even when feelings don't "morph," they may oscillate. We often swing between hope and despair, desire and anxiety. These oscillating feelings produce corresponding changes in our sense of power and of powerlessness. In our sexual life, when we feel anxiety, desire may be squelched, causing impotence (powerlessness). Of course, anxiety can also enhance desire. Fear or anxiety connected to performance (sexual, artistic, or professional) may cause a total shutdown, yet in the right dose it sometimes yields that extra frisson of excitement that enhances pleasure *and* performance. Early in her career, one gifted teacher was so overwhelmed by anxiety that she could barely speak. Years later, her much diminished but still lingering anxiety was a stimulant to her performance. Late in her career, when she was virtually anxiety-free, her performance completely lost its glitter and she was bored.

Feelings let us know what is nutrient and what is noxious; as a result, they either facilitate or impede our actions.[17] Though taking stock of our feelings is the major way to get in touch with what is good for us and what ails us, we do not always listen to our feelings. There is a kind of switch deep within us—perhaps innate, probably more often learned in the crucible of the family—that dictates whether we go with a feeling or ignore its clarion call. Thus, some of us ignore what our feelings have to say, more or less as policy.

Consider Alice, who is passionately committed to cerebral decisions, even though her feelings are exquisitely nuanced. Alice says that fear, depression, and anger are shutting her down, but intellectually she knows that it's the other way round—that she shuts down her feelings. She is intermittently paralyzed, unable to assert herself, let alone express justifiable anger. Expressing anger doesn't even occur to her until long after the event that precipitated it. Blocking out her feelings gives Alice an illusory sense of self-control, personal agency, power. But this is momentary because, although she claims to be in command, she eventually realizes that she is experiencing an emotional paralysis, a sense of being emptied out and utterly without will.

Alice's self-containment seems connected to her parents' polarized styles. Her laid-back manner appears to be a refusal to identify with her brilliant but emotionally incontinent and often abrasive father. It also stems in part form her childhood fear of what would happen if she insisted on having emotions and reactions that differed from his. Sometimes she rationalizes her style by claiming a conscious identification with her mother's quiet strength and stoicism, but at other times she sees her mother as more passive than stoic.

Not surprisingly, Alice's boyfriend, Robert, is more like her father than like her mother. He makes extravagant and effective use of his emotions, including depression, to make demands on friends and lovers, thereby controlling them—a method that on occasion comes close to blackmail. Alice thinks it's possible that she seeks Robert out not just because he revivifies her early love for her father but also because she participates vicariously in his emotional expressiveness. The result is a tilt toward a dominant-submissive relationship, with Alice experiencing herself as relatively powerless and Robert as the dominant force.

We all weigh the importance of our feelings differently. In part, it's a question of how central we believe they are to the plot of our life. Robert's behavior is frequently fueled by a sense of righteous indignation, whereas Alice seldom refers to her feelings in the anecdotes she tells. She is more detached, a good observer of others, but does not see herself as the spark that sets a plot in motion. Robert, who sees his feelings as the engine that puts events into play, gets a boost for his sense of power because he sees himself as a player initiating or controlling the action through the feelings he expresses. In contrast, Alice feels diminished because she is primarily a responder or an observer.

We may momentarily identify ourselves as powerful or powerless through objective criteria (whether we're healthy or sickly, pretty or plain, brilliant or slow, rich or poor), but our authentic identification depends on our core feelings and self-appraisals. A poor woman ennobled by love feels powerful; a rich woman, "trapped" by a seemingly glamorous life, feels powerless. To know ourselves we must become keen observers of what we feel and begin to connect our feelings to both our present and our past; and we must also let ourselves truly experience what we feel.

OVER TIME many of us learn to apply strategies of power as a way of mitigating our feelings of weakness and dependency. I've already noted that weakness often prods us to acquire power, a trajectory I will explore throughout this book. But there are some who feel as though a river of weakness flows through their lives without understanding why. A feeling of powerlessness is always with them—sometimes connected to actual adversity but at other times left over from problems they encountered in early life and the strategies they chose to counter them. Not all strategies are created equal it turns out.

A patient of mine, Brad, just entering the self-supporting stage of life, told me how surprised he was by the guilt he felt when his father gave him a new car. I inquired if he might be feeling more shame than guilt, and he burst into tears. This proved to be a turning point in his analysis. (It is another example of how guilt often feels preferable to shame.) The question triggered an overwhelming memory of feeling powerless without his father's support, followed by a detailed recounting of a series of boyhood scenes in which he had been rejected by his peers, probably because he was a sad and withdrawn child. Brad's mother died when he was young, and although his father had remarried, his stepmother never really nurtured him. He remembered how his father tried to make up for the pain and humiliation he felt at being ostracized by his peers by giving him an ever-expanding array of material things each time he came home, but this only added to his sadness and hurt. Over the years he was given name-brand clothes, cutting-edge electronic equipment, and, one particularly exciting day (several cars before the one that had prompted his tears in our therapy session), his first car. When he drove it, he said he felt as if a protective skin had been fitted around him.

A life plan, seldom completely conscious, is like a car, which both carries us along and protects us but can leave us devastated if it breaks down or, worse, crashes. The "quick-fix" power that material goods conferred on Brad was never internalized; like the car, it was a protective skin, and it was his father's to give, not something innate to Brad himself. As a result, his underlying sense of fragility and powerlessness continued unabated into his early manhood, even though by then he had achieved considerable success not only in his social life but also in college and, later, in his first job. As we discovered in subsequent sessions, what had prevented Brad from internalizing the strength of his father's support was his sense that his father resented his neediness and the stresses it brought into his new marriage. Material goods were forthcoming, but emotional goods were not.

Brad's insight into the sources of his continuing sense of weakness and the inadequacy of his and his father's attempts to remedy it was jump-started by an article he read in the *New York Times* about research on the effect of pursuing such common objectives as money, fame, and beauty. The article quoted the researchers' almost homespun or homiletic conclusion that people who valued these external goals to an unusual degree were more depressed than others, even if they had achieved their goals, because "the more we seek satisfactions in material goods [and other extrinsic goals] the less we find them there."[18] This struck a chord with Brad. He was able to link his sense of powerlessness not only to his mother's death and his ostracism by childhood peers, but also to a failure to connect with his father and the uneasiness he still felt about papering over the deficiencies in his life with material goods. With this understanding and a shift in his priorities, he began to confront his sense of weakness head-on.

Brad's boyhood humiliations and his resulting need for dependence on his father perpetuated his sense of weakness and his feeling of shame. Like him, many others are ashamed about feeling powerlessness. Recovery from these feelings does not always take place automatically, even when someone has objectively achieved power in the real world. Many of us continue to feel powerless, and this feeling can take the form of shame, low self-esteem, fear, humiliation, or lack of pride, despite outward and sometimes very real success. This paradox shows in high relief how unresolved psychological conflict can create lifelong feelings of powerlessness.

Mr. Grant, a single lawyer in his late thirties, was widely recognized as a force in his field, a subspecialty involving large-scale takeovers, which often required him to be seriously assertive. He acknowledged his eminence in his profession, gained through hard work and intelligence, as well as through early apprenticeship to a series of powerful mentors. Nonetheless, he felt that his power in business was either a charade, something he put over on others but couldn't convince himself of, or simply a matter of luck. On the eve of any anticipated professional conflict, he nearly always had one of several recurrent dreams with the same theme: (1) He is a member of an orchestra; he is sitting behind his father and is supposed to play a solo, but his violin has no strings. His father gives him an instrument with strings, but the strings are put in horizontally rather than vertically. The score is from the movie *Breaking Away* (something he feels he has never been able to do vis-à-vis his still vital, overcontrolling and undercutting father). (2) He has to sign something, but he has no pen, so he borrows A. B.'s pen. (A. B. is a former partner, a phony, possibly a crook.) The pen doesn't work; it is in four parts, and he has to put them back together again. (3) A small boy, unidentified, borrows or steals a boat with an outboard motor. He heads out to the sea and is immediately lost in its vastness. In all these dreams Mr. Grant lacks the right equipment, often because his father or another flawed father figure has palmed defective equipment off on him. These dream images—the pen and the violin, for example—are at once phallic symbols and emblems of professional achievement, clearly relating to both sex and work and demonstrating how issues of power and sex get linked in the preconscious mind.

Mr. Grant's sense of weakness was first apparent to him in adolescence, a time when his father became extremely critical of him and seemed to turn against him. Why his father did this remains a mystery, but it was this loss of his father's validation, which had initially countered his mother's lifelong rejection of him, that stamped him in his own mind as ultimately unworthy. His father's opinion may have weighed on him so heavily because for so long he had idealized his father as the counterweight to his mother's rejection. Despite his success, Mr. Grant has

retained his adolescent view of himself as a bumbler, a pose he first culti-
vated because acting the buffoon was the main way he got back at his
father for his defection. This is one way the powerless can use their infirmities to undo the powerful—and it is one of the weapons adolescents
use to bring down their parents, whether consciously or out of the deep
recesses of the unconscious. In his personal life, Mr. Grant still regresses
to "schlemiel" behavior on family occasions when his father is present.

Thus far my vignettes have implicated some inner psychological problem stemming from early life relationships as the root cause of ongoing
feelings of powerlessness. But just as often, feelings of powerlessness flow
from social issues. Many years ago, I saw an interview on television with a
dirt-poor black boy from the South who described why he had dropped
out of school. He appeared extremely dejected and said that he felt
ashamed. Why? Because he didn't have a quarter a day to spend, like the
rest of the kids. I found myself crying, even though I didn't understand
why he felt shame rather than anger or sadness. But I hadn't yet thought
through how powerlessness so often gets incorporated into our very identity. Power is experienced as exhilarating and is connected to pride, but
powerlessness—as a result of poverty, loss of a job or a spouse, illness, or
some other cause—is connected to feelings of humiliation and shame.

A sense of powerlessness is also often the product of an individual flaw
or conflict in conjunction with a cultural bias toward defining power primarily in only one way. Powerlessness of this kind characterizes Willie
Loman, the fatally flawed, tragic protagonist in Arthur Miller's *Death of a
Salesman*, the man who takes to the road "on a smile and a shoeshine." In
an article in the *New Yorker*, "Making Willie Loman," the drama critic
John Lahr recounted that Miller was once buttonholed by a theatergoer
who wanted to know what product Willie lugs around in his sample cases.
" 'Well, himself. That's who's in the valise . . . ,' Miller answered, adding,
'You sell yourself. . . . You become the commodity.' "[19] But in Willie's case,
nobody wanted to buy. The pain of his powerlessness, which speaks to us
in an utterly visceral way, has made *Death of a Salesman* the definitive
portrait of one aspect of the American psyche—the socially scripted compulsion to achieve self-esteem and personal power through success. And
the tragedy for Willie Loman is his failure to do so, or, even more, to com-
prehend what might be involved. Because Willie believes that personality
will win the day, he takes his failure as a humiliating condemnation of his
whole self. Miller described the audience's reaction to the premiere per-

formance of the play, some fifty years ago: "The curtain came down and nothing happened. People sat there a good two or three minutes. . . . Several men—I didn't see women doing this—were helpless. They were sitting there with handkerchiefs over their faces. It was like a funeral. . . . Finally, someone thought to applaud, and then the house came apart."

Perhaps the only thing that would be different if the play were being produced for the first time today is that women would be as overcome by emotion as men, because many women are now as trapped as men are by competitiveness—what Miller calls "the ultimate outer-directional emotion." (This seemed to be the case in the 1999 New York City revival of *Death of a Salesman* starring Brian Dennehy.) Ambition is the fuel that runs this country. A large segment of our culture has bought into the commodification of the self that afflicts and ultimately destroys Willie Loman. How self-worth can be generated in this culture is the unspoken question at the heart of Miller's play, and a critical issue for all of us.

BEYOND ANXIETIES and neurotic conflicts generated in childhood, a sense of powerlessness can be caused by the lurking knowledge that we and our loved ones must ultimately die. People experience this dread to different degrees and at different times in their lives. Sandy was a close friend who first introduced me to many of the nooks and crannies of New York City. He and I, as young adults, used to divide the world into people who were afraid of death and those who were not. At that time, both of us were just recovering from our childhood fear of death and, believing that anyone who had not experienced this fear was somehow shallow, we congratulated ourselves on our own sensitivity. Perhaps this was no more than putting the best face on the remnants of childhood vulnerability—sometimes a useful compensatory device. Each of us had experienced stark terror in childhood, though for different reasons, so, for us, life seemed to be a roller-coaster ride with only one inevitable destination.

At the age of two I was still nursing, my father unable to bear my tears whenever my mother tried to wean me. Around that time, I was trapped in a flood that devastated Louisville. I was rescued by boat, but I promptly developed pneumonia, requiring hospitalization (this was before penicillin). At that time parents could not stay overnight with a hospitalized child, so I was separated from my mother, delirious with fever, and traumatically weaned. Early overindulgence interrupted by life-threatening illness and trauma has led to a divide in my personality—on the one hand, self-confidence (getting to nurse for a long time connected to the sometimes mistaken idea that I could generally get my way); on the other hand, fearfulness (an intermittent anxiety that the good times would be suddenly interrupted).

My friend Sandy was a young child when his older brother was killed in World War II. His trauma was twofold: not only did he lose his beloved brother, but he felt guilty because he had deeply resented his parents' evident partiality to this brother, the oldest of their three sons. While my own fear of death receded and is now triggered primarily in response to a threat to my health, Sandy's death fear completely disappeared. He died of AIDS after a protracted illness, which he faced with great courage; whatever fears he once suffered had long since been resolved.

Confronting our precarious footing in the world shows us the limitations of our ability to control any number of important aspects of our own lives. Because we have both memory and foresight, we anticipate our own death, and this inevitably gives rise to feelings of powerlessness. Even Sigmund Freud, who relied primarily on instincts to explain human feelings and behavior, spoke in his later work of "human perplexity and helplessness in the face of nature's dreaded forces," "the terror of nature," "the painful riddle of death," "our anxiety in the face of life's dangers," and "the great necessities of fate, against which there is no remedy." Nevertheless, Freud sometimes maintained that the fear of death was nothing more than the analog of the fear of castration, thus minimizing its impact.[20] The psychoanalyst Abraham Maslow recognized that mortality is a basic human predicament, a feeling of being both "worms and Gods."[21]

Not all people counter their fear of death in the same way. Hannah Arendt wrote that in Greek civilization men sought immortality through great deeds and the hope that their memory would resound through history; on the other hand, Christianity offered eternal life as the reward for piety and belief in Jesus.[22] Some people are reassured by a belief in immortality. Others may ally themselves with a belief system, religious or not, that gives sufficient meaning to life—for example, living on in their children or putting their efforts into good works. Still others appear to be essentially untroubled by thoughts of death. But there are many who remain terrified and to whom death remains "the worm at the core" of our pretensions to happiness.[23]

But this is not the whole story about the impact of our knowledge of death. As with the ethos of the Greeks, some of our greatest cultural achievements derive from our attempt to deny or control death. Although the fear of death is sometimes paralyzing, it may also stoke our ambitions, pushing us to achieve, goading us to live more fully. John Lahr, writing about another drama critic, Kenneth Tynan, remarks: "Of the many qualities that made him an outstanding critic—qualities of wit, language, knowledge, style and fun—perhaps the most surprising was his profound awareness of death. It fed both his voracity for pleasure—for food, for drink, for talk— . . . and his desire to memorialize it." Lahr quotes from Tynan's journal: "I remember about thirty times between waking and sleeping and always while I'm asleep that I'm going to die. . . . And the more scared I am, the more pleasure and enlightenment I want to squeeze from every moment." Lahr concludes that Tynan used his writing as a hedge against this seemingly overwhelming fear, as "a way of keeping the consoling dramatic pleasures alive within himself by making them live for others."[24]

Patients suffering from overweening ambition can sometimes connect the first appearance of their fear of death to intense spurts of ambition in late childhood or early adolescence. Some consciously counter their death anxiety by striving for immortality through their achievements. A brilliant, gentle man in his forties who had been one of my college classmates tried, agonizingly, to finish his first novel as he lay dying. He was a man without children whose masterwork had not yet been shown to a publisher—a far from unique story among aspiring artists who face death early. Unfortunately, the need to counteract the fear of death and to rage against nothingness have also propelled some of the most destructive of conquerors in history.

OUR SENSE of weakness and helplessness can be intensified by difficult circumstances or by neurotic conflict, but, as suggested earlier, a fear of being powerless is a fundamental part of the human condition; it rises from the total dependency of infancy, the slightly less terrifying dependency we experience in adulthood, and our terrible knowledge of mortality. Just as gnawing are the fears and anxieties inherent in living, the inevitable day-to-day frustrations, disappointments, and sadness in our intimate lives and our work. We mourn our lost opportunities; we feel diminished or perhaps depressed by narrowing windows of opportunity. Our neurotic conflicts make us more vulnerable to a feeling of powerlessness, but they are not the sole cause of this feeling.

Unless we have some sense of being able to control our day-to-day lives, we cannot help feeling inert and at the mercy of external forces. Thus, the impulse to exert power on our own behalf or to make alliances with those more powerful than we are is an attempt to combat not just our feeling of vulnerability but also our feeling of existential fragility. Powerlessness sometimes defeats us. But just as often it mobilizes us, acting as a pivot for achievement or change. The tension between power and powerlessness in our lives determines whether or not we are able to move in the direction of internal strength and authentic power.

3

The Contradictions and Fluctuations of Power

"Power always has an untied shoelace; the very need to threaten suggests an obscure vulnerability."

—WALTER KERR, *Tragedy and Comedy*

P ower is not something we attain once and for all, but something that inevitably waxes and wanes. Several realities act to insure that power stays in flux. From the perspective of the life cycle, it is self-evident that a trajectory of power is built into the "ages of man," that is, we command power to different degrees at different stages of life. From the interpersonal perspective, we know that the exertion of power by one person over another seldom goes unchallenged; it ultimately evokes resistance from others. From the psychological perspective, we intuit that we each crave to be both dominant and submissive; our inner desires are far from unitary. From the sociological perspective, we know all too well that we are affected by life circumstances over which we have little or no control and which may enhance or impede our ability to assert ourselves. Yet self-understanding gives us the opportunity to radically expand our command of power, provided that there are new pockets of opportunity into which to grow.

LET ME BEGIN with the fluctuations of power that derive from the life cycle, a topic of mythic scope. It is ever so obvious that we start and end life as powerless. It is only slightly less obvious that the people who will ultimately wrest power from us at first appear to be helpless and dependent, whether they are our own children or the children of others. The process of a new generation taking over proceeds slowly, almost imperceptibly, and we do not like watching it happen without resisting it, because if we do, we confront our own finitude.

Most of us acquire increasing power as we grow from infancy to childhood to adulthood. Youthful optimism is partly the product of an evergrowing sense of expansiveness, mastery, and control, as we acquire new competencies and new possibilities present themselves to us. This exultation often extends to marrying and reproducing and thus taking on a sense of the power and prestige we once saw in our parents. Yet for many of us, crossing the divide from youth to parenthood introduces a new and not always welcome knowledge of our mortality. For some parents, their first glance at their newborn baby is bittersweet because they sense that the birth of their child portends their own passing: it is perhaps their first realization that they do not live outside history but are merely a part of the cycle of generations. For other parents, this knowledge is postponed until their children reach adolescence, when offspring sometimes begin their first full frontal assault on parental authority.

While it is true that the birth of a child may console us for our mortality, promising us some kind of continuity, nonetheless, as the child's life waxes, the parent's life wanes. In the later stages of the life cycle, we generally encounter a downward slope, which often mandates that we cede power and resources to the next generation. And if we are poor or ill when we grow older, the power balance with our children, now in their prime, may be completely reversed, and we may find ourselves increasingly dependent on them.

This parental confrontation with mortality at the birth of a child is a universal theme. It is part of the plotline in the tragedy of Oedipus, as related in Sophocles' *Oedipus Tyrannus*, written more than 2,500 years ago. Among its other themes, the story of Oedipus is a profound meditation on the cycle of generations. Laius, the King of Thebes, is told of the prediction by an oracle that his newborn son will kill him and will subsequently marry his wife, Jocasta. To evade this terrible fate, Laius has Oedipus's feet tied together and abandons him on Mount Cithaeron to die. Put simply, Laius sacrifices his son to preserve his own life and his own power.

A Corinthian shepherd finds and rescues the baby. Named Oedipus because of his swollen feet, he is adopted and raised by the king and queen of Corinth. Once he is grown, Oedipus consults the oracle at Delphi, whereupon he is told that his destiny is to kill his father and marry his mother. Since he believes the king and queen of Corinth to be his natural parents, he tries to avoid his fate by fleeing Corinth. On his way to Thebes, he gets into an argument with a man whom he kills, never dreaming that *this* man, King Laius, could be his biological father.

Arriving in Thebes, a town endangered by the Sphinx's spell, Oedipus saves the town by solving the Sphinx's riddle: "What goes on four legs in the morning, two legs in the afternoon, and three legs at night?" Oedipus solves the riddle by answering "Man," whereupon the Sphinx dies. This riddle is, of course, itself a comment on the inevitable toll of the passing of time. It charts man's trajectory from crawling infant through the fullness of his mature power to the encroachment on his power that an old man's cane signifies. Having saved the town and been declared a hero, Oedipus marries Queen Jocasta and they produce four children. Only when Oedipus attempts to discover who killed Queen Jocasta's husband and learns his own history does the tragedy unfold. Jocasta kills herself, and Oedipus blinds himself with her brooch.

Scholars argue about how to interpret this tale. For example, the philosopher and psychoanalyst Jonathan Lear suggests that psychoanalysts, like Oedipus himself, fail to acknowledge an essential fact about him, namely his parents' cruel and unnatural abandonment of him, focusing instead on Oedipus' crime.[1] While analytic interpretations of the Oedipus myth are extremely illuminating in decoding the relationship between father and son and the inherent conflict over who possesses the wife/mother, the Oedipus story is clearly also a metaphorical tale about power, about who gets to be King. Our inevitable conflicts with our parents are surely not exclusively the product of sexual ambitions; what we seek is the power of our parents. Oedipus acquires the crown, not just his mother. Freud emphasizes the competition between the father and the son over the possession of the mother, but fails to observe the existential tragedy that as the son grows into his strength, his father's strength begins to wane.

The Oedipal legend carries an additional message, too: it tells us how little we ultimately control our personal fate. Like the hero in John O'Hara's novel, *Appointment in Samarra*, who flees Death only to encounter him in the very place where he seeks refuge, Oedipus is unable to escape his destiny. Both stories pivot on tragic ironies that suggest how easily destiny destroys our intentions and upsets our best-laid plans.

Royal succession is a perfect theme for tragedy, because it combines the heat of the family and the mythic significance of power. Shakespeare's *King Lear* confronts head-on the conflicts and treacheries that ensue as the power of a ruler and father declines, and a succession must be established. Lear, the king of Britain, had three daughters. At the age of eighty, desiring to retire, he resolved to divide his kingdom among his daughters in proportion to their love. The two older daughters, Goneril and Regan, claimed to love him more than they could possibly express, but Cordelia, the youngest, declared only that she loved him as a daughter should. Lear felt that her answer was far too constrained and consequently disinherited her, dividing his kingdom between his other two daughters, on the condition that they look after him during alternate months. The inheritance having been passed on, neither of the two older daughters keeps her promise, and finally Lear is turned out into a storm. But the two sisters fall out and become enemies: the elder sister, Goneril, poisons the middle sister and then kills herself. Cordelia, the only truly loving daughter, who in the meantime has married the King of France, brings an army to dethrone her sisters, but instead is herself taken prisoner and hanged, while Lear dies of grief. (Jane Smiley's *A Thousand Acres* is a recent iteration of the King Lear story.)

Neither the fight over an inheritance nor the sibling rivalry that exacerbates such a fight is restricted to the tragic theater. Patricide is the oldest of stories, enacted at the literal level when, as Alexander the Great did, the prince kills his father to become king, and at the symbolic level when the young turn on their mentors and displace them. Both *Oedipus* and *Lear* emphasize the existential fact that willy-nilly the child replaces his parent, the student his teacher, the young the old.

Many businessmen and their families consult psychiatrists about conflicts between two generations or between two brothers over who should control a business, how best to preserve the integrity of the business after death, or how to protect the interests of siblings who do not work in the business. (In fact, a lucrative therapeutic subspecialty has developed to address such issues.) But fights over money often conceal deeper concerns about who is best loved. The fights that end up in the court system are often about wills that favor one survivor over another, reawakening sibling rivalries that have been thinly papered over, conflicts between one set of children and another, or between a current wife and children by a previous wife.

Even without issues of succession and inheritance, family tensions frequently arise as adolescents and young adults move toward separation and independence. Parents may be thrilled to see their children grow to independence, but that joy is more often than not tinged by the realization that as their children grow into their powers, the parents' own powers, their prestige, and their authority are on the decline. The passing of the torch from generation to generation is bittersweet. For some, maybe most parents, the reality of that process first hits home during a child's adolescence, when parents watch their children growing into a potency and beauty, a strength and a competence that they can only wistfully admire and envy.

In her novel *Lovingkindness*, Anne Roiphe describes the loss mothers feel as their adolescent daughters subtly disengage:

> What do we know about mothers and daughters? If there is a recurring myth of matricide and usurped power, who tells that story? If mothers and daughters form a unit that crackles and splits and sends particles out into the universe, particles of hate, revenge and passion, where do we hear it? Mothers are not afraid of their daughters (except for the wicked queen in "Snow White"). Our power is so oblique, so hidden, and so ethereal a matter, that we rarely struggle with our daughters over actual kingdoms or corporate chairs. On the other hand, our attractiveness dries as theirs blooms, our journey shortens just as theirs begins. We too must be afraid and awed and amazed that we cannot live forever. And that our replacements are eager for their turn, indifferent to our wishes, ready to leave us behind.[2]

Wise parents realize that at critical junctures they sometimes may have to make hard decisions for which their children may ultimately resent if not hate them. In Mario Puzo's brilliant novel *The Fortunate Pilgrim*, the heroine of the story, Lucia Santa, based on his mother, comes to an important crossroads. She must make a decision that will impact not only her family's current life but also her future relationships with her children. Her second husband—the father of the three youngest of her six children—has been hospitalized with a severe mental breakdown. When he might be coming home, she is faced with a terrible dilemma:

> Like many others this illiterate, untrained peasant woman had the power of life and death over the human beings nearest to her. On every day in every year people must condemn and betray their loved ones. Lucia Santa did not think in terms of sentiment. But love and pity had value, a certain weight in life.
>
> The man who had fathered her children, rescued her from a desperate and helpless widowhood, and wakened her to delight, was no longer of any real value to her. He would bring war into the family. Octavia [the oldest daughter] might leave; she would marry early to escape him. He would be a liability in the battle against life. . . .
>
> But beyond love there was honor, there was duty, there was a union against the world. Frank Corbo had never betrayed that honor; he had only not been able to fulfill it. And he was the father of three of these children. There was blood there. In the future years she must look these children in the eye. She would have to account to them, for he had given them life, they were in his debt. Lurking beyond this was the primitive dread that parents have of their own fate when they are old and helpless as they become their children's children, and in their turn seek mercy.[3]

Lucia Santa makes the only decision she feels will stabilize her family's safety, pushing aside the thought of what this may later cost her. She leaves her husband in the hospital, where he will eventually die. Yet she fears that her ruthlessness in doing so may forever alienate some of her children. It is no doubt this very ruthlessness to which Puzo referred when he said that whenever his own creation, the Godfather, spoke, he heard the voice of his mother.

The trajectory of the power we exert in our professional lives follows a similar—though not synchronous—arc to the one we experience in our family lives. For a while that trajectory may look as though it moves in only one direction. Our prejudice, as La Rochefoucauld put it, is that:

"One honor is a surety for more." But several things happen along the way that torpedo any such expectation. What makes the downward slope of power inevitable are age and the loss of certain skills (for athletes and dancers, and also oddly enough for mathematicians, a problem that comes sooner rather than later) or a new technology that makes what we know obsolete; a new CEO or Board of Directors; or most ironic of all, the pressure from protégés who begin nipping at our heels. We discover that just as we ourselves were ambitious on the way to the top, so, too, are there ambitious people coming along behind us. In time, someone will replace us. Either we reach retirement age or we lose our competence. Some of the saddest stories in the business world involve a useless struggles to hold on to power when the time has come to relinquish it. (Sometimes, of course, we fail in the first instance to achieve the power we want—but that is another story.)

Just as our late-life relationships with our now grown children depend on what went before, so, too, is the gradual loss of power in our work lives colored by our relationships with our bosses, colleagues, and subordinates. Those who use worldly power and domination over others as their primary mode of self-validation may find that age presents a perilous challenge if not a devastation. However, the decline of our self-worth with age is not inevitable, as I think the story of my grandfather demonstrates. But he had command of all his faculties long beyond the norm, and he belonged to a generation in which many individuals were sole proprietors of businesses, a situation that is now less common. Yet many aging people find sufficient gratification in their families, in the good fortune of their protégés (particularly if the beneficiaries of their help are grateful and not resentful), and in the pleasures and activities they continue to cultivate. They may also find pleasure, not just comfort, in the care they continue to bestow on others. Some, too, find gratification in spirituality.

THE TENDENCY to assert our own power by resisting the power of others is well-nigh universal. In fact, personal power is born together with the natural resistance we have toward any external power to which we are subject. Our resistance to external authority was the route we first took in order to establish our autonomy in early childhood. Our ability to break out of dependency is predicated on an inborn impulse to self-expression, a characteristic that is rooted in our innate predisposition to express our own will even when it means resisting parental authority.

This resistance to power constitutes one of the basic dialectics of power. It is evident not only in the relationship of growing children to their parents, but in people's almost inevitable resistance to the imperatives demanded of them by others who have authority in the social or political realms. The political and economic theorist John Kenneth Galbraith proposed that resistance to power "is as integral a part of the phenomenon of power as its exercise itself." In the political realm, Galbraith pointed out, the one regularly follows the other: "The response to an arbitrary exercise of the power to tax was an organization to dump the tea so taxed into the water; to the draft, an organization of draft resisters; to an invasion of civil liberties, an organization to protect those liberties; to male chauvinism or dominance, an organization to assert women's rights."[4]

The extreme will to power and the abuse of power invariably evoke resistance. Were there no resistance to power, all of us would be subject to those who were best at exercising it. Tyrants would inevitably prevail.

While we all share a natural resistance to authority, many of us hunger to achieve power for ourselves. We often show an impulse to overreach, to abuse our power. Yet any hubris we display invokes a resistance to our power. Hubris can bring about destruction in one's own life no less than in the tragic theatre. Such ultimately self-immolating behavior is evident in contemporary stories of those so intent on increasing not only their wealth and power but also their self-importance that they go beyond acceptable limits. Some display hubris in the reckless chances they take, sometimes borrowing to the hilt and getting wiped out in an economic downturn. When powerful people are arrogant to their associates, to journalists, or to public investigators, they create enemies, often with damaging results if the objects of their condescension decide on a course of revenge. Leona Helmsley went to jail not because the prosecutors were out for blood (people did not much care for her skinflint husband, and the Harry-made-me-do-it card could have worked) but because her former employees were. When the call for witnesses went out, a line formed down the stairs and out into the street—gardeners, maids, plumbers, repairmen, clerks, and others. That's what did her in—she had just been too mean (there's no other word for it) to too many people, particularly small people who now, at last, had a recourse.

Nations, like individuals, fall prey to hubris. Paul Kennedy writes eloquently in *The Rise and Fall of the Great Powers* "of the habit that dominant countries have of overreaching their capacity to exert military control in the world, straining their fiscal resources and hastening the demise of the empire." In his work, he portrays the difficulty that the leaders of nations have in reconciling themselves to any limitations inherent in power. Even after their decline should be obvious to them, they deny the evidence and actually hasten the process by engaging in military adventures they can ill afford, simply to prove to themselves and the rest of the world that they are still superpowers.[5]

We can take it as a rule: Given the natural resistance to power, whatever power we possess will inevitably be countered if not explicitly challenged. This is true of history's tyrants and of anyone else who has achieved success, power, money, or fame, particularly if they are arrogant. No one's power indefinitely protects them from real or symbolic attacks on their status and prestige, particularly if they have behaved disparagingly or meanly to those around them. The dominant position is fundamentally vulnerable because it breeds envy in others and leads them to covet what the dominant person has. The degree to which people gloat over someone else's fall from fortune is clear evidence of the dual attitude we so often have to powerful people—admiration *and* envy. That envy seemed evident enough in the extravagant and detailed newspaper coverage of Saul Steinberg's fall from power when his company, Reliance Capital, failed and his collection of gilded French antiques went on the auction block; most of the stories were pointedly illustrated with photographs of the Steinbergs before the fall, opulently dressed for one ball or another.

Envy is often the main reason many people in power are ultimately betrayed by those whose careers they have nourished. They become victims of patricide or matricide when a subordinate's devotion is revealed as no more than a cover for virulent envy. Consider the movie *All About Eve*, in which an aspiring actress's (the Anne Baxter character) worship of a great actress (the Bette Davis character) is a cover for her consuming desire to *be* her. Consider, too, the old Western movies about the endless challenges hurled at the reigning "fastest gun," who often, reflecting the mood of postwar screenwriters in the 1950s, wants only to settle down peacefully with his beloved.

The power position, whether in business or love, family or government, is never an entirely comfortable one, and never safe. Just as a king needed to be alert for plots to steal his crown, today's powerful must also watch their flanks. Being in the dominant power position is a surefire recipe for complications, conflict, and anxiety. Because of its fragility and inherent instability, power is sometimes more valued when we do not have it than when we do.

SOME OF THE COMPLEXITIES we experience in relationship to power are so purely internal that they are fundamental to human nature rather than institutional or situational. Part of the reason we are seldom in either a solely dominant or solely submissive position is that we have divided aspirations regarding power. Self-assertion and obedience are both critical to our developmental history; we have a psychological propensity to exert self-will even when it means dominating others, while at the same time we are inclined to submit to the will of others, particularly to someone who is an authority or who is powerful. The role these often conflicting impulses of self-assertion and obedience play in our lives—and in the world beyond our personal lives—makes our power adaptations complicated and changeable.

The evidence for the will to power—for self-assertion—is tangible enough. At the same time, most of us have a propensity to obedience that extends beyond finding ourselves in a powerless situation with no option but to comply. Side by side with our natural resistance to authority we paradoxically experience a desperate temptation to surrender to it. Drawing on Freud, the sociologist Philip Rieff argues that because love is related to the "parental fact of domination," it follows that "power is the father of love, and in love one follows the paternal example of power, in a relation that must include a superior and a subordinate."[6] Moreover, he argues, whereas Christianity proclaimed the ultimate authority to be the source of love, "Freud discovered the love of authority." Freud's genius allowed him to see the rebellion that originates in the infant's helplessness, but he also saw beyond it and saw that there is an active love of the power of the Other. Because children see their parents as what the psychoanalyst Willard Gaylin so aptly calls their "Gods of Survival," in whose power resides their safety, their sustenance, and their pride, they are sometimes reluctant to recognize any sign of weakness in their parents and may fail to express any counter will.

Our tendency to comply with external authority is demonstrated in a brilliant psychological research study, which some critics deemed immoral. Dr. Stanley Milgram, then a member of the Department of Psychology at Yale University, designed a series of experiments to examine the degree to which the average person would obey authority even if ordered to cause severe pain to someone else.[7] Milgram constructed a psychodrama in which there were three players: the lead investigator, the teacher, and the student. The lead investigator, the designated authority, wore a lab coat and told the volunteers that the purpose of the experiment was to further the cause of education and that they were to be the teachers. What the volunteers did not know was that the students were really actors. The purpose of the experiment, as presented to the volunteers, was to discover whether punishing a student for wrong answers facilitated the learning process. However, its actual purpose was to see whether the volunteers would obey authority even when they knew they were inflicting pain on someone else.

The volunteer teachers were asked to punish a student by administering a series of electric shocks of increasing magnitude each time he gave an erroneous answer. In reality, no shock was delivered, but the teachers experienced the students' cries of pain and pleas to end the experiment as real. The actor-students had been instructed to react more and more loudly as the voltage was increased, from mild grunts at the lower levels to loud cries and pleas to be released at what was supposedly 150 volts. Most of the teachers—the real experimental subjects—displayed symptoms of stress and distress, objected to the barbarity of the experiment, and begged the investigator to stop it. Yet more than 60 percent of them participated in the experiment all the way up to the upper limit, seemingly 450 volts.[8]

Milgram designed further experiments to test whether the cruelty of the teachers originated in repressed aggressive impulses—a hypothesis that had been advanced by some of his critics. Milgram gave the teachers the opportunity to shock the students at any level. When they had this choice, almost all the teachers administered the lowest shocks possible. Milgram concluded that if destructive impulses were really pressing for release, and the teachers could justify their use of high levels of shock in the cause of science, they would take the opportunity to make the students suffer. Yet there was "little if any tendency" on the part of the subjects to do this.[9]

Why did the subjects obey? Most of them rationalized their behavior as useful to society. Milgram proposed that the suppression or disappearance of one's own sense of responsibility is the most far-reaching consequence of submission to authority. He argued, "When individuals enter a condition of hierarchical control, the mechanism that ordinarily regulates individual impulses is suppressed and ceded to the higher-level component."[10]

Resist-submit; point-counterpoint. Conflicting predilections coexist in us, side by side. Oscillation between them permeates the power balances we establish in our personal relationships. In some relationships we are primarily submissive and in others primarily dominant, but in most intimate relationships our place on the continuum of dominance and submission is continually shifting. This happens not just out of necessity, but also because of our desires. We bring an internal psychological dialectic to bear and are often in conflict with ourselves about whether we should be more assertive or more compliant. But turn us loose in a group, and dominance and submissiveness stop being merely antagonists in an internal conflict. Resistance to power and obedience, taken together, propel us into group life. Here we seem to be like the primates for whom a hierarchical social organization is adaptive; aggression is directed outside the group. A predilection for both dominance and submission allows us to integrate rapidly and effectively into a hierarchical structure—familial, religious, corporate, or political. (The conflict born of our simultaneous impulses to obedience and to rebellion is a psychological antithesis that I will elaborate on in Chapter 13.)

MANY OF US are denied worldly power because of social contingencies and because of the sense of shame and helplessness that we sometimes (though not always) internalize as a result. Besides operating against both the very young and the very old, the power gradient is still, to a terrible degree, weighted against many different kinds of minorities.

The following scene from Toni Morrison's *The Bluest Eye*, written in 1970, may seem like a glimpse of another time and another place. But I recently read in the *Wall Street Journal* that a black-owned catering business would send only white employees to make initial contacts with potential customers because they felt they would otherwise lose business. The message there is the same as the message given to three little black girls in Morrison's novel, in a wrenching moment when they are brought face-to-face with the reality of their own and their families' position in the social hierarchy. Two sisters, Frieda and Claudia, have gone to find their friend Pecola Breedlove at the house of the white people who employ Pecola's mother, whom they have never heard addressed as anything other than Mrs. Breedlove, even by her own husband. As Frieda and Claudia enter the kitchen where Mrs. Breedlove is working, she tells them to wait there while she goes to get the wash. In her absence a little blonde girl wearing "a pink sun-back dress and pink fluffy bedroom slippers with two bunny ears pointed up from the tips" comes into the kitchen and asks, "Where's Polly?" When the child refers to Mrs. Breedlove as Polly, "a familiar violence" rises in Claudia: "Her calling Mrs. Breedlove Polly, when even Pecola called her mother Mrs. Breedlove, seemed reason enough to scratch her." Pecola "accidentally" tips over a blueberry pie, spattering not only the floor but the little girl. When Mrs. Breedlove comes back and sees what happened, she is angry at the three black girls, including her daughter, and turns to comfort the little white girl: "Hush baby, hush. Come here. Oh, Lord, look at your dress. Don't cry no more, Polly will change it."[11]

We may be a "classless" society by English standards, but any fifth-grade girl can tell you who's in and who's out in her crowd. The perception of the self as an outsider may of course be rooted in poverty, race, gender, or homosexuality, but it can have many other causes, some of them as subtle as personality, others as obvious as physical disabilities. But all those who have the insignia of the outsider are marked by it, for better or worse. In a way, the most profound remark about the lasting effect of social discrimination was Groucho Marx's: "I don't want to belong to any club that will accept me as a member." It's a funny line, of course, but it underscores how negatively we can be made to feel about ourselves. An old and always ambivalent if not fundamentally self-destructive mode of erasing difference was "passing"—among blacks, (such as the writer Anatole Broyard); among "chee-chees," half-caste Anglo-Indians, (such as the actress Merle Oberon); among homosexuals (such as the movie star Rock Hudson); and among other minorities. This strategy nearly always exacted a heavy price in terms of self-regard. More authentic modes of redress awaited the various liberation movements of the 1960s and 1970s.

The negative consequences of the outsider's status are perhaps more familiar than the ways it can be a surprising gift. Among other things, there is a clarity of vision that comes from minority status. In a recent book on homosexuality, John Loughery observed how early peer-pressure traumas may, paradoxically, leave their mark in beneficial ways:

> One does not have to subscribe to the notion of gay men "as a peo-ple" to feel ill at ease with the denial of all meaningful inner dif-ferences. . . . The contention of a difference-denying straight-gay sameness overlooks the truth that such was not the case for many men when they were 6 or 12 or 16. . . . They felt *touched* by a pro-found difference. And it is unfathomable that so grave . . . a dilemma would not have meaning, if only as a source of a certain kind of potential later in life. A better part of a gay man's adoles-cence and adulthood may be spent . . . in erasing or mitigating the marks of alienation, deception, and assaults . . . But the marks are there, not merely to be cultivated as a grievance or contemplated as a painful scar . . . but to be the basis for a life more attuned to other ways of seeing the world, more critical of unquestioning con-formity, more open to doubt and change than might otherwise have been the case.[12]

Loughery is making a very important observation—that "outsiders" may have unusually cogent insights into the culture's biases and fault lines and sometimes more heart than others.

Women, too, are often a "minority," even though their numbers equal those of men. Being well-placed, successful, or rich is not always the off-setting factor for women one might expect it to be. To be a women in what still is a man's world can be complicated, the usual intrigues around any kind of success being made worse, not better, by the contaminations of romance. Of course, both men and women suffer from the negative impact family can sometimes have on our psyches. But for women, there has been, and to some degree still continues to be, a bias against the achievement of their full self-realization. In the stories of the two women that follow, one fictional, the other biographical, each protagonist suffers from two mutually reinforcing grids: the relatively powerless status of women even in affluent circumstances and the specific fault lines in each of their families. Each woman comes to understand the power grid in her life in the context of a romantic trauma. In the second account (the biographical one), the protagonist ultimately achieves authentic power.

Position and wealth did not prevent the powerlessness and humiliation suffered by Catherine Sloper, the protagonist of *The Heiress*, the play based on Henry James's novel *Washington Square*.[13] The scene is the drawing room of a distinguished home in New York, where Dr. Sloper, a widower, lives with his daughter, Catherine. His wife died giving birth to Catherine. Dr. Sloper constantly criticizes Catherine as "an entirely mediocre and defenseless creature without a shred of poise."[14]

Preparing to go abroad, Dr. Sloper asks his sister, Mrs. Penniman, to stay with Catherine, mentioning her psychological infirmities and her inability to interact naturally with the world. Catherine, chagrined at her own behavior, tells her aunt that she tries to enter into conversation with her father and their guests but to no avail: "I've sat upstairs and made notes of things I should say and how I should say them, but when I am in company, I lose it all."[15] She tries to please her father, even by wearing a red dress, a color her mother used to wear. But Dr. Sloper disparages her with a pointed remark about the unsuitability of such a dramatic look for her: "Your mother was dark—*she* dominated the color."[16] Catherine shrinks under her father's incessant belittlement.

Enter an impecunious suitor, Morris, who makes Catherine feel admired and desirable, and she responds. Not surprisingly, Dr. Sloper disapproves, and he maneuvers his daughter into going to Paris with him for six months in the hope that she will get over Morris and give up her intention to marry him. But on their return, Morris is there, and Catherine remains as eager as ever to marry him. At this point the father and daughter have their pivotal confrontation.

Catherine reproaches her father for his negative attitude to Morris. He responds that their conversation puts him in a ridiculous position—thus constituting a fitting end to the most futile six months of his life, referring to their time abroad. Catherine, beginning to feel empowered, argues back that their trip was wonderful. Dr. Sloper, enraged, responds sarcastically: "Yes, that's the very word you used, Catherine. Tintoretto was a wonderful painter. The ices at the Café Riche are wonderful; almost as wonderful as Michelangelo's David! . . . You saw *nothing*, Catherine! What did Rome with all its glories mean to you? Just a place where you might receive a letter from him!"[17]

Catherine accuses her father of avoiding her in the last few weeks because she confided her continuing love for Morris. Sloper replies, "You carried the image of that wastrel with you every place we went. He blotted out any pleasure we might have had. . . . I waited a long time for my trip to Paris. I never thought I should have to see it all arm-in-arm with him. Well, there are some things one cannot do for people, even one's own daughter! One cannot give her eyes or understanding if she has none."[18]

In a flash, Catherine now understands that her father wished only to be with her mother, not with her, and Dr. Sloper confirms her suspicions: "You ought to be very thankful to me. . . . Six months ago you were perhaps a little limited, a little rustic; but now you have everything; you've seen everything and appreciated everything. You will be a most entertaining companion."[19] Finally, Dr. Sloper tells Catherine she has one virtue for Morris that outshines all the others. "What is that?" she asks, and he replies, "Your money." He, of course, intends to disinherit her should she marry Morris.

Morris, on learning this, abandons Catherine. Nonetheless she has gained something: she has seen into her father's heart and mind and understands that her father blames her for her mother's death. She grasps, too, the overwhelming impact on her of her father's belittlement, understanding for the first time the source of her own psychological stagnation. She continues to fulfill her duties to her father, but she will never be reconciled to him. Catherine is wiser, surer, but—betrayed by both her father and her lover—she is permanently wounded, worldly but embittered.

The denouement takes place several years later, after her father's death. Catherine has been transformed into a poised, elegant, knowing, sophisticated, and cynical woman. Now she turns the tables on Morris, allowing him to hope for a reconciliation—and her fortune—and then rejecting him.

Disappointment in love can sometimes have the opposite effect. The elimination of a negative emotional force can lead to flowering in late life.

We see this in the story of the publisher Katharine Graham, who found her wings only after the disastrous decline of her husband's mental health, the end of their marriage, and his suicide. In her autobiography, *Personal History*, Graham gives us an account of how she achieved authentic power relatively late in life.[20]

At first glance, Katharine Graham, neé Meyer, given the affluence into which she was born, might be expected to have felt less powerless than many other women of her generation. Her paternal grandfather was a partner at Lazard Frères. Her father, Eugene Isaac Meyer, left Lazard because of friction with his brother-in-law; made money in the market; and started his own firm, Eugene Meyer and Company, which had the first research arm of any Wall Street firm. He became a self-made millionaire, a man who ran the War Industries Board in Washington in 1917 and who in 1933 bought the *Washington Post*. Graham's mother, Agnes Ernst, was the daughter of a poor Lutheran couple, and some people suspected that Agnes married Meyer, who was short and Jewish, for his money. Graham says that when her father first made an appearance in her mother's diary, he was described "with some condescension and little apparent interest, as her rich Jewish beau."[21] But her parents established an amiable relationship and became a real couple, particularly after the family moved to Washington.

Graham was the fourth of five children. Her older sister Florence, born in 1911, was a classic beauty but grew up, according to Graham, without emotional support. Her second sister, Bis, born two years later, "lived in a state of constant rebellion. . . . She resented the power our parents had over her and met power with power in whatever way she could—and she found a number of ways." The son, born in 1915, was Eugene Meyer III, whose difficult childhood Graham attributes to "my father's unapproachability and prominence and my mother's awkwardness with men."[22] Then came Katharine herself, in 1917, and finally the youngest, Ruth, born in 1921. Of her childhood Graham writes that she was envious of Bis's nonconformist image: "I really even wanted to 'be' her. I envied her self-assurance, her independence, her daring, her willingness to cut up and roll with the family. I would have liked to be a dashing law-breaker, but I didn't have the proper instincts or the courage, and I was always scorned for passively going along. . . . I followed the rules. I was Goody-Two-Shoes."[23]

Obviously, Graham had many advantages. She was educated at the Madeira School, Vassar, and later the University of Chicago and was exposed to a life of wealth and privilege. Nonetheless, her sense of personal power was eroded by her mother's negative appraisal of her. Consistently put down by her mother, Graham believed that she was "realistic about [my] own assets and abilities. . . . [I] was not very pretty." She grew to her full height early and, feeling herself ungainly, feared she would never attract the kind of man she would find attractive. She also feared that her family would be condescending to anyone she might bring home. But she was swept off her feet by Philip Graham, a graduate of Harvard Law School who was working at the Supreme Court. He proposed within a short time of their first meeting: "He told me that he loved me and said we would be married and go to Florida, his place of birth, if I could live with only two dresses, because I had to understand that he would never take anything from my father. . . . I was incredulous—this brilliant, charismatic, fascinating man loved me!"[24] Her husband may have been sincere in his stated intentions, but they did not wind up in Florida.

Phil Graham was an ambitious man, and he became involved in her father's newspaper and eventually took it over in 1946. (Her brother, the logical heir, was committed to medicine.) In 1948 her father passed the paper on to Phil and Katharine, but he gave Phil the largest share of the stock because he believed that "no man should be in the position of working for his wife."[25] Graham found herself totally in accord with this plan. Phil later expanded the company's holdings to include television stations and *Newsweek*.

For Graham, her husband was "the fizz in our lives," dazzling to one and all: "His wit, great energy, soaring imagination and fervent desire for excellence . . . were so strong that I ignored the fact that he was frequently using that wit at my expense."[26] From the very beginning, Phil and her mother conspired to deprecate her. Of her marriage she wrote: "Always, it was he who decided and I who responded. From the earliest days of our relationship, for instance, I thought that we had friends because of him and were invited because of him. It wasn't until years later that I looked at the downside of all this and realized that, perversely, I had seemed to enjoy the role of doormat wife. For whatever reason, I liked to be dominated and to be the implementer. But although I was thoroughly fascinated and charmed by Phil I was also slightly resentful, when I thought about it, at feeling such complete dependence on another person."[27] As Phil became more powerful and sought after, Graham settled even more firmly into the role of supporting her man.

But Philip turned out to be psychologically unbalanced. Some twenty years after they were married, he suffered the first of a series of manic-depressive episodes, which included not only abusive behavior toward Graham but infidelity. Eventually, he proposed not only a divorce but that he buy out her interest in the paper. She was willing to give him the divorce, but she refused to give him the paper. This was the turning point in Katharine Graham's life. Her determination was total: "I was not going to lose my husband *and* the paper. And if my husband was firm in his decision to leave me, then I would fight to keep the paper."[28] But he broke off his affair and, rapidly deteriorating, returned home to be taken care of by Graham. Shortly thereafter he killed himself.

It was then, in 1963, that Graham took on the presidency of the *Washington Post*. At first, she saw herself as a kind of interim manager; then she reluctantly assumed the role of publisher, in 1967, and, finally, the position of chairman of the board of the Washington Post Corporation. Gradually, she came to acknowledge her own gifts. Thus it was only in midlife that she first began to achieve independence and exercise her own potential—largely, she suggests, as a result of two insights. One insight was the way male colleagues condescended to women, herself included, and the other was her budding grasp of feminism.

Graham tells of a dinner at Joseph Alsop's house, followed by the customary separation of men and women after the meal. At that point, she told Alsop that she was going to leave quietly "when the women were dismissed."[29] He argued that the separation was merely to allow the men to use the bathroom, but she said this was nonsense and she was going home to read. She did it intuitively, not as a political statement: "I had no intention of starting a revolution, but my action did indeed trigger a minor social coup, as news of my innocent suggestion spread. Because I was regarded as a conservative on these social issues, my stance was particularly effective. The illogic of expecting women to leave while men held meaningful discussions became obvious and the practice gradually broke up all over town."[30] Graham's friend Gloria Steinem was an important influence; Steinem, more than anyone else, "changed my mind-set and helped me grasp what the leaders of the movement—and even the extremists—were talking about."[31] Gradually Graham began to look at the way women were being treated even within her own company.

Looking back with amazement on her own passivity, Graham depicts her earlier self as saturated with the prejudices of her time. Circumstances brought her to a crucial decision—to fight for the *Washington Post*. She was, of course, rich and well-connected. Still, one has to admire her for taking a stand in her middle forties, and then embracing changing ideas about the roles of men and women and charting a new life course. Her marital crisis appears to have precipitated a reorganization of her psyche, allowing her to achieve what I would describe as authentic power.

Graham's story is riveting in its depiction of the way powerlessness and deference can infuse a woman's life even when she is born into a world in which privilege and power are taken for granted. It traces the winding, often painful road away from her mother's and husband's negative appraisal of her and toward a new trust in herself. Though her story has a glamorous setting, many other women have followed the same road over the past thirty years. Graham's capacity for self-determination and her assumption of power took wing, in part, on her dawning awareness of the constraints that had been placed on her in her most intimate relationships. But I would speculate that the seeds of her autonomy may have been there all the while, born in her childhood admiration and envy of her sister Bis's self-assurance, independence, and daring.

EVEN IN THE BEST of circumstances, power can be challenged and eroded and needs to be reasserted, renegotiated. But neither is powerlessness etched in stone; it, too, stands ready for renegotiation. Powerlessness can be overcome through events that impact what we know and what we feel. When the power of feelings—sometimes even the paralyzing feelings of anxiety and depression—get connected to knowledge and insight, they can become the fuel that leads to assertion and even to rebellion. As J. B. Priestley remarked of the fifteenth-century Pope Alexander VI, who initiated the practice of censorship virtually almost as soon as books were invented: "Power, which has its intuitions, recognized its enemy."[32] Knowledge coupled with emotional insight can lead to radical change.

Censorship is crucial to maintaining an unjust rule, for when the oppressed learn too much about the nature of their oppression, the seeds of rebellion are sown. This is true not just of the political world but of families and interpersonal relationships in general. Parents, spouses, and governments sometimes conspire to control knowledge, fearful that knowledge can lead to insurrection. And censorship is practiced on the personal as well as the public level. No less than Pope Alexander, those in power—whether a tyrannical mother, a dominant husband, or a nineteenth-century mill owner—see knowledge as threatening to the status quo, just as the majority of slaveholders preferred that their slaves remain illiterate. In the end, it is up to the powerless, the dispossessed, the victimized to speak out on their own behalf.

In his play A *Doll's House*, written in 1879, Ibsen provides the women's movement with one of its heroines, Nora Helmer. A *Doll's House* turns on an emotional and intellectual insight, through which Nora reorders her understanding of her past life in a way that will forever alter her future. In contrast to *The Heiress*, A *Doll's House* shows us that such insight may be the basis not just for new knowledge but also for a new beginning.[33]

As the play opens, one Christmas Eve, Nora returns home from a shopping spree bearing gifts for her beloved husband, Torvald, and their three children. A surprise visitor awaits her in the parlor, an old friend she has not seen in many years. Mrs. Linde, an impoverished widow who has returned to her hometown in desperate straits, envies Nora's comfortable life—a happy marriage, a lovely house, and a successful husband who has just gotten a promotion at his bank.

But Nora confides to Mrs. Linde that she is greatly troubled. Many years ago, when her husband was ill, she forged the signature of her recently deceased father on a bank loan to get the money she needed to take Torvald to Italy—a warm climate was his only hope for recovery. She has been secretly repaying the loan ever since. Now, however, Nils Krogstad, an employee at Torvald's bank who is about to be dismissed because of his disreputable past, has discovered her secret and is threatening to expose her unless she uses her influence with Torvald to help him hold on to his job. Nora is terrified about what will happen if Krogstad tells.

When Krogstad sends Torvald a letter revealing the secret, Nora's self-recrimination is so profound that she contemplates suicide. As she has feared, Torvald flies into a violent rage, blaming Nora at least as strongly as she blames herself, despite the fact that the forgery was committed to save his life. He "magnanimously" declares that he will not divorce her, because he wants to avoid a scandal, but that she is to live in their home as a pariah, cut off not only from him but from their children, so that her immorality will not be passed down to them.

Under the influence of Mrs. Linde, with whom he has fallen in love,

Krogstad explains in a second letter that he has destroyed the evidence of Nora's forgery. Now that Torvald realizes he won't be ruined, he forgives Nora and promises to love her as his own little wife once again. But Nora finds herself unable to forgive him—not because of his initial reaction but because of his about-face. She sees that he is not idealistic or noble but merely self-interested and conventional. At the play's end, Nora declares that Torvald is a stranger to her, and she cannot spend one more night in his home. Though he pleads with her to stay, she leaves, slamming the door behind her.

This play portrays what I call a change moment, a place in time when one's sense of self is significantly altered by a sudden shift in understanding, coupled with emotional insight, and resulting in an altered sense of oneself in the world.[34] The same potent combination of knowledge and feeling emerges in successful psychotherapy, when patients come to understand the sources of their conflicts both emotionally and intellectually. These conflicts almost invariably encompass issues of power and powerlessness.

Nora's slamming of the door—as has often been remarked—reverberated not only in the theater but in a new social phenomenon, the early women's movement. Nora's insight continued to reverberate in the consciousness-raising of the 1970s. From a few scattered groups of women meeting in living rooms, talking honestly about their dissatisfaction with their lives—love, family, work, and sex—and experiencing the revelation that their unhappiness was shared by many others and was rooted in their status as second-class citizens, the power of the movement grew to a tidal wave that transformed the social landscape of the late twentieth century.

Let me turn now from the theater to a true story of one man's journey, a religious conversion that had profound personal and social consequences: the story of Malcolm X, as told in his autobiography.[35] Born in 1925, Malcolm Little was the son of a Baptist preacher who favored the back-to-Africa movement of Marcus Garvey. In 1931 his father was run over by a streetcar, and the suspicion was that he had been murdered by white racists. Though Malcolm's mother struggled to keep her children together, her health declined and the welfare system separated the children from her and from one another.

Malcolm's life soon deteriorated, and as a young man he became a criminal, an addict, and a pimp. Just before he was twenty-one, he was convicted of theft and possession of a gun. Paradoxically, his imprisonment saved him, because in prison, he was converted to Elijah Muhammad's Nation of Islam. His brother Philbert, who belonged to the group, had urged him to join. His brother Reginald also wrote to him, telling him not to eat pork or to smoke cigarettes—and this would be a way to get out of prison. Malcolm ignored Philbert but listened to Reginald because he thought Reginald was on to a scam. Only later did he realize that his renunciation of pork and cigarettes was his "first pre-Islamic submission." All his siblings conspired to convert him to the teaching of the Honorable Elijah Muhammad. In the beginning, Malcolm was intrigued by the potential power of the scam. What he wanted was to get out of jail. But his grab for the power of the hustle gave way to his search for a more authentic power.

Elijah Muhammad taught that "the key to a Muslim is submission, the attunement of one toward Allah." Just as important was "true knowledge of the black man," an important heritage. Malcolm X eventually underwent a real conversion. "I remember how . . . reading the Bible in the Norfolk Prison Colony Library, I came upon, then I read, over and over, how Paul on the road to Damascus, upon hearing the voice of Christ, was so smitten that he was knocked off his horse, in a daze. I do not now, and I did not then, liken myself to Paul. But I do understand his experience." Not only was Malcolm "saved," but he turned his energies to furthering the cause of his people through religion and political action.

Malcolm X found autonomy and purpose through submission to a higher authority. And, very importantly for him, he was also able to reach back to the aspirations of his long-dead father and reestablish continuity with him. The Autobiography of Malcolm X remains a virtual bible and a source of inspiration for young blacks—it was one of the cultural influences that promoted black pride and black power and that ultimately fed into the civil rights movement.

Change moments are moments of emotional and intellectual insight that alter one's perception of external or internal reality, of one's role in one's own suffering, and of the relationship of the self to the other. Then, the negative feelings that create a sense of powerlessness and low self-esteem can sometimes become the impetus for a turnaround. Such turning points can reconfigure the self and the world so dramatically that they may be experienced as discontinuous with what has gone before.

Just as personal turning points can come about through a major reorganization of how we understand our past life and relationships, revolutionary social movements can also be spurred by new knowledge, releasing powerful surges of emotion. Knowledge often leads the oppressed to see and understand the excesses of those in power. The emotional response to that knowledge motivates people to act on it. In addition to the woman's movement and the civil rights movement, other kinds of information processing has fueled other movements in our time—for example, the gay rights movement. One source of this "information processing" is the moral insight that frequently accrues to minorities, allowing them to see critical flaws in the culture around them. By virtue of being an outsider, one possesses a gift of vision sometimes unavailable to the insider. This is, I believe, one of the points John Loughery is making in his exploration of what it means to be homosexual.

When the vision of the outsider is put at the service of cultural analysis, we start to hear profound discourses about the social function of exclusion. And once people start analyzing such issues, many of the culture's fundamental assumptions about itself become visible for the first time and may start to crumble—and with them the status quo. What minorities bring to the table is the habit of skepticism, the willingness to question power arrangements in which they have no investment, and a deep mistrust and dislike of the motives of those who have kept them down.

Just as personal change depends on discontent (the power of the emotions) coupled with new ideas or information (the power of knowledge), so too are the powers of emotion and knowledge critical to social/political change. Hans Morgenthau, a theoretician of political power, proposes the ideal dialectic between truth and power: "Truth, by unmasking the pretensions of power, at the very least disturbs the powers-that-be; for it puts power on the intellectual defensive. . . . Truth may even challenge the *status quo* of power on the level of practical politics if it is supported by sufficiently powerful interests. Once those interests have won the struggle for power, yesterday's truth becomes today's ideology, justifying, rationalizing, and covering up for the new powers-that-be. Then a new cycle begins and truth again challenges power."[36]

Yet, as Morgenthau acknowledges, many intellectuals have sidestepped the function of speaking truth to power, sometimes by conveniently separating themselves from the political sphere—a strong temptation, for at times it may be in one's self-interest to remain silent. The self-isolation of intellectuals from the political sphere has a long history. Morgenthau recounts how Leonardo da Vinci, reproached by Michelangelo for his indifference to the fate of Florence, replied that the study of beauty occupied his whole heart. Morgenthau also recounts what Goethe said about power, that "the political song is an ugly song" and that one can pursue the good, the true, and the beautiful within one's own chosen sphere.

Yet this is not always the case. Change moments do take place and have important reverberations, sometimes personal, sometimes social-political, sometimes both. Rosa Parks won't give up her seat in the front of the bus. Kaboom. Oedipus *will* find out what is causing the plague, though he is warned not to go there. Kaboom. Katharine Graham leaves the dinner party when cigars are passed around and the women move to another room. A small Kaboom (the dinner-party revolution).

While analysts and psychotherapists often think of change as internal, patients don't define progress as primarily psychological. (Except for those determined to stay neurotic; they become all too good at greasing the wheels in just this way, spinning out insight after insight, but never getting the traction to act.) Patients think of change as doing something of which they have been frightened. The powers that be are against them. But just as every revolution in history had to start somewhere, with a specific individual and a specific act, so, too, does personal change find its echo and then its reinforcing momentum in the change an individual's behavior has on the behavior of others. If you do something different, then maybe your oppressor or your opponent or your clinging dependent or your withholding boss will do something different in his stead. The psychoanalyst Avrum Ben-Avi in the face of a chronic stalemate a patient reported in his personal life asks: "Well, is she going to change or are you going to change?"[37] The upshot of this remark is that the patient might as well go first. And, so it is with personal behavior, too. Refusing to eat the first cookie guarantees you won't wolf down the whole package.

Though I have been considering the way our power must inevitably erode, I am also insisting that the contradictions and fluctuations of power can work in our favor for long stretches of time. They work not just for the person who has power but particularly for the person who does *not* have power. For such a person, the ironic homily is that one should go ahead and act. These are the very people the gods of fluctuation and contradiction are so often waiting to smile upon.

The power of specific feelings—disillusionment, resentment, rage, hopelessness—if they get connected to insight or knowledge can lead to radical change. Re-visioning, the act of looking back with an eye to reinterpreting the present, may be the prologue to a radical attempt at change, whether personal or political. Such a drive to a truer reinterpretation of the past is part of our deep-seated impulse to survive, a refusal to live within the limitations foisted on us by circumstances.

PART

Interpersonal
Power

TWO

4

Powers of the Weak and Powers of the Strong

"Conventional books on power tell us a lot about the powerful. . . . To understand the workings of power as a relationship one must also consider the situation of the weak. . . ."

ELIZABETH JANEWAY, *Powers of the Weak*

The happiest of our personal relationships depend on an intuitive connection, on the mutual and mostly benign efforts to let our desires be known while remaining responsive to our partners' desires. Mother and child may be so exquisitely attuned that it is difficult to say who wants what from whom, who initiates and who responds. Similar entwinement and empathy can be found in other pairs too, whether they are lovers, friends, or creative collaborators. But in every relationship, the partners' wishes will sometimes diverge. In negotiating such differences, we either try to influence our partner or allow ourselves to be persuaded. Whatever tactics we use, we are willy-nilly involved in power.

The ability to negotiate power is at the heart of every successful relationship. In the most fulfilling relationships, the mechanisms of arriving at a power balance remain out of sight, the blend seamless, with sufficient gratification on both sides. If we grew up respecting and identifying with the nurturant power of our parents, we are more likely to form a healthy sense of our own agency and to relate to others through care and cooperation. A respect for agency as it exists both within ourselves and in others serves as a counterweight to the temptations of submission or domination, and sometimes enables us to form relationships based on the co-sharing of power. This generally works best when there is a tacit agreement to control different aspects of our joint lives.

When it comes to negotiating the power balances in our relationships, we favor specific tactics that fall under the rubric of the powers of the strong or the powers of the weak. The powers of the strong, including the prestige and authority of one's position as well as recourse to threats, intimidations, bribes, and force, are self-evident. The powers the weak exert are often subtle and do not always look like power maneuvers, even though they can be extremely effective. They include submissiveness, deference, ingratiation, manipulation, and vicarious power obtained through attachment to a powerful person.

I must introduce a caveat here. Appearances of strength or weakness may be deceptive. Someone who commands power in the world and utilizes the powers of the strong does not necessarily feel strong. A brilliant investment banker, a man who had been an unathletic, bespectacled teenage boy, extremely shy and deferential, terrified of rejection by other boys and particularly by girls, achieved power in the business world by virtue of his mathematical brilliance, analytical abilities, and subsequent success on Wall Street. Yet he never overcame his early life feelings of ineptness. Though he is dominant in the professional domain and controls the financial fate of many of those around him, he still harbors a sense of internal weakness. His still-conflicted sense of his own power, a residue of his awkward adolescence, leads him to a perpetual display of one-upmanship. His behavior, predicated on his need to appear smarter than anyone else, has made him feared, which is a kind of power, but it has also made him unpopular, limiting his professional and social mobility. He senses that his peers dislike him but does not know why, and he feels ill at ease in many settings. Nor does he feel comfortable with women, harboring the suspicion that it is his money rather than his person which is the draw.

Analogously, the weak may not be so passive, suppressed, or ineffectual as meets the eye. They often command the strong. In F. Scott Fitzgerald's novel *Tender Is The Night*, the psychiatrist Dick Diver saves and then marries his psychologically disturbed patient, Nicole. While Nicole's life appeared to have been stabilized by Dick, in reality both their lives are structured around her. As the story evolves, it is Nicole, the fragile sick one, who is more prepared for life: "Nicole had been designed for change, for flight, with money as fins and wings. The new state of things would be no more than if a racing chassis, concealed for years under the body of the family limousine, should be stripped to its original self."[1] He on the other hand—the charming, engaging, energetic doctor—is fatigued, emptied out, destroyed, and destined for obscurity. During their relationship, despite surface appearances, she has gained strength while his has been eroded and his underlying weakness revealed. Just as in sexual encounters, where it is generally agreed that "bottom" rules, the submissive person often triumphs in a dominant-submissive relationship.

The Powers of the Strong

Dominance constitutes a psychological relation between those who exercise it and those over whom it is exercised.[2] Occasionally, we have all wanted to control the actions and minds of others. Sometimes all we want is the *possibility*, particularly if we anticipate that others will comply with our wishes without them being articulated.

The economist and political theorist John Kenneth Galbraith proposed that the powers of the strong be classified in four categories: *coercive power*, exerted through implicit or explicit commands and bolstered by physical threats only if "persuasion" fails; *compensatory power*, exerted through the offer of compensations or advantages; *conditioned power*, exerted through the invocation of traditional authority and belief; and *charismatic power*, exerted through personal magnetism. Dominant individuals, like submissives, may also resort to manipulation, deceit, and treachery.

Coercive Power

In ongoing relationships, a dominant-submissive gradient is common, sometimes operating out of the awareness of both participants because it is consonant with prevailing attitudes—for example, between husband and wife, parent and child, employer and employee. Subtle forms of domination may go unnoticed: one person may control others through the sheer volume of words, filling up every conversation so that no rejoinder is possible, while another takes the air out of the room by profusely demonstrating his or her feelings. One partner may not even recognize the other's dominant tactics until a significant moment clarifies it. In Susan Isaacs's novel *Longtime No See*, a widow reconnects with a past lover of some twenty years earlier, and catches a very subtle form of domination. Facing him over drinks, the widow observes: "His eyes were still on mine. Over the years since we'd parted, I'd recalled so many details about Nelson, but this I'd forgotten, his ability to win any staring contest in the world. Never actually a contest: Nelson didn't appear to be holding your eyes to confront you, the way an animal does to establish dominance. At least it had never seemed that way then."[3]

Only when a preexisting balance is upset will the dominant partner make his or her priority explicit: "You're talking to your *husband*." "*Never* talk back to your mother." "You forget I'm the boss at your peril." The dominant partner may belittle, shame, or bully the other person, or, worse, freeze him out. If these ploys fail, he may up the ante and resort to threats, punishment, and even physical violence. However, the dominant does not generally need to take such explicit and punitive action; his potential to do so is what gives him ascendancy.

In the business world, the boss exerts control through the threat of firing his employee or stinting on a bonus. Here the use of raw power can be counterproductive. When the boss is on a rampage, the employees whisper behind his back. "He's losing it." And it is possible he is—losing not only his temper but also his authority and power. Losing it, in the sense of giving way to excesses of rage, threats and even physical violence, can be observed at many levels (from a spouse having his or her way one time too many to great powers exhausting themselves in needless wars).

Coercion can also be expressed through withholding. The heroine of Aristophanes' play *Lysistrata* brings peace during the Peloponnesian War by persuading the women of Athens to withdraw their sexual favors until peace is achieved. A wife or husband may withhold sex, but much more potent is the threat of abandonment.

Compensatory Power

In contrast to outright domination, compensatory control is achieved by offering benefits, advantages, or rewards. Parents frequently try to control their children's behavior with bribes, or through the implied promise of future rewards. This technique sometimes teaches adolescents to insist on rewards for compliance and prizes for performance.

Galbraith writes that middle- and upper-class husbands traditionally maintained their dominance by giving their wives tangible rewards—clothing, jewelry, cars, housing, entertainment, and participation in social occasions.[4] Such financial power of persuasion was bolstered by the belief that the husband was innately the more powerful partner, insofar as "the masculine will was by nature stronger than the feminine will." The wife's compliance was further motivated by her wish for a secure place in the world at a time when single women were regarded as failures, and married women were dependent on their husbands for financial security. The belief that male superiority and female submission were part of the natural order formed the basis for an ongoing male hegemony.

In both the business world and the social world, money, position, and access (extrinsic sources of power) confer dominant status. To appear to be powerful—to give the impression that one is in the position of affording entrée to a job, a club, or a world—elicits deference and often acts to make one influential, even if no concrete benefits are bestowed.

Conditioned Power

Social compliance is mediated through belief systems that are communicated in ways large and small—through our schools and places of worship, through the movies we see and the books we read, through what our parents told us and showed us, through what I have described elsewhere as our shared cultural unconscious.[5] Some degree of conditioned power is necessary to the coherence of any society. Social compliance is seen in our willingness to abide by the judicial system and pay taxes (although, as Galbraith notes, even these practices have their vociferous opponents). Conditioned power is so natural to us that we fail to recognize how much we are affected by it, when in fact it influences many of the most personal decisions we make about how to live our lives. The recent reexamination of traditional male dominance shows how deeply an entrenched belief system impacts on our everyday behaviors and choices.

Many people believe that the strong should protect the weak from potentially corrupting knowledge. Thus, parents censor what their children see and some husbands keep the intricacies of their business lives to themselves to spare their wives any unnecessary worries. But it is worth noting that the most obvious examples of culturally sanctioned dominance are almost necessarily those that are already in the process of unraveling.

Very few of us are astute enough to see through to the culture's hidden assumptions when they have as yet to be challenged.

Charismatic Power

Charisma can be totally independent of holding a position of power. Most observers describe charisma as an inherent animal magnetism, and one has called it the "naked capacity of mustering assent."[6] People who possess it almost automatically command our deference. The energy emanating from a charismatic individual is almost tangible. Nonetheless, a complex relationship exists between charismatic people and those they inspire. There are some people who seem to require a charismatic figure to whom they can attach themselves. In pursuit of such a figure, they may move from one guru to another.

Charisma is part of the political process, and those who possess it are given the edge in any debate or contest. When a politician is said to be boring, what we usually mean is that he or she lacks charisma. Well-intentioned President Gerald Ford jumps out as an example. However, charisma is not always an asset pure and simple. Suppose a young man, a charismatic editor, is brought into a publishing house to shake things up. He may or may not prove able to do the job, but in the beginning his rivals will regard him with fear and enmity because they have felt the playing ground shift. (Here again one sees the natural resistance to power in all its guises.) Generally, charisma is not enough in and of itself. In the end, it must be backed up by skill and talent, sometimes of a demagogic nature.[7]

Manipulation

In addition to the four categories just considered, there is manipulation. We might think of manipulation as one of the powers of the weak, and often it is; but it is also the modus vivendi of some of our most powerful figures. Acutely sensitive to interpersonal cues, they know how to use others' emotions, needs, and weaknesses for their own ends. Self-proclaimed down-home country boys, for instance, often go to great lengths to disguise their shrewdness—the veritable wolf in grandmother's clothing. The quintessential American version of humbleness and self-deprecation has become an art form among American politicians. An insider once noted the interaction between two masters of the game: "Ike, one of the better political generals the Army has produced, may have sometimes out-country-boyed Lyndon Johnson when (majority leader) Johnson didn't know it. Ike, too, was a fine actor and not a bad manipulator of men."[8] This political prototype goes back to one of our boy heroes, Tom Sawyer, who, when his Aunt Polly insisted that he whitewash the fence as a punishment for playing hooky, figured out that if he made it look like great fun he could con his friends into taking their turns.

Manipulation can be played in a self-deprecating register. In *David Copperfield*, Dickens explored humility as a disguise for manipulation in his character Uriah Heep: "His hypocritical assumption of humbleness, his damp bony hands, his fawning hatred of those he has deceived, his calculated dependence upon their loyalties and affections, his ingenuity in spinning his web, make him despicable and dangerous. . . . Uriah Heep can worm his way into the confidence of an experienced man of affairs, generally get the upper hand of his weaknesses, and reduce him to subservience."

The Powers of the Weak

Indebted as I am to Galbraith for his delineation of the powers of the strong, I am also indebted to Elizabeth Janeway for her labeling the powers of the weak as such.[9] Just as the act of domination employs specific tactics, so, too, does the act of submission.

Why would someone seek a submissive adaptation? Sometimes, it is for practical and situational or even political reasons—as it is for members of marginalized groups, who have neither the wherewithal to exert power directly or the strength to oppose others' demands. Submitting is the primary response available to them, and they deploy it in the hope of avoiding harm or achieving concrete benefits. At various times, women, blacks, and the poor have mobilized submissiveness as an adaptive response to their subordinate situation.

Submission in intimate relationships may go unnoticed by both parties because it is part of the mores of a family or a national culture, a product of conditioned power. With few exceptions, the Victorian wife deferred to her husband, as a duty. In such a case, the submissive person mobilizes the powers of the weak to adapt to social custom because of realistic concerns—not because of any deep-seated psychological motive.

However, subordinates may react in two opposite ways. Some focus on how to limit the extent to which they are restricted, controlled, and dominated; this is another example of the natural resistance to authority. They may yield outwardly but not inwardly, hence the anthem of internal withholding mobilized by women who are reluctant sexual partners: "You may have my body but not my soul."

Others fail to mount any resistance, even to outrageous demands. They may actually fail to put up their hands in self-defense. This basic fact of life needs to be noted. Why should this be so? Sometimes a pervasive deference originates from an internal injunction to fulfill the expectations of someone else. This can be the result of the anticipated intimidation by a parent lest one not comply, a fear that gets transferred to subsequent intimate relationships. Other times the submissive person's reluctance to contest power may be motivated by realistic concerns—by the recognition that resistance will simply evoke greater aggression. That is, the failure to resist power may be the only adaptive response available.

Submission is often effective because some dominants respond protectively to it, or at least cease their aggression. While we know that in the face of domination we are motivated to back down, the opposite is equally true. In the face of submission, we are motivated to ease up. This is what makes true sadism so exceptional: it feeds off the very thing that inhibits aggression in most people. There's no reason to assume that we are not basically constructed the same way as other animals in terms of our innate responses to signals of submissiveness, and in most confrontations between members of the same species, submissiveness halts aggression.[10]

However, submission is not always a defensive ploy. The most interesting thing about submission is that it can be deployed as a power maneuver, although one expressed in the "passive" voice. Then the submissive is no more than a submissive manqué, utilizing the powers of the weak as a means to control others. Submission becomes a strategy that, like domination, consists of a series of psychological maneuvers aimed at controlling or manipulating someone else. People who apply these tactics can achieve strong influence and sometimes even control of a lover, friend, or business associate who has real power in the external world. Then submission becomes an effective, though indirect route to power. Taken together, these tactics constitute the "powers of the weak."[11]

Sometimes, too, a submissive actively seeks a dependent adaptation out of a sense of internal weakness, allying themselves to someone who is seen as a greater power in order to achieve vicarious power and patch over a sense of personal neediness. When this predilection gets eroticized, the submissive person may go so far as to taste the pleasures—and the peculiar powers—of masochism. Then submission is a powerful, ever-ready motive of its own.

Here, then, are four separate motives that may lead us to invoke the powers of the weak: submission as a necessary adaptation to the power structure we inhabit; submission as a self-defensive maneuver in a personal relationship; submission as a strategy for controlling others; submission as a way to borrow someone else's strength. The tactics that we use can also be classified in four categories: dependency-submissiveness; ingratiation and flattery; manipulation; and the mobilization of vicarious power.

Dependency and Submissiveness

In any structured society, certain people are defined as "dependents" on others. Beyond any assigned social role, dependency can be learned as a career path in the course of one's upbringing. A wealthy and overprotective mother forbids her daughter to participate in any household chores, and teaches her that it is a sign of good breeding to be waited upon. The girl grows up without any basic skills, and with a sense that she must be served, her dependency rationalized as superiority. This adaptation can be narcissistically gratifying and experienced as its own kind of power, in which service is exacted from the external world. Such learned helplessness is a continuation of the childhood fantasy: "I do not have to do that; it will be done for me because I am special." A crisis arises only when the child becomes an adult and is cut loose by her parents. The upshot may be a breakdown, as the helpless individual sinks into hypochondriasis or some kind of emotional collapse in a last-ditch coercive effort to regain dependent gratification.

Submissiveness is often the product of fear; a wife may assert herself, but fearing that she has pushed too hard, plunges headlong into a major abandonment anxiety, and decides that a compromised, obedient relationship is better than none at all. In her early life, she may well have felt diminished by the attitudes of other family members, who judged her as somehow inferior. Why should such a child suppress her anger at being made to feel inadequate rather than fight back? Everyone needs a place to be, to feel safe. Especially for children, the family home is their sanctuary, their cave, and they need to secure a safe place somewhere in that cave, even when it's not a place of priority.

Ingratiation and Flattery

Weak expressions of power include ingratiation, flattery, minute ministration to the needs of the other person, and the elevation of the other's priority over oneself. A little boy batting his eyes at his mommy gets her to buy him the remote-controlled racing car that his father thought was too extravagant. And the graduate student who constantly quotes his professor and dances attendance on him may well get the coveted position as teaching assistant. Both maneuvers depend on flattery and ingratiation, and—like the appeal of helplessness or the provocation of guilt—they are roads to power.

In some cases, the need to please may take precedence over one's independent activities. A woman ingratiates herself with her boyfriend by taking exquisite care of him. She cooks every dish that he loves to eat, entertains his friends, makes few demands, is profoundly interested in the minute ups and downs of his well-being, and is afraid to make any requests of him. Here, she substitutes ingratiation for coercion or force as her major means of control. This pattern of behavior not only permeates her romantic life but extends to all her other relationships. Over time she feels that she has lost touch with her innermost desires in her frenzy to please others.

Ed, a masseur in his twenties, is unable to set limits for his clients, paradoxically leading to a big turnover among them. One of his clients, John, is very domineering; when Ed arrives for an appointment, John keeps him waiting but still insists on his full time. Ed is then late for his next client, who eventually fires him. Ed also falls prey to overbearing clients in other ways—he offers favors that fall outside the domain of his responsibilities. His ingratiating manner and his need to please extend to his friends and neighbors as well. For example, his next-door neighbor, Al, had a kink in his back and asked Ed to work it out. Al then asked for a second appointment but failed to show up. The next evening, Ed saw some-one go into Al's apartment for a party he had not been invited to. When he saw Al the next morning, he felt uncomfortable but said only, "Oh, we'll make our appointment some other time."

In treatment, Ed stumbled over this story at first, rationalizing that he was the nice one. But once he admitted to himself that he was angry at Al, he was able to understand that he had made himself the butt of his neighbor's scorn—a very painful insight. Even so, it was a long time before he found the origins of his behavior in the role he played in his own family. The oldest of three children, he was taught by his mother that he must always oblige his father who was ordinarily a good man but periodi-cally went on drinking binges, during which he would explode in anger and sometimes beat the children. Ed was taught to suppress his own will and to keep the family peace. Ed did not know why he was more suscepti-ble than his siblings to his mother's blandishments, but he had become the designated family peacemaker. Only after his encounter with his neighbor was he able to see the role he played in those incidents that left him feeling simultaneously virtuous and humiliated.[12]

Manipulation

Like the strong, the weak also resort to manipulation. Some of us torment and control our parents, and—later on—our lovers by making them feel responsible for us and guilty if they do not bail us out. A child may get into trouble so that his parents are forced to rescue him. Children of the rich may be ruined because they are allowed to use negative assertion—a kind of pseudo power. Their parents buy them out of trouble—"We're saving you just this one last time"—halting any impetus their offspring may have to develop inner guidelines and real strength. But although a child may use helplessness or acting out to control his parents, this does not generally lead to any sense of authentic power.

Chronic invalids who control their nearest and dearest from the sickbed are a classic example of manipulation through powerlessness. Fans of The Sopranos know that Tony's mother was a classic manipulator. A wife who has "married down" may recite to her husband a long litany of the hardships she endures on his behalf. A mother may remind her chil-dren how much she has sacrificed to give them an education or how she stayed in an abusive marriage to keep the family intact. In such cases, self-sacrifice and moral superiority are invoked to induce guilt.

A submissive person may deceive a dominant person in one way or another, but this strategy, too, creates a sense of self-impoverishment. Our ability to disguise our feelings allows us to manipulate other people, but at a price. The manipulative person sacrifices not just autonomy but self-respect. Then, too, because we know that others can disguise their true feelings, we often question how authentic their manifest feelings are. (Part of the reason we exult so much in babies and dogs is that the feelings they express are almost always genuine.) But let us not too quickly scorn the time-honored device that can sometimes be useful, even if we don't altogether endorse W. C. Fields's comment "If it's worth having it's worth cheating for." These tactics sometimes bring their own delicious thrill, and perhaps one ought not go a whole lifetime without ever knowing the pleasure of putting something over on someone else. Indeed, Mark Twain may have been suggesting that we reserve authenticity for emergencies: "When in doubt, tell the truth."

I do not mean to imply, however, that the majority of those who invoke the powers of the weak choose them deliberately. Some individuals are so genuinely helpless that they have real disorders of powerlessness. They lack what the psychoanalyst D. W. Winnicott identified as a sense of healthy "omnipotence," the indispensable capacity for self-generating action and creativity needed to connect oneself with the world.

Vicarious Power

In childhood some of us do not attempt to wrest power from our parents, and instead shelter ourselves under the umbrella of their power—or, later in life, under the power of parental surrogates. We look to them for safety, protection, and the warmth of their aura of strength. In conversation, as in behavior, we stand ready to extol the power of our protector, whether boss, spouse, parent, or older sibling. Insofar as we can induce our rescuer to depend on us, even exploit us, we achieve a kind of security. We have a sense of permanence and importance if we are indispensable to someone powerful. However, the corollary of depending on vicarious power is that we worry about losing our connections to those on whom our power or well-being depends.

Ironically, the people we choose to lean on may themselves be looking for an outside source of power. A single lawyer, in treatment with me some years ago, was often referred to by his colleagues as "the Godfather." In addition to controlling the professional lives of the many people who reported to him, he provided all kinds of professional perks for his "congregation," from high-paying speaking engagements to job recommendations and numerous personal favors. People looked up to him as a power figure, whose beneficence was part and parcel of his great sense of personal well-being and security.

But this particular godfather turned out to be a godfather manqué. He used the godfather role to patch over his underlying sense of powerlessness and weakness, the sad legacy of a childhood spent in poverty with a passive father and a mother who was a chronic invalid. Needy of an external source of power himself, he had risen to prominence in his field by using his brilliance to attach himself to a series of more and more influential lawyers until he made partner. Now this practice is so common as not to be worthy of much note. What betrayed his underlying dependency were his relationships with a series of women who were without exception the daughters of even richer, more powerful men than he had become, men he could relate to as surrogate fathers. In my view this pattern is always noteworthy. Paradoxically, but perhaps self-evidently, my seemingly powerful patient was looking for his own godfather, real or symbolic, to look after him. One measure of his growth over time was that when he married he chose a woman who was quite substantial, though she, like him, came from a circumscribed background. With her, he came to internalize a feeling of genuine power.

Reliance on vicarious power can sometimes be relatively innocuous. One moderately shy woman told me that the only time she felt comfortable at parties—certain that people would want to talk to her—was when her husband was a CEO; his power encompassed her, so that his employees and their spouses would approach her and initiate contact. In contrast, others are unaware of their dependency on vicarious power and are surprised to discover how differently they are treated when their circumstances change. The daughter of a famous writer, who had grown up surrounded by egotistical writers who appeared to dote on her, was shocked when they dropped her and her mother shortly after her father's funeral.

The Psychological Landscape
of Power

How we come by our "choices" or "preferences" in the way we exercise power is the result of temperament, early experiences, and the conventions of the world we inhabit. Beginning in early childhood, thinking about power relationships—consciously or unconsciously—takes up a considerable amount of time. Even a small child has an intuitive though as yet unarticulated sense of her place in the world, an understanding that there is a hierarchy of power, an awareness that her ability to control her life rests not only on learning how to exert her own power but also on learning how to relate to and influence or manipulate the power of others. Childhood teaches us many of the basic power maneuvers.

We soon learn that there is just so much we can do to control others and that there are repercussions for our willfulness. From infancy on, we encounter opposition to our natural desire to have our own way, and this results in a clash of wills between us and our parents. If we failed to find a comfortable balance of power with our parents or our siblings, we will continue to create similar skews in our adult relationships. The present ricochets off the past. For instance, one young man chooses to argue with his male friends if a difference of opinion arises, but with his girlfriend, he will simply walk the other way, believing that she will capitulate out of fear that he will break off the relationship. He learned these responses from his father and mother, respectively, before he was five years old.

If we were overcontrolled or browbeaten, we may identify with the aggressor and resort to control, coercion, or manipulation to get our way. We may also be preoccupied with the opposite—how to avoid being restricted, controlled, dominated. In the latter case, we are the underdog.

Then there is guilt. If we pursue our wishes despite our parents' objections, we do not always get off scot-free. We may become so fearful of their disapproval, punishment, and their possible abandonment if we follow our bliss that we transfer this fear to our later relationships.

Our ancient relationships don't simply impact on our current ones but are perpetuated in an underground life of their own. The power balances we arrive at in our adult lives are complex not only because they are cocreated, but because our current relationships are inevitably infused with echoes—introjects—of our early life relationships. In an autobiographical story, "Mama and the Meaning of Life," the existentialist therapist and gifted writer Irvin Yalom tells of a dream in which he is wired up in a cardiac unit and thinks he's dying.[13] Leaping out of his bed, he darts off to the Glen Echo amusement park, where he takes his place in line for the House of Horrors. Much to his surprise, he sees his mother in a group of onlookers and calls out to her, "Mama! How'd I do? How'd I do?" In the context of the story, this is a shock. His mother had been dead for more than ten years, and, in fact, Yalom was emotionally estranged from her ever since an incident that happened when he was eight years old and she took him to the movies. Whether inadvertently or purposely, she started to sit down in a pair of empty seats next to a much-feared neighborhood tough guy. When the tough guy told her the two seats were saved, she scorned him and sat down, thus, permanently condemning Yalom to his enemies' list. But she had no awareness of this at all, no concern about what her sangfroid was going to cost her son. Yalom never forgave her. He went on living with his mother year after year "on terms of unbroken enmity. . . . She was vain, controlling, intrusive, suspicious, spiteful, highly opinionated, and abysmally ignorant. . . . Never, not once do I remember sharing a warm moment with her. Never once did I take pride in her or think, I'm so glad she's my Mama." Clearly, too, there were additional reasons for their estrangement—her haughty, cavalier attitude permeated their relationship.

Yet the dream tells another tale. Even though Yalom "divorced" his mother at an early age, she lives on in him. He invokes her to pass judgment on how he has made out in life: he wants to know if she's proud of him. Yalom is in thrall to *her* judgment of him. And why not? In our early lives, we *are* the powerless ones; our parents are our generals and judges. The power of Yalom's mother has continued to exist in a subterranean place and now, when Yalom is in his sixties, it explodes into consciousness.

Why does she surface now? Yalom doesn't say, although he hints in another story that many of his current concerns are connected to intimations of mortality, and he confesses that he fears death. Perhaps his fear of death, as in the dream, leads him to reconsider his life. What impact has his maternal dybbuk had on his life? She has certainly affected the scope of his ambition, and she has probably affected his sense of inner power or powerlessness.

Yalom's story dramatizes something that is true for all of us: the voices of our early childhood stay with us throughout life, though we are not always conscious of them and even though the speakers may be long dead. These voices grant or deny us recognition and shape the power strategies we subsequently "choose."

One of my patients, a professionally successful man, who remembered his mother as being very overbearing, always told me with great gravity what his wife thought and how she interpreted his motivations. Even when he was angry at her, he disavowed the legitimacy of his own feelings by taking her interpretation of events as the literal truth—and denying his own agency. The only way he managed to maintain his sense of a separate self was to take a mistress.

Those who avoid expressing what they feel in favor of stressing what a partner feels are giving power to the partner. The origin of this kind of relationship is sometimes to be found in the truce a child makes with an overbearing parent. Children apparently conclude that even though a parent feels a need to dominate and control, the parent is a protector, someone to depend on. Someone who continues such an accommodation into adulthood is left with a sense of self-doubt, vacillation, and mistrust of his own feelings. The result is a generalized sense of powerlessness, almost invariably in intimate relationships though not necessarily at work.

In the course of growing up, we learn how power is distributed among those closest to us, and we develop an ability to intuit how this may affect us, even when we are not directly involved. For instance, as an adolescent Laurel inadvertently discovered her mother's complex relationship with the mother's sister, Laurel's Aunt Dorothy. Lying in bed one morning, she overheard a conversation between her mother and their next-door neighbor. Her mother was bragging about Dorothy. Laurel immediately understood that her mother believed she held a privileged social position because of her wealthy and socially prominent sister. At the same time, however, her mother felt disadvantaged vis-à-vis Dorothy. Laurel generalized from this an understanding of how connections to powerful people may confer prestige in one context while causing feelings of inferiority in another. Such a bifurcated emotional response is almost inevitably the dilemma of the spear-carrier, the acolyte, the dependent relative, and—often—the wife of a successful husband. For Laurel, the price paid by her mother seemed too high, and out of her shame for her mother she conceived the ambition to be important in her own right. One might say that the conversation she overheard led to a moment of recognition. There may well be something about power, and about our natural aptitude for fitting ourselves into power relationships, that makes such moments of recognition likely. Sometimes, too, we read in the eye of someone else how we have been appraised—as strong or weak, competent or helpless, a life force or a weak reed.

A primary arena in which power is first learned, then continually negotiated and renegotiated, is the relationship between siblings. The poet Sharon Olds writes of her sister, "Hitler entered Paris the way my sister entered my room at night." Olds goes on to describe how this older sister sat astride her and peed on her.[14] She doesn't tell us what their present relationship is, but writing the poem may have served as a partial redress of the humiliation inflicted on her in childhood. (Not surprisingly, many writers say that they are inspired by revenge.)

Olds describes a primal confrontation, but we often find subtler ways of asserting power over our brothers and sisters, especially when we are younger or weaker. We learn how to get them into trouble with our parents, for example. At the dinner table, a little girl quietly kicks her big sister under the table to provoke the older sister to hit her, eliciting the predictable wrath of their mother. Or a younger brother snitches on an older brother. For the psychoanalytic critic and scientific historian Frank Sulloway, sibling rivalry, not the Oedipus conflict, is the engine of history. He believes that unconventionality is a trait of younger siblings and is developed because they need to differentiate themselves in order to avoid competition with the firstborn.[15] Ultimately, though, our rivals and competitors are also our companions and co-conspirators. Unwilling to lose our affectionate ties to our siblings, many of us learn how to negotiate friendly relations with them.

We also use friends to work out issues of control and power in early childhood. In games of war or games that involve hiding and catching, we are flexible—alternating the roles of attacker and attacked, hunter and hunted. We learn the concept of taking turns, which helps mitigate against quarrels over priority while still allowing each of us a taste of it.

In early childhood we may also learn patterns of powerlessness, especially if our parents consistently undercut us and denigrate our attempts at mastery or independence. Sometimes it's not even active undermining that creates this sense of powerlessness; rather, it's neglect. A boy of three makes himself a nuisance trying to break into the circle of his seven-year-old brother's friends. This pattern becomes set for life, as he begins to feel perpetually outside and disadvantaged, irremediably less powerful than his brother, whom he tries for years to imitate. This dependence on his brother developed because his parents never looked after him or protected him, leaving him to seek his brother's unreliably protective wing. Sometimes he would be his brother's sidekick, but too often he was an unwanted tagalong. Nor did his brother grow up unscathed; unresolved guilt over what he feels was mistreatment of his brother, which he now tries to make up to him, has led to bouts of self-abnegation in his own intimate life.

The uses we make of our childhood strengths and weaknesses are complicated and do not always play out in any linear way. Michael Korda has noted that in the business world, men who were bullies at school "often develop a very sophisticated repertoire of bullying techniques in adult life, though they may eventually find themselves at a disadvantage if they meet a more powerful bully." On the other hand, those who were persecuted by bullies and learned how to deal with them by "flattery, cunning, and a display of weakness, usually go on using these defenses against adult bullies with the same success." Korda concludes that the most successful power players in business (or other arenas) can do both, and "don't mind looking foolish or weak when it's useful—a certain amount of ego destruction is not a bad thing."[16] Here Korda demonstrates how the powers of the weak can sometimes be invoked to triumph over the powers of the strong.

Our adaptations during adolescence are not necessarily predictive of our adult lives. Those who were popular in high school may use their gifts to advantage in later life. But sometimes a high school student, popular simply by virtue of mastery of the dating game or excellence in team sports, fails to develop internal resources. It's no surprise that in movies depicting class reunions, the nerd almost always turns out to be the winner, often the CEO of a computer company. This theme also appears in a short story by John O'Hara in which a high school football player reaches his pinnacle on the playing field, with his life going straight downhill from there. Being popular often depends on superficial social skills, such as wearing the right clothes and looking "in." But being popular can be so gratifying in the moment that it interferes with the career dreaming so often connected to future success.

Gender, and our parents' response to it, may dictate many of the power tactics we will favor in early and later life. Some influences begin in childhood but continue to affect us into adulthood. Much is written in popular psychology—and in this book—about how we come to identify with one or the other parent and how we are shaped by key experiences of our early lives.

Some new research suggests that specific patterns of dominance and submissiveness related to gender may begin with interactions between mothers and infants. The researcher and psychoanalyst Daniel Stern found evidence for this in a video of a mother and her young son, which he analyzed frame by frame.[17] The boy, about nine months old, is sitting on the floor playing with a wooden puzzle. His mother moves him into a position where they might play together. The boy picks up a piece of puzzle to put in his mouth. His mother says "no" and restrains his arm, remarking, "Puzzle, not to eat." (This is a typical thing mothers do. To preclude an inappropriate activity, they give an explanation. They say "This is a leaf. It's not to eat. We don't eat leaves.")

The child says "Uh." He again picks up the puzzle. The mother reiterates, "No. Not to put in your mouth." There is a pause. He says "Uh" again, and his mother says "I said no." He does it twice more. She makes her disapproval known again, and she becomes more and more serious in her need to override him. She turns her head toward him and scowls with her eyebrows. Her voice loses its musicality and sounds more stressed. She says "Don't yell at your mother. I said no." But her response is not yet intense.

The two have entered a kind of game that will escalate until one or the other backs down. The mother's voice hardens. The child says "Uuhh." The mother turns, pulls back, softens. She's quiet. Her vocal tension is gone. She's almost sexy, conciliatory; she raises both eyebrows. At that point she says very musically, "I said no." But the boy has won. They both seem to understand the point they've reached. Her hand is on his arm, but she doesn't stop him. This is the turning point, and he overrides her. With a grunt of satisfaction, he puts the puzzle in his mouth. She says "Does that taste good? Its only cardboard." But as soon as he defies her and gratifies himself, she shows contempt.

In his microanalysis of the video, Stern considers the mother's behavior before she says no. Her son looks at her, knowing what's coming. They don't appear to be negotiating anything new. Stern suggests that the baby is learning the point at which he can ignore what his mother is saying. He theorizes that the mother is both rejecting her son and teaching him how to overpower her, thereby inducting the boy into a male pattern charac-teristic of their subculture. In that culture, men fail to listen to their wives and often betray them, only to feel overcome by guilt, depression, and self-loathing. Not only is the boy being raised as a little chauvinist, but there is something to observe in the mother's scorn as well.[18] All this is occurring outside conscious awareness.

Sometimes parents know exactly what they are trying to convey. Sam tells a not uncommon story of growing up in a tough neighborhood in the Bronx. One day when he was about eight years old, he came home crying and told his father that he had been threatened by a neighborhood bully. The father told Sam to go back out there and beat the hell out of the bully or Sam would get the beating of his life. More frightened of his father than of the bully, Sam did as he was told. For him, this worked out well—he licked the boy and felt the beginnings of masculine pride. But a frailer boy might have been psychologically crippled.

The writer Robert Timberg tells a similar story—that of James Webb, a marine who fought in Vietnam and later became secretary of the navy and a novelist of the Vietnamese experience. According to Timberg, Webb's life course was set early: "[Webb] is, as those who know him read-ily attest, a warrior, the descendant of warriors, an American samurai for whom the ultimate test is combat. . . . He started early. When he was four, his father, a veteran of WWII and the Berlin Airlift, would clench his fist and hold it out. 'Are you tough?' 'Yes, I'm tough.' 'Then hit my fist.' Jimmy swung, crushing the knuckles of his tiny hand. 'Is that as hard as you can hit? Hit it again.' The boy swung again. Same result. 'Are you tough?' 'Yes, I'm tough.' 'Then hit it again.' He swung again. By now he was sobbing. 'C'mon, c'mon, you're tough. Hit my fist.'"[19] James Webb, like Sam, was taught a hard lesson about the way men must act to hang tough.

Many boys are still taught to tough it out, but girls are more often advised to be polite and considerate, and to please. When my own sons (who are now thirty and twenty-seven) were in grade school—at a time when the women's movement was well under way—I was astonished to discover that at the picnics of their progressive school in New York City, boys were sent off to play ball while girls were asked to pass cookies.

I do not contend that boys are by virtue of hormones or training more knowledgeable about power, but rather that the two sexes will be likely to adopt different tactics of power—boys will learn more direct modes of power, while girls will more likely use indirect modes. Men who raise their voices are generally considered commanding; women are considered shrill. Aggressive men are considered good leaders; merely assertive women are still too often regarded as witches if not bitches. Thus, gender shapes our understanding of both interpersonal power and personal power, often mandating which power modalities we use.

Power Balances

While many of us might prefer relationships based on sharing power, many relationships formed around a dominant/submissive gradient are lasting, and even gratifying, provided that the gradient is not too steep. Even two dominant individuals may have a stable, though stormy, relationship, as exemplified in the movies by the great romantic dueling couples like Katharine Hepburn and Spencer Tracy. Perhaps the least functional pairing occurs when two submissives come together: then, neither partner can be relied upon to choose a direction, to push the envelope.

Convention sometimes dictates the way our power relations are structured. A traditional upper-crust woman in a traditional society may defer to her husband while controlling her children and servants.[20] Her daughter grows up to do the same. Sometimes, however, our traditional attitudes about power can undergo dramatic transformations when we are pressured by feelings for our loved ones. The movie *Billy Elliot* tells about a working-class English boy in an extremely manly culture who discovers that he wants to become a ballet dancer. Billy's father is a coal miner who does backbreaking work just to get by and whose life has been made more precarious by a ruinous strike. He compensates for his relative powerlessness by sharing the macho companionship and pursuits of his fellow miners and through his iron-fisted control of his family. Horrified to discover his son's newly found passion, which he sees as unmanly if not effeminate, the father puts up a stiff macho opposition. And manliness is all he has got. The triumph of the film is its portrayal of his conversion from abhorrence of Billy's passion to support of him in his search for self-expression and autonomy. The father's love permits him to view the world and the possibilities it holds for his son more broadly, and to radically change his ideas about what constitutes real strength.

The balance of power can shift, sometimes within the course of a single conversation, particularly when it becomes clear that one person wants something more than the other one does. If she wants to get married more than he does, for instance, he holds the power. Change can also take place if one partner changes dramatically; thus if an overweight wife loses twenty pounds, her husband may sit up and take notice. External changes, like a promotion and a monetary windfall or the loss of a job or severe illness, also shift the balance.

Our personal psychology is sufficiently complex that we often find ourselves in different power positions in different relationships. Stories of extremely powerful businessmen, feared by their rivals and their allies, who become mesmerized and dominated by a woman, are so common as to be clichés. The dominant woman in such a relationship may herself personify or embody a cliché—the power behind the throne, a femme fatale, a dominatrix, an invalid wife. A teenage girl, whose friends' parents admire her good nature, tyrannizes her mother in private: she is unyieldingly dominant and controlling with her mother while socially she is agreeable, pliable, and sunny. A much-decorated soldier, fearless in battle, is excruciatingly shy on a date. And so on. The relational strategies we adopt are context-related, suggesting that we all harbor the dual impulses to dominate and to submit.[21]

The underlying balance of power between two people is not always self-evident. The participants may deceive themselves, both rationalizing that one is more powerful when it is the other way around. This pattern is more common when the wife is the real power. People may even remain unaware that there is a power balance in the relationship until it breaks down, or until it is called to their attention by a child or by an outside observer.

Whatever balance we achieve, internal changes on the part of one partner can result in dramatic and often disruptive shifts. For instance, dealing successfully with a drug or alcohol problem, which should prove a boon to a relationship, may actually become disruptive. This occurs when the power balance was organized around the unconscious gratification both partners derived from the fact that one of them was playing the rescuer. Many bad marriages endure precisely because of the gratification that comes from the "strong" partner's ministering to the addicted "weak" partner. Even when the healthy partner is suffering, she may be getting pleasure from her presumed saintliness and moral superiority.

Success of one partner can threaten a relationship. When a husband writes his first book, in the time when he does not yet know whether it will be a success or a failure, or a wife is expecting an important promotion, the spouse may be afraid of losing the relationship. This insecurity—and the implication that the spouse's failure would be preferable to marital strain—may cause a crack in the bond.

Shifts in a power balance can result from a moment of recognition. A generally passive woman unexpectedly asks her husband why he came home so late without calling. Ordinarily, she never questions him, but now she can read guilt in his eyes; she knows he is having an affair. While she may feel humiliated, she is empowered by knowing the truth. She has acquired leverage, and her husband can no longer look down on her for not seeing what he is up to. He will need to reevaluate his opinion of her; she will need to address the fear that made her blind. Power is renegotiated when an adolescent goes to work and earns his own money, or when a powerful man loses his job and is no longer the family's main or only breadwinner. But when the balance of power changes, the resulting disequilibrium may be conducive to growth. One must always remember the lesson of the women's movement: the traditional power equilibrium based on male dominance, while it may have stabilized a relationship, sometimes hobbled the individual development of one of the partners.

Although power struggles may intensify over time, they may be resolved, sometimes in ways that surprise both partners. Consider the wife who doesn't work and her high-salaried husband who doles out small amounts of money to her. This leads to bickering that begins to erode their bond. One such wife got a job as soon as her children had left home. Once she controlled her own money, she no longer needed to ingratiate herself with her husband, nor did she need to complain about his stinginess. Her ability to assert herself forced her husband to see how destructive his need to control her had been to their marriage. Changing one's own behavior is almost always the most effective way of getting someone else to change.

If we fail to find a workable balance of power in a relationship, it may deteriorate into an overt struggle, which often takes the form of accusations and blame. John Cheever gives a terrifying example of his parents attacking each other at the breakfast table:

"Leave me alone, just leave me alone is all I ask," says she. "All I want," he says, "is a boiled egg. Is that too much to ask?" "Well, boil yourself an egg then," she screams; and this is the full voice of tragedy, the goat cry. "Boil yourself an egg then, but leave me alone." "But how in hell can I go boil an egg," he shouts, "if you won't let me use the pot?" "I'd let you use the pot," she screams, "but you leave it so filthy. I don't know what it is, but you leave everything you touch covered with filth." "I bought the pot," he roars, "the soap, the eggs. I pay the water and the gas bills, and here I sit in my own house unable to boil an egg. Starving." "Here," she screams, "eat my breakfast. I can't eat it. You've ruined my appetite. You've ruined my day."[22]

Here the power struggle seems to have become an end in itself rather than a way of working out a conflict or redressing an imbalance. The struggle has taken on a life of its own and is being pursued ruinously.

Paradoxes of Power

When we successfully exert our will, the outcome may nonetheless create more discomfort or anxiety than pleasure. If the dominant party uses coercion to effectively control his partner, he may feel diminished by needing to employ it—a kind of catch-22. The rich man with his new trophy wife wonders whether it was his wallet that has actually bagged the prize. An extremely competitive and dominant businessman feels cut off from the people under him and vigilantly guards against hostile moves by competitors and envious employees—thus the expression "It's lonely at the top."

Another fault line in dominance is its fragility. Because the permanence of the power position depends on bringing the subordinate's will into some kind of correspondence with one's own or warding off rivals and marauders, the problem the dominant individual faces is how to hold onto power, how to forestall one or another kind of insurrection. In the business world, a naturally dominant person may sometimes choose to take the position of second-in-command on practical grounds, either because he recognizes the essential superiority of the person in the number one position or because he intuits that he will last longer as the number two and may still have the option of moving ahead later. A senator may figure out that he will have a more enduring public career than someone who makes a disastrous bid for the presidency.

Those who are powerful in business or government do well to broaden the base of their power, heeding the excellent metaphorical advice that one should always belong to more than one club. Some, however, turn their attention to the insignia of power—memberships on boards, country estates, classic cars. These symbols are meant to reinforce power and often create a false sense of security, an expectation that one's status will survive the loss of one's original source of power.

Charismatic power also has limitations; it does not always sit easily with its possessor. A friend of mine, a powerful intellectual, charismatic speaker, and adviser to four presidents—told me about the one time he permitted himself to hold an audience in his sway and felt what it would be like to be a demagogue. As a refugee from Hitler, he was horrified at the hypnotic effect he had on the crowd and never again permitted himself to sound an emotional rather than a rationally persuasive argument in his subsequent speeches. His reluctance to exert such charismatic power was certainly based on moral concerns, but there was also a psychological component. My friend, although well-known, even famous in some circles, was more comfortable in a secondary role than in a dominant one. This was true in his personal and professional relationships and was related to his need to disidentify from his overbearing father, a prototypical family dictator. But he was totally free of any inhibitions in his creative life, and in an irony unnoticed other than by himself and a few intimates, was thought to be one of the most "powerful" thinkers of his day.

A charismatic individual may come to deplore the obligation to shine. An acquaintance of mine, much celebrated as a charmer and a great wit, bitterly laments feeling that he always has to sing for his supper.

Some people, sensing the intrinsic paradoxes of power, conclude that the dominant partner in a relationship, who by definition needs a subordinate on whom to exert power, is no more free than the subordinate and that, consequently, there is but little autonomy in the dominant power position. Sad to say, the master requires a slave.

Paradoxes abound. Authentic power can grow out of the soil of weakness. While honing one's emotional subservience to an overbearing parent (or to a latter-day surrogate) generally leads to a loss of self-determination and to a sense of powerlessness, it sometimes can be turned to good account in one or another service business, where one must be exquisitely attuned to the feelings, desires, and egos of the client. One woman sees herself as a self-guided approval-seeking missile and is so viewed by her intimates. But her ability to read what clients require, honed out of years of needing to please, has made her a formidable magnet in attracting new business for her company, certainly one kind of power.

There is an echo of this kind of power in a recent interview with one of the hot leading actors of the moment, Brendan Fraser.

> Interviewer: "What are your anxieties?"
> Fraser: "Probably just not pleasing people."
> Interviewer: "You have that one? That one sucks."
> Fraser: "Yeah, but you *should* have that one. Through making it work for other people, you find a way of making it work for you."[23]

Even when such powers are highly effective, they may be less than satisfying to the person who is exercising them because they are expressed in the "passive" voice.

Given the drawbacks to both the dominant and the submissive positions inherent in bickering relationships, the co-sharing of power should be ideal. This is frequently but not always the case. If cooperative relationships are so constructed as to be completely even-steven, they may become dysfunctional in crisis situations where someone must take the lead. Moreover and more usually, many relationships that appear "cooperative" mask a latent dominant-submissive interaction: the cooperation is revealed to be a sham when the submissive person finally insists on having a say in what is happening. We can perhaps better understand such pseudo-cooperative relationships through a comparison to some research findings describing modes of group interaction among the flight crew in the cockpit of an airplane.

The cockpit crew is a small, highly structured, group, in which crew effectiveness is impacted on by a number of socio-psychological, personality, and group interactional variables.[24] Two kinds of breakdown can occur in communication. One kind occurs because of a lack of cohesion and bickering within the group, so that group members are unable to coordinate their actions. The other kind occurs because there is too much cohesion. The phrase "too much cohesion" is a gloss on the submissiveness of one of the partners. To the degree that a copilot is psychologically subservient or submissive to the captain, he may fail to alert the captain to potential trouble, or he may try and not be heeded—either way resulting in a catastrophe in the air.

The researchers H. Clayton Foushee and Robert L. Helmreich reported on a number of airplane crashes that proved to be connected to the psychological relationship between the pilot and copilot.

> In 1982, a B-737 experienced difficulty taking off in a snowstorm in Washington, D.C., failed to maintain an adequate rate of climb, and crashed into the 14th Street Bridge. The cockpit voice recorder . . . tragically documented the cause as the breakdown in the group process. The co-pilot made repeated subtle advisories that something did not appear quite right (engine set at substantially less than normal takeoff thrust due to a partially ice-blocked probe, causing false, high-thrust readings on the engine gauges) and these advisories were, for whatever reasons, not attended to by the captain. This message again did not go unnoticed by the NTSB [National Transportation Safety Board], which recommended that pilot training include "considerations for command decision, resource management, role performance, and assertiveness," implying that the primary cause was the co-pilot's lack of assertiveness and possibly a general hesitancy among subordinates to question superiors forcefully.

Eugene Tarnow, another researcher, exploring the problem of excessive obedience on the part of the copilot, quotes a firsthand report of a first officer's difficulty in communicating with his captain.

> I was the first officer on an airline flight into Chicago O'Hare. The captain was flying. . . . On our approach, Control told us to slow down to 180 knots. I acknowledged and waited for the captain to slow down. He did nothing, so I figured he didn't hear the clearance. So I repeated, "Approach set slow to 180," and his reply was something to the effect of, "I'll do what I want." I told him at least twice more and received the same kind of answer. . . . [Despite

many more attempts to intervene, the first officer was continually rebuffed.] Finally, however, the captain responded, "You just look out the damn window."[25]

Tarnow, too, believes that a captain's excessive need to maintain control in conjunction with a copilot's lack of assertiveness and a general hesitancy among subordinates to question superiors lies at the root of many crises in the air. (This is reminiscent of Stanley Milgram's leader/teacher/student research!)

Subsequently, the airline industry used these data to develop an intervention called crew resource management training to address specific attitudes and behavior on the part of the cockpit crew. This training has resulted in fewer miscommunications and missed communication in the cockpit.[26]

This kind of research has now been applied to other professions; for example, investigating teams have been looking into problems in communication among health care workers in operating rooms and intensive-care units. Although this work is still in progress, one conclusion so far is that intensive-care staff, like cockpit crews, advocate hierarchies, whereas surgical teams are less likely to do so. However, those in charge almost invariably believe that there is better teamwork than those who are lower in the hierarchy: "Surgery generally reports good teamwork with anesthesia but anesthesia staff do not necessarily hold a reciprocal perception."[27] The point here is that relationships which appear egalitarian to the dominant member may in fact be steeply hierarchically structured. Such a relationship can stifle any independent thinking on the part of the crypto-submissive person, even in life-and-death situations.

Thinking about cooperation within the family in the light of these research findings helps us to understand how family decisions can be contaminated by the inability of one member to assert an independent point of view. In essence, what seems to be cooperative is not—the appearance of concordance has taken precedence over independent judgment and over the adjudication of differences of opinion.

We can readily see how marital or family decision making may be damaged by an individual's inability to assert an independent point of view. I often hear stories from patients about how the good parent failed to protect them against unjustified chronic criticism by the bad parent. Sometimes, the good parent may even fail to protect the child from physical abuse at the hands of the bad parent. In essence, manifestly stable power balances—even those construed as egalitarian—do not guarantee good decision making or healthy relationships.

Deference to a spouse apparently crippled the initiative of one onlooker who might otherwise have intervened to save a life. When Kitty Genovese was murdered in Queens, New York City, in 1964, she was within shouting distance of thirty-eight apartments. Twice her assailant ran away, apparently fearful that the police might intercede if the neighbors responded to Genovese's screams for help.[28] The third time, he came back and finished stabbing her to death. All the occupants in the thirty-eight apartments were subsequently interviewed. Some said that they thought what they were hearing was no more than a lovers' quarrel. But one occupant stands out. A woman said that she had asked her husband to call the police. He answered that it was none of their business, and she acceded to his judgment. Yet the interview with her suggested that she had not yet recovered from having relinquished her own judgment and autonomy. She said that she regretted not having listened to her heart.

Like agreement, stability is not always a good thing in a relationship. Some researchers, for example, divide marriages into four different categories: unsatisfactory but stable, unsatisfactory and unstable (that is, the marriage terminates), satisfactory-stable, and satisfactory-unstable. Thus a good marriage may end whereas a bad marriage may endure. In part this is because sadomasochistic relationships give gratification on some unconscious level, with at least the promise of stability, so that they continue despite the fact that the partners torture each other mercilessly.

Good relationships depend on sensitivity to what our partners say and do, and sometimes on being able to give in or compromise. Insisting on having our own way each and every time is demoralizing for our partners. In the end, however, in situations of real moment, each of us must find the courage to listen to our own heart and mind. Authentic power in the interpersonal realm encompasses both the capacity to compromise and the strength to hold firm on important issues. This kind of balance is a prerequisite for a gratifying, comfortable, functional relationship—and so, too, to the maintenance of our self-respect and an inner sense of possessing authentic power.

5

Power in
Intimate Relationships

*We are biologically programmed to find other human beings the
most important objects in the world.*

MIHALY CSIKSZENTMIHALYI,
Flow: The Psychology of Optimal Experience

Our involvement in relationships
is not optional. We begin life completely dependent on our parents or
other caregivers. We grow and develop with their love, encouragement,
and guidance and with their affirmation of us as valued individuals. As we
grow older we become more consciously preoccupied with how we interact with others, focusing not only on our past and present relationships
but also on hoped-for relationships in the future. Our involvement with
our intimates (or our hope for such involvement) is evident in our
moment-to-moment stream of consciousness, in which we replay, daydream about, worry about, or happily anticipate our interactions with
them.

At first glance, intimacy on the one hand and dominance and power
on the other seem to be diametric opposites. In almost all the primates,
attachment seems to diminish dominance and aggression. But in
humans, matters are much more complicated. For us, in fact, intimate
relationships are intrinsically connected to power in two important ways.

First, the achievement of an intimate relationship empowers us. Feeling important to someone we are close to provides a sense of belonging and security, and the mutual recognition necessary to our self-validation. The feelings we share become the very bread and honey of life.

Second, power issues are woven into the texture of our intimate relationships. We worry about the stability of our relationships; we wonder if we said too much or too little, if we were insensitive or even offensive, if we pushed too hard or not hard enough. We assess our impact on others and theirs on us—did we seem too interested or not enough? Will a friend or lover disappoint us or overwhelm us? Who is on top? Who is in control? Here we are dealing directly with power issues within a relationship. Even when an intimate relationship is long established, we still ponder how to sustain it—how to keep it from fading away or becoming too large in our lives. If we feel controlled or stifled, we may plot how to escape. In the most successful relationships, we manage these power issues automatically, without much conscious awareness.

INTIMACY DEVELOPS in infancy and evolves throughout our lives. But it is not easily defined. To a large extent, intimacy, at least in its contemporary connotation of the mutual exploration of inner life, is a distinctly modern concept. Moreover, what people experience as intimacy varies a great deal and depends on their individual value judgments and preferences.

As typically defined in the dictionaries, intimacy means close familiarity or a close association or connection. I prefer the novelist Marilyn French's less formal take on it: "Mutual pleasures are the sacred core of life, food, bodily warmth, love, and sex. These things are sacred because they are necessary, because they confer pleasure in the giving and in the receiving so that it is impossible to say who is giving and who is receiving. They satisfy the profoundest needs, and in their satisfying satisfy two."[1] There is sexual intimacy and there is emotional intimacy, and the two may or may not go together. There is the intimacy of kin, of lovers, of friends and the intimacy of those who work together closely.

There is a difference between an intimate moment and an intimate relationship, the latter requiring some ongoing attachment or commitment. In contrast, an intimate moment may take place between virtual strangers during some intense experience. Anonymity, in such a case, may itself open the gates for intimacy and then intensify the experience; a classic example is the brief heightened emotional charge that can take place between two strangers on a plane. Such an encounter may be the prelude to an intimate relationship, or it may be no more than an instant of mutual understanding. People who are frightened of an ongoing intimate connection because they fear losing their independent self may be more comfortable with brief, intense encounters as a form of intimacy.

What each of us experiences as intimacy depends so much on individual preferences and ideals that we all describe it differently. This is evident in the story of Simone de Beauvoir's lifelong liaison with Jean-Paul Sartre, as recounted in Deirdre Bair's biography of Beauvoir.[2] These two brilliant people, stars of the French philosophical and political world, viewed their love as a primary, essential relationship for more than fifty years, even though they had no sexual contact with each other after the first eight or ten years and never lived together. Throughout all those years Sartre confided to Beauvoir every detail of his sexual life with other women, sometimes asking her to intercede to promote or break off his current romance. He even asked her to befriend his sexual partners. All this caused Beauvoir enormous pain. Nevertheless, she made sure that Sartre felt no discomfort in confiding in her. Apparently she was willing to pay this price to preserve her relationship with him—or perhaps this was how she defined intimacy. In contrast to Sartre, she kept her own sexual adventures private, because she was concerned for his welfare and did not want to cause him pain. And with the exception of her relationship with the American writer Nelson Algren, she was never as deeply consumed by her passing affairs as he was with his.

Here is a situation in which one partner tells everything and has no concern about the effect of his words on the other. His partner tells him little but is deeply concerned about the effect of her actions on him. Is this truly an intimate relationship? To put it another way, can one hand clap? Perhaps my question reveals nothing more than my own biases about what constitutes intimacy. Maybe stopping short of total commitment suited both of them. They appear to have had an amazing ease of intellectual exchange, and they both insisted on the primary importance of their coupledom, despite Sartre's desire, late in life, to marry a young Algerian woman. Friends of Sartre and Beauvoir dissuaded him from doing so in order to prevent the private and public hurt—the humiliation really—that the marriage would inflict on Beauvoir. Sartre compromised by legally adopting the young woman.

Intimacy comes in many forms, and we must respect its variety, if it does not involve too much harm. Sometimes the partners' emotional investment in an intimate relationship may be strikingly unequal. For Beauvoir and Sartre, intimacy was by most contemporary romantic standards seriously flawed, but it assuaged many needs for both. This raises questions: Is compromise possible? Is intimacy in one area worth shortcomings in another? For Beauvoir and Sartre the pleasures of the bed were replaced by a meeting of minds and a committed friendship. Yet even there her connection to him appeared greater than his to her—but perhaps not.

No one can be sure how successful and how genuinely intimate the relationship between Beauvoir and Sartre really was. It certainly contained elements of intimacy bought at the price of independence and of independence bought at the price of intimacy. Their story cautions us that relationships must be examined on their own terms; one needs to know a great deal about the players before making a judgment. Psychoanalysts are often amazed at the compromises people make and still achieve, however imperfectly, real happiness in life.

Intimacy is perhaps best understood in terms of its absence. Lacking it, we feel cut off, lonely, isolated, and empty. If we have achieved it and then lost it, we feel as if we have been sealed off, exiled from some blissful state. We want to be connected and through that human connection to feel alive, joyful, our true selves. We want to be close to another human being and confident that we are hearing and being heard, understood and understanding, loved and loving. We want to touch someone physically and know that someone is there, is real, knows us and is present with us in the moment. The paths of intimacy are always turning and twisting, and in today's complicated world they become increasingly tangled, overgrown with myths and misconceptions. A continuing failure to be close to someone else is a perfectly good reason to seek therapy. And many people do, with the achievement of intimacy as their expressed goal.

Intimacy has unfortunately become a buzzword in popular culture, a focus of much self-help literature that urges us on to the pursuit of an elusive perfect togetherness. These days, women perhaps more than men have been led to believe that intimacy entails a mutual exploration of inner life—why he likes his mother better than his father, why she gave up motherhood for her career or her career for motherhood, why he gets headaches and she is prone to accidents, why he likes company and she likes solitude. In this voyage of mutual discovery, exploring the *why* is itself the act of intimacy.

But intimacy is more than just knowledge, more than just talk. Talk, in fact, may sometimes prevent real intimacy. Our almost exclusive emphasis on verbal intimacy tends to obscure intimacy's fundamental nature, which always has a quality of empathy, of caring and sharing; knowing may be optional. Intimacy may be found in enjoying a private joke; hugging or exchanging approving looks; showing pride in each other; ordering pizza at two in the morning or remembering when we used to; worrying together about a child or the outcome of a breast biopsy; watching a basketball game. Just as fundamental to intimacy is the pleasure in being alone together, with no words needing to be spoken.

For a group of my college friends, intimate friendship was defined as a group sitting around a kitchen table slicing salami and talking, alternating between gossip and deep "intellectual" questions. (Calling ourselves the Salami Cutters, we reinforced each other's pomposity. But if not then, when?) We generally share with friends our feelings and our overlapping interests. But many friendships are based almost exclusively on shared activities.

Long-term friendships are part of a structure that we depend on not just for safety and companionship but also for affirmation. We take pleasure in reminiscing with a friend about important events and relationships in our lives. Some of us share with friends secrets that we don't reveal in other kinds of close relationships. (Spouses don't necessarily want to know about our past loves in any great detail.) Close friends are the people with whom we check out our decisions, anything ranging from how to handle a work crisis to our ambivalence about forthcoming marriages or impending divorces, to whether to jump a city or stay put. In addition, friends are our memory bank, and we turn to them when we lose contact with the flow of our own lives. While we generally think of deep friendships as primarily same-sex, they can also occur between a man and a woman, particularly if the two have shared some formative experience. When I went to medical school, few other women were in my class. I felt privileged to form meaningful friendships with three male classmates—such friendships were not as common in the 1950s and 1960s as they are today. (They may have been possible because two of the men were married and I soon introduced the third to the woman he would marry.) Yet some things are probably discussed most easily with friends of the same sex, particularly the body and its pleasures and problems. But whatever their gender, we are blessed when we have among our friends some with whom we have maintained close ties for decades.

Intimacy has many facets, but it always depends on letting down barriers. Such trust between two people is seldom easy to achieve and we suffer when it disappears or fails to grow. Our culture emphasizes romantic intimacy, and this tends to obscure the importance of other kinds of intimacy—between parent and child, between siblings, between friends, between coworkers. It also obscures the fact that the sequence and nature of our intimate relationships tells us a great deal about ourselves.

OUR CAPACITY for intimate relationships is established in early life. The work of the English psychoanalyst John Bowlby helps us understand the lifelong effects of early relationships on the child's future capacity for intimacy.[3] Bowlby found that if healthy adult relationships are to be achieved, attachments must be formed in early life. However, he was careful to distinguish attachment from dependency. Instinctual satisfactions like being fed are different from attachment. Attachment becomes evident only when a child recognizes that her mother or another primary caregiver is distinct from others and begins to protest separation from *that person*. Attachment is person-specific; it is based on recognition and preference, and on the knowledge that we are recognized in return.

Bowlby systematically watched babies who were abruptly separated from their mothers. He described the sequence of their responses: first they protested with angry cries, and then, when the mother did not return, their anger turned to despair and the babies became quiet, sad, withdrawn, and still. In infancy, we begin to exercise our capacity to be a separate self, to reach out to specific others and have others reach out to us. This is not a matter of physical need alone. Bowlby found that babies who were fed but not loved did not thrive; many became ill and died. In short, love is vital to the strength we gradually acquire.

At seven to nine months of age, the infant begins to know that her mother is a separate being, not under her control. And here arises the possibility of real mutuality. The infant seeks attunement, mutual recognition, peekaboo, songs, smiles reflecting smiles; she seeks a mother who understands when she is hungry or tired or has had enough tickling. These are the bare bones of a relationship that the child seeks. The connection to her mother is developing well when she recognizes that her mother is someone separate and still someone close and dependable.

But closeness is only part of it. As babies grow into toddlers, they must also push away and be allowed to follow their own independent needs and whims. At first, though, the two poles of desire—interrelatedness and independence—seem confusing. Just as a child begins to express a wish to be independent, she becomes aware of her mother's inner life and of her need for her mother. The child who feels loved, whose mother is in tune with her feelings, will be increasingly independent, forming a real self in the crucible of her toddler years.

The infant researcher and psychoanalyst Daniel Stern, using his frame-by-frame analysis of videotaped interactions between mothers and infants (which I discussed in Chapter 4), has extended Bowlby's insights. Stern found that while children are becoming independent of the mother, they still want to preserve relatedness, attunement, and mutual recognition with her. Stern calls the baby's earliest sense of mutuality *core relatedness*, reserving the term *intersubjectivity* for the baby's emergent awareness, at seven to nine months, that separate minds exist, which may or may not share her emotional state.[4] Real intersubjectivity is contingent on the child's recognition of her mother as having a mind of her own; attunement and mutuality relate not only to her recognition of her mother's difference from herself but to her ability to respond to her mother's feelings. In true intimacy, the child not only recognizes the inner life of other human beings but also develops an ability to empathize with them and to tolerate if not negotiate differences.[5]

In adults, as in children, intimacy includes satisfaction of needs (the mother feeds the infant, the husband nurses his sick wife, partners give each other sexual and sensual pleasure), but it also encompasses shared moments in which we are aware of one another's feelings.

This need to be recognized within the mind of another, understood intuitively long before psychoanalysis was ever a gleam in Freud's eye, was poignantly captured by Pascal:

> We do not content ourselves with the life we have in ourselves and in our own being; we desire to live an imaginary life in the mind of others, and for this purpose we endeavor to shine. We labor unceasingly to adorn and preserve this imaginary existence and neglect the real.[6]

Our deepest sense of self-worth rests on how we feel we are appraised by those we let truly know us. To be known and *still* be loved may be the greatest gift of all.

Because we are inextricably intertwined with other people early in life, our well-being and our sense of self are forever bound up with others. This is true not only because others are a source of dependent gratification but, just as important, because we first learn who we are in connection with them—our knowledge of ourselves is always tied to our intimate relationships. The pleasure we take in relationships is such that they may come to supersede the pleasures of the flesh; our happiness in being connected to another person takes priority over pleasures experienced more narrowly.[7]

The path to intimacy is not always free of problems. Toddlers and children who fail to acquire the ability to be on their own, to do it themselves, lack a sense of being self-starters, of achieving agency and personal power. The resulting dependency always carries the curse of feeling powerless. Here, then, is the first glimmer of our need to balance interpersonal relationships with our desire for personal power. Our simultaneous need for autonomy (self-assertion) and mutuality (intimacy) is at the core of our emotional life, sometimes erupting into a painful internal conflict about what our priority is or should be.

Conflicts between these two poles of development occur all along the way. The natural push to be independent sometimes clashes with the need to be close. However, the strength to explore the world and be in touch with it depends on a child's ability to keep the mother's image in her mind; to acquire this ability, a child must be allowed to be both independent and dependent. If we are not assured during our early years that we can both go away from and return to our mother, then in our adult lives we may tend to shut off the need for mutuality or the desire for independence. Either way, we cannot be authentically intimate with another. Both our interpersonal world and our sense of autonomy become skewed. We either become dependent or suffer from an exaggerated need for independence.

Not only babies swing between mutuality and autonomy. As men and women, we need just what we needed as two-year-olds: independence and self-enhancement as well as closeness, care, the folding of our body into another body, the wrapped-up, protected self that can almost become part of another. Intimacy and the demands of autonomy must be balanced. Most of us come close, then back off; we want to be loved but not swallowed. Even in the best relationships, intimacy waxes and wanes.

Troubles related to this fundamental tension between intimacy and autonomy create some of the summer squalls and the winter storms that disturb our relationships. He wants to watch the football game. She wants him to plant bulbs in the yard with her. They both want to be together but not necessarily at the same time. Intimacy is delicate. It occurs when both parties' wishes come together, but we cannot command this. He needs to prove his independence just as she needs interdependence. She has to work on the afternoon when he wants to be caressed. No wonder so much goes wrong. No wonder we are so often caught in a conflict, with one person moving toward the other just as the other is moving away.

Thus we are condemned to an endless tug-of-war between equally compelling pleasures—those attached to mutuality and those that confirm the self as separate and autonomous. Mutuality may be a prerequisite of autonomy, but the two represent different aspirations. As a result, some degree of betrayal is almost built into the conflict between a couple's simultaneous needs for intimacy and autonomy.

The dichotomy between intimacy and autonomy may underlie Freud's observation that mental health can be defined as the ability to love and to work. Love empowers us through recognition; work empowers us through independent action. Throughout life, we must keep balancing our need for connection with our need for independence, and we must arrive at compromises. Unfortunately it is often difficult, and sometimes impossible, to reconcile these different aspirations; each set demands our time and consumes our devotion. This inherent propensity to conflict affects not just lovers but also parents and children and all kinds of intimate pairs. This means that we must continually negotiate and renegotiate our intimate relationships. This, sadly, is the human condition.

WE TEND TO THINK that an affectionate, intimate relationship is a bulwark against issues of domination, submission, and aggression. We are sometimes surprised when the first conflict arises with a lover or our child. Yet, as I have said repeatedly, all relationships are laced with issues of power and are subject to disappointment, discontent, and even rupture.

People expect to find stability when they marry; they would do better to expect change—especially in the balance of power. Change can come so rapidly that one half of a couple becomes rudderless—or, rather, leaderless—at least until he or she is able to establish personal power. One senses that this was true for Anne Morrow Lindbergh.[8] She was famous early in life as the wife of Charles Lindbergh, and later in life as a writer, beginning with the publication of *Gift from the Sea*. When she first met Lindbergh, she wrote in her diary: "I felt the whole world before this to be frivolous, superficial, ephemeral." She married him two years later, and they were described as a blissful couple. But four years into their marriage, their twenty-month-old son was kidnapped and killed. The Lindberghs went on to have five more children, but something was changed for Anne. A. Scott Berg, in his biography of Lindbergh, describes their marriage as "a complex case history of control and repression, filled with joy and passion and grief and rage." He recounts problems that erupted in their marriage, among them Lindbergh's frequent absences and his bossiness, argumentativeness, and emotional remoteness: "After the birth of each of their six children, Lindbergh would take his wife away on long plane journeys, some lasting weeks, as a way of 'weaning' her from her children. He was angry at her displays of emotions (even after the kidnapping and murder of their child) and he would scold her if she complained she was having trouble with her writing."

Anne Lindbergh's idealization of her husband diminished over time; she seems to have been most estranged from him when he became infatuated with the Nazis in the early 1930s. She found solace in a brief encounter with the aviator and writer Antoine de Saint-Exupéry, but he was already married and also had a mistress. Later, in 1956, she had an affair with Dana W. Atchley, a renowned internist at Columbia Presbyterian Hospital.[9] But she stayed in her marriage and after several years Atchley became simply a friend. By that time she had anchored her identity in her writing and in her deep involvement with her children and grandchildren. According to Berg, she concluded: "I must accept the fact that my husband is as completely different from me as he can be." Though the Lindberghs sustained their connection, their love was buffeted by triangulation (his resentment of her attachment to her children) and by his need to both control her and be independent of her.

Triangulation is the introduction of a third person into an intimate relationship. Throughout our lives, we need to integrate our one-on-one relationships with ties to a third person; thus almost any relationship is triangular. Triangulation is with us from the beginning of life: first, in a three-way bond between us and our mother and father. It is ubiquitous, involving a child and parents, siblings and a parent, an adulterous pair, three friends, or three colleagues. It may sometimes stabilize a relationship but will just as often be disruptive. As with the Lindberghs, the marital bond may be strained by the conflicting claims of children. The balance of power may then become unstable—the father fearing that the baby comes first, the mother needing her husband's support all the more now that she must contend with caring for the baby. (It is sometimes helpful in working out these conflicts to remember that we ourselves were once intruders who triangulated our parents' relationship.)

Triangulation appears in a multitude of situations. Two women who are intimate friends may find themselves uneasy when their husbands join them. One of them suddenly experiences her friend as slightly distant, as though the friend is damping down her affection so as not to offend her husband. Now her friend appears less than a free agent, too subservient to her husband.

Intricately brokered and long-established balances of power between friends may be disrupted by a triangulation that is perceived as betrayal. Monica and Jane had been extremely close friends since high school (where I first met them). After college, they moved to the same city. They spoke to each other by telephone at least once a day, enjoying mock fighting and wisecracking. They were consistently helpful to each other, providing delicacies for each other's dinner parties, dressing out of each other's closets, and detailing for each other the delicious minutiae of their individual adventures. Their relationship was so close that Monica's husband came to resent Jane, who was unmarried, and sometimes he insisted that they entertain without inviting her. Jane retaliated; knowing that Monica did not want her to be friendly with Monica's former boyfriend, she nonetheless invited him to a dinner party without telling Monica. Monica heard of Jane's "betrayal" through the grapevine. Jane was probably getting back at Monica for excluding *her*, though she may also have hankered for her friend's old beau. Monica and Jane had enjoyed many pseudo fights in which they safely vented their anger, but this was different. Their quarrel escalated, and they stopped speaking.

Although they miss each other desperately, neither of them will make the first move to reconcile. They live in the same neighborhood and run into each other in shops or at the movies. Monica sees Jane, Jane catches sight of Monica, but they both avoid eye contact. Each is waiting for the other to make the first move. Monica describes it as a power thing: "It's an in-your-face standoff. I want the friendship, but she has to capitulate. She's in the wrong, not me. I know she wants to make up, but she has to do it straight-out. She has to make the first move." Jane feels unable to do this, even though she acknowledges to herself that she was perhaps wrong to invite Monica's old beau without telling Monica. Jane will not initiate a reconciliation because she refuses to vacate her position of power, her freedom to do as she likes. Power and pride, like anger, are the stuff of everyday life.

Other conflicts may arise in our relationships because of competition, failures of empathy, intense separation anxiety, issues of trust and mistrust, power struggles, disillusionment, or isolation.

Competition between friends, lovers, or parents and children can create tension and sometimes lead to a rupture. Two young fashion designers, each of whom appreciated the other's talent, set up their own business and did well until a recession caused them to dissolve their partnership and take separate paths. Going their separate ways implied blame and was the first inkling of an estrangement. One started a new company and made substantial money within a few years; the other joined an already established company and made less money. Their different degrees of success intensified their estrangement, and they drifted apart.

Problems related to competition often arise when friendships originate in mentoring. The friendship may be full and rich, but when the protégé no longer needs the mentor and moves into an equal or even a superior position, the mentor tends to pull away, feeling somehow humbled. Time, as well as tact on the part of the former protégé, may sometimes repair the damage. Even between husbands and wives, when one consistently commands a table the quieter partner may feel irritated and jealous.

Failures of empathy occur in even the closest of intimate relationships. The partners may see intimacy differently, one taking therapy as a model, the other not wanting to share fantasies, dreams, or ambitions. Privacy also may be regarded differently, with one person not wanting to divulge personal information, regarding it as a breach of confidence, while the other feels that spontaneity is being checked. One marriage broke up because the husband told his best friend about a slightly aberrant sexual practice that his wife enjoyed. Even without sharp differences, one partner will sometimes feel misunderstood, however slight the provocation. Misunderstandings may be compounded in relationships between men and women, who, as Deborah Tannen suggests, use language differently and, as many believe, may even inhabit two different cultures.[10]

Some degree of conflict is inevitable in almost all relationships. Freud was skeptical about the durability of an unambivalent intimate relationship, observing that "the evidence of psycho-analysis shows that almost every intimate emotional relationship between two people which lasts for some time—marriage, friendship, the relations between parents and children—contains a sediment of feelings of aversion and hostility which only escapes perception as a result of repression. This is less disguised in the common wrangles between business partners or in the grumbles of a subordinate at his superior."[11] Disappointment, irritation, competition, and envy threaten harmony, mutuality, and intimacy, leading one partner to feel less important than he or she has been. To repair the damage, we must acknowledge our sometimes less than noble feelings and apologize, or, alternatively, hold firm, asking for a change on our partner's part. Sometimes we need to search our hearts for forgiveness.

Many problems concerning intimacy derive from internal feelings of weakness—separation anxiety, fear of abandonment, suspiciousness, a sense of insecurity, or an impaired capacity to trust. All these problems result in the misuse of interpersonal skills, a kind of squandering of assets, that exacerbates the sense of powerlessness.

Separation anxiety, expressed as extreme dependency or clinging, can erupt into, and subvert a relationship with a lover, children, friends, or colleagues. Early in a love affair, a woman with separation anxiety constantly calls her lover on the phone, just to chat. He tells her that she is interfering with his work, and when she is unable to control her obsessive need for contact and reassurance, he ends the relationship. She convinces herself that the problem was his fear of intimacy, not realizing that the problem was her own excessive need for contact and reassurance. Her underlying fear is that people will disappear from her life, and she tries to prevent this by clinging. Her use of the powers of the weak, now run amok, precipitates her rejection—a case of a self-fulfilling prophecy.

Similarly, a mistrustful friend or lover may engage in a series of provocations to test the authenticity of a relationship. A woman suspects that a friend is distancing from her, so she calls at odd hours to see if the friend is home and free to talk, until she becomes a nuisance and gets dumped. An insecure man may fly into a rage over the smallest of slights—if, say, his girlfriend is fifteen minutes late when he was eagerly awaiting her arrival, or when she overcooks the pasta which he likes al dente. He attributes such lapses not to chance but to her hostility. Yet after his blowup he fears rejection, and he begins to plead for understanding, toleration, and forgiveness. An insecure woman always feels rejected and hurt because she thinks her boyfriend is inattentive—he forgot to call, he is undemonstrative, he spent too little on her birthday gift. Rather than discuss her grievances, she resorts to sarcasm, scorn, or screaming. She runs out of the house, hoping to be pursued, but when he fails to oblige, she suddenly becomes contrite, begging to be forgiven, promising never again to behave so badly. These ploys—whether they draw on the powers of the weak or the powers of the strong—are attempts to control our partners, to force a response from them.

The psychoanalyst Peter Lawner notes that such confrontations are "tests" which come "from both a lack of trust and from a *typically masked wish and striving to reopen the issue of trust* ... from the unconscious (and often conscious as well) expectation of disappointment by the Other but also from a wish to question whether one's pessimistic expectation in the relationship could be mistaken."[12] People who engage in testing in their personal lives usually also do so in other situations—with their friends or with their therapist, for instance.

If trust is an ongoing issue, a person's relationships are likely to be characterized by roller-coaster emotions, uneasiness, and uncertainty. However, some people whose capacity to trust is impaired may improve, particularly if they are fortunate enough to find a partner who is willing and able to respond empathically to a barrage of tests.

Power struggles based on priority and control are threaded through our closest relationships in the same way as conflicts between intimacy and autonomy. Lovers who achieve happiness and stability have by definition arrived at a workable balance of power. The balance is often so subtle and so apparently automatic in its operation that neither the lovers themselves nor outside observers notice it. (However, sometimes the lovers' perception is not the same as that of outside observers. In one female-dominated relationship with which I am well acquainted, both husband and wife assert that the husband is the controlling force. Both are more comfortable agreeing that their relationship conforms to the prevalent cultural expectation—male dominance and female subordination.) Sometimes the balance of power is disrupted because it is maladaptive—from the beginning, one partner has been made to feel like a second-class citizen whose wishes and needs never have priority.

While many power struggles reside in the character structure of the protagonists, others are a product of specific circumstances. Byron and Janet met in school but have been geographically separated for several years. Until a few months ago, they were monogamous, but Janet decided that the long-distance relationship left her feeling lonely. She initiated a breakup, but then she had second thoughts and called Byron to ask for a reconciliation. He readily accepted. Together again, they decided to reestablish their monogamous relationship. For her, the relationship is business as usual. But Byron wants to talk out what happened. Janet adamantly resists any such conversation. Byron resents her refusal and feels closed out, controlled. Finally he confronts her: "This is no relationship if you can't talk out what happened. I'm leaving." He is on his way out the door, when Janet realizes that she has to capitulate or the relationship will end. "Stay!" she pleads, and Byron comes back. They sit down and begin to explore why they separated and what their feelings were during the separation. Not only do they talk out the history of their relationship, but the balance of power between them shifts to Byron, at least for the moment. However intricate, varied, and surprising lovers' arrangements to achieve a balance of power may be, the only criterion for judging them is whether the lovers feel satisfied that neither is being unduly exploited.

Unlike the struggle between Byron and Janet, some power struggles are intractable. When love is on the wane, power manifests itself in a tug-of-war. For example, when the expectations for passionate love are unfulfilled, the wish to give to and sacrifice for the beloved deteriorates into disappointment, self-justification, resentment, and a desire to receive. Mutuality is then replaced by a struggle for priority. An embattled lover may no longer be committed to the couple but may instead decide to provide for himself. Ron, a former patient, is an example; here he is speaking of his wife:

When I first met Janice, I believed that still waters run deep—that underneath her shyness she was a supportive, passionate woman possessing many of those qualities I wanted in a wife. But what I first saw as a kind of timidity that my marrying her would cure turns out to be rigid isolation and withholding. The more I try to break through, the more she recedes into herself. I thought I was doing a lot of introspection to see how I could change, but it's been the cover story for getting Janice to change. What I was really trying to do was to seduce her as validation of my own masculinity. Now I'm more ready for authentic self-exploration. That leaves Janice free to go her own way, to split. She's been complaining about pressure from me all along, so maybe my separating myself in this way will allow her to look into herself. If she doesn't change, I'll find someone else. I hope she does, but if she can't I will move on. Heads I win. Tails I win.

Either way he wins—how different from the lover's plaint. One has only to hear these words to realize that he is no longer passionate. He is hopeful, yes; committed, perhaps; sensible, certainly. But he is no longer in love. And here we see one more way in which power comes into romantic love: as the sadder-but-wiser last act, as insight takes over and starts clearing the stage as we get ready for the next drama in the theater of our lives. When love is over, personal power begins to reassert itself.

Many difficulties in our relationships are specific to our personal histories. Our intimate relationships—with friends and lovers—serve as a map of our past and tell us how we may have been as babies or children in relationship to our parents.

One man describes his mother, who was divorced early, as almost invariably depressed, bitter, and blaming. She feels perpetually victimized—neglected by her parents, abandoned by her husband, wronged by her employer, slighted by her children. His mother taught him that happiness was a pipe dream, that relationships are difficult if not impossible. He rejected her view and dedicated himself to proving her wrong. But he appears to have married a woman whose attitude to life echoes his mother's. He has spent most of his marriage trying to do for his wife what neither he nor anyone else could do for his mother, all the while becoming more and more depressed himself.

Men and women whose parents were depressed may try to rescue others rather than simply being with them. If a mother's depression goes beyond a certain threshold, her baby or young child may become disorganized with regard to forming an attachment. Some people later resolve this by a reaction formation, becoming caregivers is their relationships. Others may become overcontrolling. Both responses are maladaptive attempts to undo or reverse history.

A few of us fail to form intimate relationships. Here the problem is not a conflict between mutuality and independence, or any of the conflicts inherent to intimacy, but the process of establishing intimate ties. A lack of trust in the human environment—a fear that others will deceive or betray us—diminishes some people's ability to open up. Too much wariness and self-protectiveness prevents others from breaking through the barriers they put up as armor. Or their compensatory need to dominate or control another person may make it impossible for them to serve as a mirror of the other's inner self, the tender reflection that is a basic requirement of intimacy. A person who cannot trust others must choose either isolation or the domination of others.

Those who fear that they will be engulfed by another person have somewhat different problems from those who cannot trust others. Mistrustful people, although they fear betrayal, may still actively seek connections. The budding love affairs of those who fear engulfment lack emotional depth or intensity. I'm not talking about a husband or father who slips out every weekend morning to go to the gym and then to the office. Rather, I mean someone who never has come close, who has never nurtured or been nurtured. This person surrounds himself or herself with a moat to protect against the dangers of intimacy. For those who fear personal contact, isolation is a protection against the damages that might occur with closeness—the disappointment, vulnerability, attacks, more pain.

Some people retreat into isolation as a consequence of childhood trauma. They may have been abused, may have been ill and often hospitalized, may have had a parent who died suddenly, or experienced one or another of the other myriad disasters that can be the human lot. (It is worth noting, though, that such a trauma can also open the human heart.) People who are indifferent, aloof, afraid to let another person get close may well have been deserted as babies, or responded to only erratically. They may have received only impersonal, unloving, inconsistent care. Men and women who have hidden their feelings and disguised their needs are also often depressed, fearful of their own anger and the anger of others.

The normal evolution of mutuality also can be subverted by too much intrusiveness. This too can create a fear of engulfment. The psychoanalyst Jessica Benjamin, using Daniel Stern's framework, describes how a mother unduly sensitive to her baby's unresponsiveness can be experienced as overwhelmingly intrusive:

> The mother who giggles, jokes, looms, and shouts, Look at me! to her unresponsive baby creates a negative cycle of recognition out of her own despair. . . . Here in the earliest social interaction, we see how the search for recognition can become a power struggle: how assertion becomes aggression . . . The child loses the opportunity for feeling united and attuned, as well as the opportunity for appreciating (knowing) his mother. He is never able to fully engage in or disengage from this kind of sticky, frustrating interaction. . . . Even as he is retreating he has to carefully monitor his mother's actions to get away from them; even withdrawal is not simple.[13]

One woman, painfully fearful of intimacy, said that until she was eight years old her mother had insisted on wiping her after each bowel movement and inspecting the product. That practice ended only when she threw a tantrum. Some people who have been similarly violated early in life avoid intimacy because they equate it with being intruded upon, infantilized, or controlled.

An almost complete retreat into isolation may be the aftermath of certain kinds of parental abuse. I am not referring to people who enjoy being alone from time to time; I mean those who avoid intimate contact altogether. For them, too, isolation becomes a protection against the damage that closeness can cause. Such isolation may stem from the paranoia of someone who has suffered physical or sexual abuse.

GIVEN THE MYRIAD PROBLEMS that can beset intimate pairs, no relationship could survive if modes of healing were not part of the psyche. Sometimes, after strife has torn them apart, a couple's intimate rituals have a healing effect, even if they don't explicitly discuss their quarrel. In the film, *East Is East* George Khan, a Pakistani immigrant, is married to Ella, an Englishwoman, who runs his fish-and-chips shop.[14] They live with their six children in a lower-middle-class section of Manchester, England. George is an old-fashioned patriarch who believes it is his duty to control the lives of his children. While Ella is deferential, she is also able to maintain her dignity and her sense of self. George encounters problems with his sons, who have a sense of English freedom along with the Pakistani ideal of respect for parents. But George and Ella's marriage remains tender and respectful, particularly because of Ella's sensitivity and tact. In a frenetic household, the couple's evening tea is a moment of quiet intimacy. Ella always asks George if he would like a cup of tea, and he invariably answers "half a cup."

A crisis arises when George arranges marriages for two of his sons with two Pakistani sisters they have never seen. The two women turn out to be remarkably ugly, and their mother makes insulting and derisive comments about the Khans' crowded household, presided over by an Englishwoman. Ella defends herself and her children; the other family leaves abruptly, in anger. George is so enraged that he threatens Ella physically, and their children intervene to protect her. It looks as though the marriage is over. Ella flees, and George appears defeated.

But the next day Ella is in the fish-and-chips shop and George appears. Neither apologizes, but Ella asks George if he would like a cup of tea, and as usual he answers "half a cup." The healing process is under way.

Despite the many disappointments and the inevitable friction that intimacy breeds, it often survives and in many instances deepens and grows, especially if the partners are capable of some mutual adaptation. One great pleasure of intimacy, as described by the psychologist D. W. Winnicott, is the ability to be alone together.[15] Winnicott held that the ability to be alone as an adult is fostered early in life by a caregiver who permits the child to be alone in his or her presence. Being alone together not only is a pleasure but can also bring about healing when grievances arise. Because being alone together allows an individual to recover naturally from feeling overwhelmed by the demands and signals of the partner, it is enormously advantageous to the long-term survival of intimacy. George and Ella found this kind of moment in their tea ritual.

ROMANTIC LOVE presents a special case of intense intimacy.[16] Whatever we may think of it, romantic love is the single most powerful passion in many people's lives. People generally assume that it will inevitably fade, but it may in fact have an outcome that is either redemptive and exalting or utterly destructive. Perhaps as a way of taming it, reducing it, even denying its existence as a singular and extraordinary force, psychologists sometimes depict romantic love as no more than a nucleus of physical passion around which a cluster of other feelings—admiration, respect, affection, intimacy, commitment, and approval—cohere. In our culture, passionate love generally comprises both carnal desire and affectionate bonding. But its defining purpose is ultimately neither sexual nor companionate. It is not reducible to sexual passion, and it is more than a mature commitment to affectionate bonding.

What distinguishes passionate love from sexual love or affectionate bonding is the lover's intense longing to merge with the other person. This nucleus—the wish for fusion—draws the other feelings to it. The Italian sociologist Alberoni describes passionate love as "a terrible force . . . that . . . makes each of us irreplaceable and unique for the other. The other, the beloved, becomes what only she can be, that absolutely special one. And this happens even against our will, even though we continue for a long time to believe that we can do without the one we love and can find that same happiness in another person."[17]

An authentic love relationship can be achieved only through mutual choice; both participants must be sovereign. If someone of high status falls in love with someone of lower status, the difference in external power is obliterated. Thus it might seem that romantic love is an exception to the generalization that all relationships have elements of power. But even romantic love is never completely free from the influence of power. In fact, passionate love intensifies both the empowerment and the distortions of power found in all interpersonal relationships.

Lovers achieve power through the formation of a couple, a new incarnation of the original, powerful parental unit. They are empowered through the mutual identifications they form, and as a consequence they transcend the boundaries of their former selves. They are often freed from old patterns, habits, and other rigidities of character. There is also power in recognizing that their dreams of passionate love have come true. These are but a few of the reasons that falling in love is often accompanied by unusual spurts of energy, growth, and change, and by a sense of richness, abundance, and inner strength.

At the same time, romantic love creates a major paradox centered around the issue of merging. The aim of romantic love in its most complete form is clear: the lover seeks union with the beloved. The longing in passionate love is to unite, to merge, to transcend the self. Lovers seek the union, or mythic reunion, of souls and bodies that belong together because they are two halves of one whole. So intense is this impulse to merge that it may take precedence over all other considerations—even happiness.

Merging, however, is fundamentally at odds with another aim of love. If we achieved a complete merger, it would annihilate both partners' identities. Therefore, love, which is committed to preserving the beloved as well as the self, cannot ever reach its goal. As Hans Morgenthau puts it:

> If love is a reunion of two human beings who belong together, that reunion can never be complete for any length of time. For, except in the *Liebestod*, which destroys the lovers by uniting them, it stops short of the complete merger of the individualities of the lovers. It is the paradox of love that it seeks the reunion of two individuals while leaving their individualities intact. A and B want to be one: yet they must want to preserve each other's individuality for the sake of their love for each other. So it is their very love that stands in the way of their love's consummation.[18]

This paradox is one of the great dilemmas that destabilizes love through the lover's insistence on doing away with separateness, either through self-surrender or by the domination of one by the other.

Some degree of self-surrender is a necessary component of merging; indeed merger is an epiphany intrinsic to passionate love. Since the barrier to merger is the self's boundary, what is sought is self-transcendence, a renunciation of oneself as separate. We say, "I lost my heart to him" or "her," but what we mean is that we have dissolved, one into the other. Thus, there is a striking overlap between the language of love and that of religion.

While the impulse to surrender oneself—as part of the impulse to merge—must be regarded as an essential part of passionate love, it can be realized for only brief moments. In such epiphanies, achieved most often though not exclusively during sex, the lovers experience their separate selves as mingled and enriched with no compromise of the essential autonomy and integrity of either. Transcending the boundaries of the ego enlarges and enhances the self rather than obliterating it. Intermittent self-surrender, then, can be a form of self-assertion; giving oneself can be the ultimate expression of one's free will. Rather than being demeaning, it is experienced as empowerment. This may be because the lover is surrendering more to the power of love than to the power of the other.

Self-surrender, though, may go too far. In intermittent merging, the lover seeks a new, expanded joint identity; but the impulse to merge may be debased into a different kind of surrender, in which the lover seeks to submerge his or her identity in that of the other. Such a surrender is extended in time rather than intermittent, and one-sided rather than mutual; it is, perhaps, best described as submerging, rather than merging. The lover is seeking not so much to transcend the self as to bolster the self, to make up for weaknesses in his or her own personality.

Between merger and enslavement, one sees different kinds of self-surrender that are more sustained than intermittent moments of merger but involve elevation of the self—not masochistic degradation. The self finds meaning in service to the lover and perpetuates the connection through the powers of the weak. Though the lover has surrendered part of his autonomous identity, he may hold onto his own self-identity and his pride in himself as the full, nurturant giver. However, when pursued past a certain point, surrender impoverishes the self rather than enriching it.

The lover may lose his pride and become no more than an appendage to the beloved.

The other side of the coin is the will to possess. To some degree, possession is always a component of love; as a consequence, love unleashes primitive urges and fantasies, especially a devouring hunger for the beloved. Domination and conquest are mobilized to satisfy that hunger. This is the meaning of Socrates' comment: "As wolves love lambs, so lovers love their loves." Lovers feel that only when they possess the beloved will they be completely fulfilled. But while they mobilize the powers of the strong, going so far as to exert tyrannical power over the beloved, they become enslaved to their own hunger.

Possessiveness and enthrallment—power in the form of domination and powerlessness in the form of surrender—are part of passionate love. Morgenthau remarks: "An irreducible element of power is requisite to make a stable relationship of love, which without it would be nothing more than a succession of precarious exaltations. Thus without power love cannot persist; but through power it is corrupted and threatened with destruction."[19]

While the wish to possess is almost always part of love's hunger, when it is propelled by a sense of powerlessness, it will pervert love. The lover who desires possession is prepared to obstruct any force that might come between him and his beloved. He feels justified in his claims on the beloved and his excessive need that she belong totally and exclusively to him. The force of this passion is not dissimilar to the omnivorous claims an infant makes on his mother. The lover believes that the beloved is obligated to him, and, in fact, owes him whatever he wants. This can lead to a violent sense of betrayal if his wishes are not met.

While domination may ensure possession, it destroys love. By asserting his own superiority, the lover may undermine his beloved's self-determination and agency and ultimately do away with the original reasons he desired her. One patient, consistently disparaged by his mother, sought validation from a series of women who, he felt, had special qualities. But in attempting to overcome the shame his mother had engendered in him, he undercut each woman's confidence and no longer saw her as worthy of his idealization. Then he would reenact the process with someone new. For other lovers, love can be experienced only as longing; if the object returned their love, this would be seen as submission, which automatically elicits devaluation. Jean-Paul Sartre cuts to the core of the lover's dilemma when he suggests that the lover wishes to possess the beloved as an object and yet simultaneously wishes that she remain a free subject—able to love him of her own free will.

Another reason why domination to ensure love is doomed is that the beloved's spirit remains inaccessible. Spirit becomes visible only through behavior; hence, the primary goal in domination must be to govern the other's behavior. But this is never enough for the insecure lover, who fears that the other is saying, "You may have my body but not my soul." Thus the lover may try to make the spirit of the other visible in the body, so that there can be no secret refusal, no withholding. When domination is thus "metaphysicalized," the body is not simply a vehicle *for* spirit; it is identified *with* spirit. If someone attempts to use power as a means of transcendence, it often takes the form of sexual domination, as can be seen, for example, in the Marquis de Sade's writings.

Possession through domination can never be entirely satisfactory. The desire to ensure possession and to guarantee union may result in the most extreme acts of love: the lover, in a desperate attempt to extinguish all possibility of the beloved's independent thought or actions, may kill both of them—thus literally enacting a perversion of the *Liebestod*.[20]

I HAVE DISCUSSED INTIMACY throughout this chapter as though it is generally a good thing. But psychoanalysts know that certain forms of intimacy are not always good for your psyche. Intimacy can be corrupted by distortions of power. Love may be obsessive, between lovers or between parent and child. An obsessive parent, feeling that his or her own fate depends on the child's unfolding life, can spiritually suffocate the child. Here, intimacy may be achieved, but the child is stunted. The smothering parent and the smothering lover—both are capable of closeness but incapable of separateness. Human suffering follows in their wake. There may be the subjective sense of togetherness in a sadomasochistic relationship in which each partner understands and echoes the other's needs, but the resulting drama does not free or nourish anyone. In some relationships, a partner with an exaggerated need for connection may let the other person take over: "I am not important, but my husband, my wife, my lover is everything. We are so close that I am really him, or her." This kind of intimacy is a travesty; it acts as a bludgeon although it is ostensibly in the service of happiness.

Intimacy is not a skill like word processing that can be taught in class-rooms. It depends on a delicate exploration of the inner world—its style, its disappointments, its illusions, its wrinkles. Formulas for breaching walls, one's own or those of others, tend not to work. Yet intimacy can sur-prise us by appearing suddenly and unexpectedly. However difficult the experience of closeness with another mortal, it is worth the struggle and the pain. The more flexible we are, the more we can enjoy a variety of forms of intimacy with a range of different people, and the richer our emotional lives will be.

6

Sex, Gender, Hierarchy, and Power

"What a man did only for God, a woman did always for a man."

KATHERINE ANNE PORTER, *Collected Essays*

Although sexual liberation had its beginnings in the first half of the twentieth century—in the first wave of feminism, the free love movement, and the flapper era—it really came into full flower in the 1960s. It was soon followed by the first stirrings of gay liberation at the end of that decade (Stonewall was in 1969) and the new women's movement of the 1970s.[1] All three flashed across the cultural landscape only to recede to some degree after achieving partial acknowledgment. There were smaller movements, too, that of the cross-gender (or transgendered) movement and of a sadomasochistic subculture. But by the 1990s, a spate of books—including *The Decline of the Male* and *The End of Masculinity*—described the reputed threat to the male psyche posed by the women's movement.[2] These books proposed that the empowerment of women and homosexuals brought about a parallel dislocation in the male psyche that marked the diminution if not the end of male heterosexual dominance.

All of these developments impact on the way sex is understood and practiced, and they also have ramifications for the gender ideals or "norms" we strive for.[3] Not only our theories but our sexual behaviors and gender roles have changed, accompanied by changes in our sense of power and powerlessness, pride and shame. Women and gays feel more empowered at least to some degree, and men reportedly less empowered. Utilizing insights from the various liberation movements, theorists of women's studies and queer theory have addressed questions about sexual politics, the complex relationships among sexual preference, self-identity, and sexual object choice, and how patriarchal values influenced power issues in sexual relationships and on normative definitions of gender.[4] The basic assumptions fueling these liberation movements have inevitably influenced the way psychologists and psychoanalysts understand power as it relates to sex and gender.

Sex and Power

Personal sexual power is based on orgasmic pleasure. Orgasm, like a runner's "high," is a natural opiate, leading to ecstasy.[5] But the function of sexuality is broader than the momentary pursuit of pleasure or the relief of discomfort. Self-stimulation in infancy provides essential pleasure that is not dependent on others. The ability to produce pleasure and orgasm at will, through masturbation, gives an adolescent a sense of self-sufficiency and power.

Given the correlation between sexual pleasure and power, it is no surprise that a man's failure to achieve an erection is called impotence, which, by definition, means a lack of power. In women, however, the inability to be aroused is called frigidity. The word *frigidity* seems to focus more on the woman's failure to respond to a man than on the loss of her own sexual pleasure. *Frigid* means cold, not powerless; it implies an accusation rather than a diagnosis. Yet, during many eras, women were socialized to avoid sexual arousal and orgasm, one of life's greatest pleasures, consolations, and sources of autonomy. Such deprivation mandated one kind of powerlessness.

The psychoanalysts Kurt Eissler and Heinz Lichtenstein suggest that there is a direct link between sexuality and identity.[6] Arguing that orgasm, when viewed in its relationship to the ego, must contain a meaning and function beyond attaining physical pleasure and reducing tension, Eissler suggests that it serves as an affirmation of personal existence.[7] And Lichtenstein sees nonprocreative sexuality as serving the evolutionary purpose of establishing a primary identity.[8] Viewed in this light, the cultural suppression of female sexuality can be seen as an instrument of male dominance, not just as a guarantor of paternity.

The sexual domain, though presumably designed for pleasure, bonding, and procreation, is a major vehicle for issues of power and powerlessness. Sex often becomes an arena for issues of control and power struggles, fantasized or enacted, and for the expression of love, hostility or dependency, and domination as well.[9]

The inherent connection between sex and power is made explicit in the many everyday metaphors that use sexual imagery. Justin inherits half a million dollars from his cousin, who disinherited ("stiffed") his live-in girlfriend to leave his money to Justin. Justin, feeling quite noble, decides to divide his inheritance with her. Justin's father, Morgan is furious, screaming at him, "Weak power, so Goody Two-Shoes, definitely limp-dick." There is a power component in expressions such as "taking" or "having" someone, or being had, and it is explicit in sadomasochistic imagery. Sexual fantasies are often infused with images that resonate with power issues: being seduced, seducing, being overpowered, overpowering. Sexual designations—tops and bottoms, stone dykes and femmes—also have clear power connotations, describing power issues between the participants. Then there is the individual or joint "fuck you" to the world that is implicit in the fantasy, or reality, of deliberately violating prevalent taboos.

Two people participating in any joint act may each construe his or her own role as the more powerful one. But this is particularly true in the sexual domain, because every sexual act is saturated with the participants' preconscious and conscious fantasies. Consider a woman performing fellatio on a man. It is possible that from her point of view, she is in control, able through her technique to bring her partner to orgasm at will. He, on the other hand, may believe that she is subservient, dedicated only to his pleasure. Or alternatively, both may feel powerless, she humiliated to be servicing him, he feeling passive and unmanned by a powerful woman. Clearly, how one feels and how one is viewed by one's partner may not be the same.

In sex, one partner may choose to focus on his or her own orgasmic pleasure, on control, or on delivering pleasure or pain to the partner as alternative ways to express power. Thus, some men are famous for postponing their own orgasmic pleasure in order to make a woman crazy with desire. And some women who fail to experience orgasm nonetheless do achieve a sense of power through the deft execution of sexual techniques that alternately tease and gratify a man and thus increase his sexual pleasure.

Considerations of interpersonal power enter our sex lives in our choice of a sexual partner, in the question of how sexual pleasure and reciprocity are parsed, and in the many control issues that permeate even a "consensual" sexual act. The question of who controls the timing and frequency of sex as well as the choice of, insistence on, or refusal of a particular kind of sex act can become the basis for a power struggle. If a power struggle is resolved so that one partner is dominant over the other, the submissive partner may experience a sense of powerlessness that extends beyond the sexual domain. Traditionally, women have been the powerless partners. Those who didn't want sex most often resorted to the powers of the weak—pleas of headaches or illness—to say no. And a woman's sense of her intrinsic powerlessness was often confirmed by social conventions. Even as late as the 1950s and 1960s, some analysts told their female patients not to insist on an orgasm, lest they undermine their husbands' sexual potency. Thus they endorsed the cultural convention that being female was one of the single most powerful determinants "in the shaping of a life consigned to organized subordination."[10]

Nonetheless, sexual attractiveness has been one of the powers that many women most prize. Here a woman's sense of power comes not only from the pleasure of sex but also from the sexual allure and magnetism that allow her to hold sway over men, sometimes very powerful men. Catherine Zeta-Jones, a more than competent actress in her own right, leapfrogged to fame only when she married Michael Douglas, an older man who was one of Hollywood's power brokers. Her personal canniness was evident in her choosing to play a role in the movie *Traffic* while noticeably pregnant, thus displaying her cutting-edge sensibility. Yet, for many, derivative power has a particularly poignant quality because it is a substitute for more enduring kinds of strengths. Someone who has been a life-long beauty, even if happily married, feels her power diminishing as her sexual glow begins to fade, though this may not happen until her fifties and for some exceptional women not at all. A few femme fatales may still be going strong at seventy-five; Mae West may well have been one of them. While women who possess an unusual power to elicit desire in men may not experience authentic power, women who lack this quality or who feel that they are in some way unattractive nearly always suffer a blow to their self-esteem.

There are men, too, who trade primarily on their sexual allure, but they seem to be fewer in number. What is experienced as sexy in men is not so much physical magnetism or allure as power—hence Henry Kissinger's well-known remark that power is the ultimate aphrodisiac. (Fantasies about male movie stars are inspired not just by their physical allure but by their status.) Lack of sexual attractiveness does not hit men as hard as it hits women, because by and large men are prized primarily for other attributes. However, some homosexual men suffer from concerns about their physical desirability as much as women do.

The way we feel about our physical selves (and sex organs) and our power to attract admirers affects whether or not we feel powerful. Some less than beautiful women and some less than handsome men nonetheless view themselves as devastatingly attractive; their expansive self-confidence can sometimes recruit others to their perception, while some attractive men and women may have an extremely negative physical self-image. Not just our feelings about our overall attractiveness but also about our genitals and our secondary sexual characteristics may cause us pain—women worry about the size of their breasts while men worry about the size of their penises. The only generalization to be made is that the pride we take in our physical selves is generally connected to a sense of power, and the shame we feel to a sense of weakness and powerlessness.

Female Sexuality

When I was in college and the first calls for sexual freedom were being heard, one of my more politically "progressive" and sexually experienced girlfriends told me that a guy had asked her to sleep with him. Regarding herself as a liberated woman, she couldn't think of a good reason to say no, except that she had no sexual interest in him. What she was struggling with was the idea that sexual liberation *mandated* sexual participation. I had to persuade her that being truly liberated meant following her own desires, not someone else's. Authentic personal power is always correlated with the freedom to exercise choice.

Of course, there were many potential benefits for women in sexual liberation. But they depended on the woman's willingness to demand sexual pleasure for herself. As a result of sexual liberation, women became far more aware of the need to insist on their own pleasure and could relinquish the view that their primary function was to serve men. This shift meant that a woman was free to demand adequate sexual stimulation, to renounce the idea that the man's orgasm terminated the sexual encounter, and to feel less inclined to fake an orgasm in order to please him.

Another shift in power made possible by sexual liberation was that women became capable of initiating sexual encounters, taking the risk of being refused or being thought too bold. A woman could act as an agent in her own right, rather than serving as the object for a male subject. This was an extremely important change, giving women power not only in the workplace and the home, but also in the realm of the erotic. It means that women no longer value themselves primarily as the object of sexual desire, but are more willing to express themselves as the desiring subject. How dramatic a change this is sometimes becomes apparent when we look at movies from different eras.

Susan Bordo, an academic and writer, observes that you only realize "what's been forbidden when it's finally permitted."[11] For her, the degree to which movies have generally played to the male gaze rather than to the female gaze became clear when she saw *The Bridges of Madison County*. She applauds Clint Eastwood, "who began his career as a 'screw you' action hero and wound up directing and starring in one of the best 'women's movies' of all time." Eastwood tells the story of the lonely housewife and itinerant photographer almost entirely from the heroine's (Meryl Streep's) point of view, "focusing on her desires, conflicts, and anxieties (rather than the hero's, as was the case with the book). [It] made me aware of what I'd been missing. . . . After she's had her bath and dressed—and it's still not clear between them what's going to happen— she places her hand on his shoulder during a phone call. That's all—a hand on a shoulder. But the film has been so finely tuned to her as a sexual subject . . . that the erotic charge of the gesture is almost unbearable. My sister and I, watching the movie, gasped in unison"[12] For Bordo, the film's power comes from its taking the female gaze as its reference point.

Bordo observes that although the 1960s were a time of female liberation, bringing women "the pill, the Beatles, Helen Gurley Brown and Gloria Steinem, they drove the male-body-as-sex-object underground." In the 1950s, movies like A *Streetcar Named Desire* (with Marlon Brando),

Sweet Bird of Youth (with Paul Newman), and *Picnic* (with William Holden) had focused on "female desire in the *plots* of the films" and exploited the plots "to allow the camera to lavish erotic attention on the actors' gorgeous faces and bodies." In the movies of the 1960s and 1970s, women, "liberated" from sexual repression, became the sole focus of the camera's erotic eye, while the " 'beautiful men' virtually disappeared."[13] In these movies, women reverted to their traditional role as objects of desire, while the actions of the men set the plot in motion—and that is the essence of power. Perhaps these movies constituted a kind of wishful thinking on the part of the old order, part of the resistance that is bound to accompany such profound shifts in the power balance between the sexes as had been put into play.

As for what could explain the "gaze" being expressed in those fifties movies Bordo cites, what she doesn't note is that two of them—*Streetcar* and *Sweet Bird of Youth*—are film versions of plays by Tennessee Williams. Is it possible, in part, that the gaze directed at the male as sexual object came to women courtesy of a gay sensibility? My hunch is that it may well be so, and that gay liberation and women's sexual liberation are linked. The cultural importance of *A Streetcar Named Desire* to gays is underlined in the homage Pedro Almodovar pays to Tennessee Williams in his recent film *All About My Mother*.[14]

The musical play *Dirty Blonde*, which depicts a budding romance between two present-day fans of Mae West, explores West's rise to stardom, showing how she was coached by homosexual men to flaunt an exaggerated sexuality. What better way to describe Mae West than as a campy rendition of an old-fashioned male homosexual fantasy, strutting her stuff and intimating an almost limitless appetite for the pleasures of the flesh? Some female impersonators still "do" Mae West. While earlier generations of women were impacted by gays in this incarnation of femininity, subsequent generations of women have responded to a later evolution of the gay male sensibility. One contemporary mode of femininity—as bone-thin if not anorexic, elongated, sometimes dressed in skinny pants suits—was the fantasy creation of a cadre of male homosexual designers, including Yves Saint Laurent. And is it any surprise that some of the scripts for the television series *Sex and the City* are written by gay men? Some of the plotlines, with very few alterations, could be played by gays looking for gays. Gay aesthetics have also permeated male heterosexual styles and culture, in part through Calvin Klein's ads for men's jockey shorts.

The ability to initiate sex and to insist on sexual gratification, and the concomitant ability to act as agent rather than object in realms beyond the erotic, were not the only changes set in motion by sexual liberation. Shame about the female body and its functions—menstruation, pregnancy, childbirth—were diminished, to be replaced by pride. To take one example, consider the change in the way pregnancy is experienced and perceived. When the movie star Demi Moore appeared on the cover of *Vanity Fair* in 1991, voluptuously pregnant, wearing nothing but a green silk/satin peignoir and high heels, she was immediately understood to be proclaiming pride in her pregnant body and declaring that her sexual allure was undiminished. By so doing, she was challenging the longstanding view of sexuality and pregnancy as mutually exclusive—a view that had been shared by men and women alike. The idea that the pregnant female was beautiful caught on instantly, vanquishing the embarrassment many women had felt about being fat, awkward, and ungainly. I was in Rio de Janeiro a month or two after the Moore *Vanity Fair* cover came out and was astonished to see another pregnant naked woman in exactly the same pose on the cover of a glossy Brazilian magazine (surprised not only that the idea of the power of the pregnant belly had traveled so far so quickly, but also at the transferability of new sexual symbols from culture to culture). These iconic images remain a subject for photographers. For example, the *London Sunday Express* ran a photograph of the pregnant singer Melanie Blat singing and dancing onstage, her abdomen not only bared but tattooed.[15] A Pea in the Pod, a line of maternity clothes, showed a sexy, naked pregnant woman in its ads. And in February 2000 the cover of *Vanity Fair* featured a beatific, pregnant Annette Bening with her dreamy-eyed husband, Warren Beatty, on his knees, resting his hands and cheek on her belly. This last example may actually be telling us just as much about revisions in our ideas of masculinity, for here we have a man who, along with Jack Nicholson, was for many years the very emblem of rampant male sexuality (and dominance), but on this cover he was suddenly domesticated and submissive.

At the same time that sexual liberation for women is proceeding, there is a retrograde effort by evolutionary psychologists—"evo-psychos" as the science writer Natalie Angier calls them—to promote theories about the greater vigor of male sexuality. Angier sardonically points to the essential illogic in their argument: "Women are said to have lower sex drives than men do, yet they are universally punished if they display evidence to the contrary. . . . Men have the naturally higher sex drive, yet all the laws, customs, punishments, shame, strictures, mystiques, and anti-mystiques are aimed at full hominid fury at that tepid, sleepy, hypoactive creature the female libido."[16] She observes that if women were fundamentally hyposexual, it would be superfluous for men to go to such lengths to control women's exposure to sexual advances.

Male Sexuality

Some men still view females as receptacles for the purpose of growing babies or sating male desire. It is not easy to give up the myth of phallic omnipotence and supremacy. The image of the "large, powerful, untiring phallus attached to a cool controlled male, long on experience, competent, and knowledgeable enough to make women crazy with desire" has longstanding and very deep roots in our culture.[17]

Some feminists say that this image is infused with hostility, even sadism. Some years ago, Kate Millett, in her book *Sexual Politics*, examined how an all-conquering male sexuality is depicted—and celebrated, to the detriment of those being conquered—in some serious fiction (works of Norman Mailer, Henry Miller, D. H. Lawrence, and Genet).[18] And in *Against Our Will: Men, Women, and Rape*, Susan Brownmiller declared: "Throughout history, no theme grips the masculine imagination with greater constancy and less honor than the myth of the heroic rapist. As man conquered the world, so too he conquers the female. Down through the ages, imperial conquest, exploits of valor and expressions of love have gone hand in hand with violence to women in thought and in deed."[19]

While both Millett and Brownmiller are brilliant analysts of the sociology involved, they fall short of a real understanding of the psychology of male sex and power. The operative word in Brownmiller's analysis of the male stereotype is *imagination*. Any comprehension of male sexuality must also take into account the more or less unconscious fears underlying men's conscious wishful fantasies and their frequent enactment.

Male fantasies cover over, or deny, men's sexual fears, some of which are pervasive. With regard to performance, men worry about getting it up, keeping it up, and satisfying their partners, because there is a fundamental difference in sex: men cannot hide a failure to achieve an erection, whereas there is no certain way to gauge a woman's sexual arousal or orgasm. Thus it is difficult for a man to be sure that he is a good lover.[20]

Some men fear sexual impotence, and this fear can lead to actual impotence. The popularity of Viagra establishes that the idea of the ever-ready male is more myth (or fantasy) than reality. Experiences of sexual inadequacy may be more frequent now, when so much of the traditionally male turf is of necessity being ceded to women.[21]

Even men who are confident about their performance are sometimes so intent on demonstrating their ability to gratify a woman that their own participation lacks spontaneity. Such men may feel comfortable pursuing their own pleasure only after they have brought the woman to orgasm; they may be able to attain full erection only when the woman is sated.

Perhaps the most striking feature of the male's sense of inadequacy is his belief that other men truly possess the macho sexuality he aspires to, making his own endowment and skills appear even more meager. The overestimation of other males' potency may have its deepest roots in the small boy's awe of his father's superior sexual endowment. Many men appear to suffer, too, because of their idealization of the male experience during adolescence, the only time perpetual randiness and readiness appear to be the rule.

To compensate for their sense of genital inferiority, their anxiety about performance, and their fear of women's rejection or infidelity, many men resort to fantasies of power. In these fantasies, through utilizing denial and reversal, the penis emerges as all-powerful, performance as extraordinary, sexual partners as plentiful, and dominance and aggression as reparative themes, reversing what the fantasizer believes to be true. Such fantasies fuel men's project of male dominance and female subordination. The crossover between power and sex in the male psyche was underscored in Michael Lewis's book *Liar's Poker*, in which he reported that the most successful investment bankers were referred to as "big swinging dicks." For lower-income men, macho swagger and macho fantasies compensate for feelings of subordination in the male economic hierarchy.

While men's macho sexual fantasies are in some ways adaptive, insofar as they counteract underlying fears, they can also aggravate an already pervasive sexual anxiety by reinforcing the belief that other men are living the fantasies instead of just imagining them. Unlike many other cultural chroniclers, I believe that anxiety over performance and prowess is much more basic to male sexuality than its reputed aggressive content, because of feelings of weakness and fear of inadequacy that are engendered early in life. Not only is a boy subject to castration anxiety—a result of fear that his father will retaliate for the boy's rivalry—but also, as some French psychoanalytic theorists have suggested, because he may have suffered an even earlier blow to his sexual narcissism due to his inability to win his mother's sexual love.[22] In other words, the boy's fear of his father and the threat of castration are not the only factors in his renunciation of his mother. He also withdraws from his erotic "investment" in his mother because he feels he does not have the genital endowment to compete for her.[23] He senses that his mother rejects him in favor of his father because his penis is too small. Many men never recover from this literal sense of genital inadequacy. It appears that they are therefore destined to suffer lifelong penis envy. Indeed, a boy more often than a girl suffers from penis envy.[24]

As a consequence, many aspects of men's sexual insecurity involve body image. The same body hatred that so often afflicts women can be seen to afflict men as well and is reflected in the varieties of body modification that men are increasingly seeking. The number of men engaged in bodybuilding has increased dramatically. Some men also take steroids, to increase their musculature and strength or simply to look like muscle men.

In *Maxim* magazine, Richard Farmer told the writer Rebecca Gooch about his own attempt to remake his body: "As a kid I always had this image of myself as being small. Although I was never puny, at five feet nine inches I felt short compared to my father and brothers, who were all over six feet. On top of that, being the youngest of four, I always felt I had to do that much more to get noticed.

Even at fourteen years old, I knew that the more powerful you were, the more recognition you got. I figured that although I might be shorter, I didn't have to be smaller, so I started Olympic weight lifting at the gym for a couple of hours after school four times a week. . . . After awhile I even found that I enjoyed that lingering soreness in my developing muscles the day after a heavy workout. I knew that meant I was breaking down muscles and forcing them to grow. I was getting stronger every day."

He soon realized that the men whose bodies he most admired had an open secret. They were "on the juice," a code name for steroids. And so he too went on the white tablets. Whereas Farmer had once been disgusted when he looked at pictures of bodybuilders like Arnold Schwarzenegger, he gradually began to admire the muscle men. Within weeks his arms, which had been "stuck" at 14.5 inches, had grown to 17.5 inches in circumference: "Those muscles felt totally different from normal muscle because they were constantly engorged or loaded with blood. They didn't give when you squeezed them, they were iron-arm hard and laced with veins. I thought I looked awesome. And like the model with outrageously oversized silicone tits, I didn't care whether it was synthetic or not. I just loved turning heads. . . . After a while, you couldn't not notice me!"

When Farmer took a break from steroids, as he was advised to do, he felt himself "deflating like a burst balloon." So he decided to skip the breaks. Although obsessed, he rationalized that he was dedicated. He graduated to bodybuilding contests: "The competitors would spend every offstage moment eyeing each other like bitchy fashion models. I'd starve and dehydrate myself to help define my muscles. Other guys resorted to laxatives. I once saw three guys share a suppository just minutes before a competition."

But the warnings to take breaks turned out to be valid. His muscles started to detach from the bone, and his ligaments were stretched as thin as cobwebs. One day as he was walking up the stairs, his leg gave way and his kneecap shattered. At age thirty, he was desperately ill. He had a fever, spent twelve weeks in the hospital with gallons of pus being drained from his leg, and developed necrosis: "I'd been trying to turn myself into a musclebound freak but ended up looking like a monster." Finally healed, he put himself back together and found himself through a Chinese system of meditative exercises called T'ai Chi Chuan. Five of his bodybuilding buddies are now dead.[25]

In the same issue of *Maxim*, a man calling himself "Preacher" sent a letter to the editor describing a "medical breakthrough": "Now, about this penile enlargement surgery crap. I'm a biker—tattoo, bunch of broken bones, all that. When I was a young buck hanging around the Bay Area and working an AFL-CIO job, I was introduced to a technique by a patch holder in a Bay Area club that I want to share with you. You take a padlock that weighs approx. six to eight ounces, put a fat rubber band on its shackle (the part that opens and closes), and wear it on your schlong. . . . You do it about 15 to 20 hours a week and you do this for a *couple of years*. I know other bikers who have told their sons about this when they hit puberty, and I sure as hell woulda liked to have been told about this by my father when I was that age. It can move your dick from being six and a half to about nine inches. Anyone, and probably at any age, can do this. It does require some perseverance . . . but then so does anything worthwhile."[26]

Many men feel that their penis is inadequate in either length or girth. This is a concern that appears even more widespread than women's doubts about the size of their breast. (It may more closely approximate women's concerns about gaining weight.) Both heterosexuals and homosexuals agonize not just over physical endowment but over their performance as well. There is one significant difference: heterosexuals feel much more threatened by the appearance of another man's erect penis—probably because of a fear that sexual innuendo is involved. And just as women are now having breast-enlargement surgery and liposuction to counteract their anxieties, some men are opting for penile enlargement, an increasingly booming business. Dr. Gary Rheinschild, a specialist in penis enlargement, reported that he performed more than 3,500 penile enlargements in a single year. His stated ambition is to make penis enlargement "as common as breast implants."[27]

Women's sexuality, long viewed as passive and submissive, is now recognized as powerful in its own right, while male sexuality, so often considered invincible, is now seen to have its vulnerabilities. Yet cultural stereotypes do not disappear overnight and many men, as well as women, still enact them in fantasy, if not in reality.

In the English play *Closer*, Patrick Marber's four-character drama, one of the two men, Larry, speaking to one of the two women, is explicit about men's use of fantasy: "You give us imagery and we do with it what we will." This emphasis on imagery is meant to imply that the reality of the woman herself is not essential to male desire and may even be a detriment to it. *Closer* was reviewed as "the latest in a series of anti-romantic comedies from England about the joylessness of sex . . . which has also become a commonplace in hip America."[28] The same negative view of sex is found in movies like *In the Company of Men*, *Happiness*, and *Friends and Lovers*.

Perfect sexual communion may be an ideal beyond the reach of most of us. Liberated, carefree sex—the promise of sexual liberation—has not been achieved for either sex, in part because sex envokes so many primal battles in the struggle to achieve autonomy. Given that sexuality first develops in the relatively dependent, helpless child, it is unlikely that sex can ever be completely free of connotations of submission and dominance. At the same time, it is certainly possible that being female will not invariably have connotations of submissiveness. In other words, the limitations to sexual liberation—meaning liberation from power as a contaminant—reside not in the biological nature of sexuality, nor exclusively in cultural and political arrangements, and certainly not in the gender difference, but in the universal condition of infantile dependence. It may be that the consequences of dependence, a lingering sense of powerlessness, and the need to overcome it through the enactment of one or another kind of power form the substance of tragedy; this thought, of course, echoes Freud's pessimistic assessment of the human condition.

Gender and Power

Freud's theory of gender, that man is born but woman is made—the theory that whereas masculinity is natural to boys, femininity is a result of the little girl's retreat from assertiveness when she discovers that she is castrated—has proved untenable because we now understand that it is inaccurate to view gender attributes as natural in boys but compensatory in girls. Boys and girls begin to diverge in behavior, mannerisms, and interests as early as twelve to eighteen months, long before they discover the differences in their bodies. Working with intersexed children, the sex researcher John Money and his colleagues at Johns Hopkins found that the first, crucial step in children's gender differentiation, in viewing themselves as either masculine or feminine, is their self-designation as male or female, which generally but not always develops in correspondence with the child's biological sex, and the corollary labeling of the child as male or female.[29] Differences in gender role result from many diverse antecedents—biological differences, power relations, scripting, socialization, the sex-discrepant expectations that shape fantasies and cultural myths, as well as genital awareness and Oedipal dramas as described in classical psychoanalytic theory.

This is by no means a full account of the complexities of gender. Relatively recent investigations have found that gender identity is not just dichotomous, either masculine or feminine. Like biological sex, and like the sexual impulse, gender has many different configurations, mandating that we address the different varieties of masculinity and femininity, leading some to refer to a multiplicity of masculinities and femininities.[30]

We also now know that aspects of gender role can be modified as a result of cultural changes. As mores change and the repressive barrier shifts, different behaviors become acceptable.

Female Gender

Why did women agree for so long to be the Other, to give up their agency in order to accommodate the male will? As in any other area, the sharing of power depends on a dialogue between self-assertion and recognition of the other's sovereignty. Some theorists argue that women raise their daughters to receive approval for submission; if the girl asserts her will, approval is withheld. To the degree that the girl acquiesces, her striving for autonomy is disavowed or split off. The primary way she then experiences agency is at one remove, through identification with a powerful man on whom she comes to depend not only sexually but psychologically.

While this scenario may accurately reflect some mother-daughter interactions, it is one that is embedded in a social system that assumes men are de facto the possessors of power. In fact, female passivity, submissiveness, and compliance, sexual or relational, began to recede as the women's movement gained momentum—and this shift has occurred despite the fact that child rearing arrangements have remained much the same. The source of female submissiveness, it turns out, is not the mother but male hegemony, conveyed to us from infancy on by what John Kenneth Galbraith calls conditioned power, belief systems that I have described elsewhere as a shared cultural unconscious.[31] The fact that male power and female submission are part of our social fabric has done more than the mother-daughter bond to undermine female agency. The incentive for female compliance has been that submissive girls might find it easier to get married than self-assertive, uppity women.

Nonetheless, gender liberation, like sexual liberation, has a long prehistory, reaching back to the birth of romantic love. If, as Stendahl posited, romantic love depends on an idealization of the love object, women had become objects of admiration by the time of the appearance of the courts of love during the Middle Ages. And, in part, it was the freedom to exercise choice in their own marital destiny that set women on the road to authentic empowerment.

However, liberation as a conscious pursuit and political enterprise is the fruit of the labors of women like Mary Wollstonecraft in England,

Elizabeth Cady Stanton and Susan B. Anthony in America, and Simone de Beauvoir in France, among others. All these women had been politicized through participation in earlier causes. As the critic Vivian Gornick observed, each had been "an ardent partisan of a powerful social movement" (the Enlightenment, the Anti-Slavery Movement, and Existentialism, respectively) before they became feminists. Each of them, "living a heightened life inside the visionary politics that had sparked her intellectual being, came, in turn, to see that she was 'only a woman.' "[32]

Perhaps only after these women had grasped that the powerlessness of some other group—black slaves, for example—resulted not from the inherent limitations of the slaves themselves but from the needs of the slaveholders, could they turn their attention to the strictures in their own lives that rendered them powerless. The contribution each then made to feminist understanding turned, appropriately enough, on an application of a central insight of the movement to which she was devoted. Wollstonecraft, from the perspective of the Enlightenment, passionately urged that women become rational beings; Stanton and Anthony, with their experience of the Anti-Slavery Movement, urged that every woman exercise governance over her own inviolate self; Beauvoir, as a proponent of Existentialism, urged that women cease to be the Other.[33] Only then did it become possible for them to discern that men's dominance of women was cultural, not natural (that is, not hardwired). But they also realized that, unlike slaves, who were compelled to submit, the compliance of women had been obtained through collaboration.[34] Women had been conditioned to see their nature as inferior (this is an example of conditioned powerlessness), and only when they recognized their own role in their subordination did change became possible.

Consciousness-raising is necessary but not sufficient for the fomenting of revolutionary changes. The 1963 publication of Betty Friedan's *The Feminine Mystique* in the United States raised consciousness but did not launch the women's movement.[35] As the sociologist Cynthia Epstein observes, ideas do not generally trigger social change until they become grounded in a political movement. Thus *The Feminine Mystique* resulted in "cultural awareness, not a call to arms." That call came three years later in the form of the National Organization of Women (NOW). As Epstein notes, the idea of NOW originated not with Betty Friedan but with a black woman lawyer, Pauli Murray, who "proposed that they form an 'NAACP for women,' " Murray urging that they invoke the model of the civil rights movement in the women's movement.[36] Only an organization based on a revolutionary insight can muster the power necessary to over-turn entrenched models of conditioned power.

Of course, even before Betty Friedan and before NOW, women sensed their lack of personal power, but were not able to get beyond the provident "by nature" argument. Nonetheless, in movies made before the woman's movement, one can identify women's wish for empowerment. The film critic Molly Haskell says that she personally cherished "the heroic or contrary images of women that went against the grain of oppression—either slipping cunningly through the cracks of a patriarchal world order or defying it outright. As glorious monsters, Muses, femmes fatales, worker bees, queen bees, sweet and sour dames, movies were full of women in convention-stretching roles."[37] The fantasy life of the disenfranchised resonates with such subtle intimations of power. We use movies and other fictional forms to access heretofore buried desires. In many cases, works of art not only reflect and disseminate change but help to initiate it.

And that change has been very profound over the past thirty years. The morphing of the female gender role is obvious in the following scene, which I observed at 7 P.M. on a Saturday night: A young woman walking down the street in front of me is talking on a cell phone. "Where am I?" I hear her say. "Here I am at Seventy-Second Street, just coming up on Columbus, and I was just thinking I'm free tonight and I was wondering if you guys might have any plans." For this woman, somewhere in her middle twenties, to have the freedom to try to get something going at the last minute on a Saturday night is a great advance from thirty or forty years ago. Back then, a woman would have been embarrassed not to have a proper date—one for which she would have been invited at least a week in advance—and she would be concealing, not revealing, that fact.

But to whom was the woman on the phone talking? Did the phrase "you guys" refer to guys literally, or to some combination of men and women, or even to women alone? It could be any of the above, for "you guys" has become generic; it does not identify the sex of those it addresses. But it *is* a designation that implies power. Consider how unlikely it would be that someone talking to a group of men or a mixed group would ever refer to them as "you gals." In essence, it's still a compliment for a gal to be a guy—she thus moves from a lower-status to a higher-status group—while it would be an insult to call a guy a gal. A friend of mine, a Spanish translator, makes a similar observation about gender designations in Spanish. She notes that the question "Hombre, qué pasa?" tends in conversation to lose any connotation of gender.[38] As Haskell writes, "we are all, in some measure, more comfortable with maleness than with femaleness."[39] For what other reason might this be than the fact that power still accrues to maleness?

Conversely, what of the denomination *girl*? Generally, to call a woman a girl is a put-down.[40] In the 1970s feminists expended a great deal of energy on deleting that word from the language. (Remember Gary Trudeau's cartoon celebrating the birth of a baby woman?) But just as the word *nigger* is horrendous if used by whites while sometimes acceptable if spoken by blacks to blacks (because they have co-opted it to denote strength), girl is becoming acceptable and even rebellious if used by females. At a conference in Lima, Peru, a group of us went to a museum that had dual collections of Aztec gold and weapons. One of my most ardently feminist friends exclaimed, "A *girl* museum and a *boy* museum!" "You go, girl" is the new rallying cry as some younger women, self-identified as feminists, have begun to redefine the meaning of *girl*, to attach to it both a woman's strength and her frivolity. Thus the Spice Girls used their mantra "girl power" as a slogan for uppity femininity.[41] The idea is that the liberated female need not shape her image according to male models of power but can create her own model, which can, if she likes, embrace the fun and zaniness of being a girl. As one observer commented, "It's [not] a diminishing of one's power but a whole source of power."[42] In a postliberation world, opposites coexist, so that a woman can be professional and sexy, serious and silly.

But the new assertion of "girl power" does not effectively challenge the everyday language and behavioral biases that give priority to males. We may still introduce married couples as Mr. and Mrs. I've never seen an envelope addressed to "Mrs. and Mr." Most women still take their husband's name and even if they don't, it is the husband's name that is almost always passed on to the children. No matter who owns a car, driving it is still generally considered a male prerogative. This is an obvious expression of male status, given that driving a car makes most of us feel in control (think of the expression "in the driver's seat"). Such practices show how strongly hierarchical our culture remains and how we are conditioned to accept that hierarchy through our lifelong immersion in symbols that confirm the priority and strength of maleness and the corresponding weakness of femaleness.

Paradoxically, although women's emancipation may have begun with romantic love, the current female gender role stuckedness has a lot to do with the high social valuation placed on marriage for women. In an article in the *New York Times*, Felicia R. Lee reported that "conversations with more than a dozen single women in their twenties, thirties and forties" revealed that although most of them had successful careers, they still "admitted to a nagging little voice inside their heads that says they want a man to take care of them." In her view, "The princess of the city seeks a millionaire and the rich nerd wants a Barbie Doll with an adoring gaze, interior package optional."[43]

The bias toward males as being more powerful (possessors of higher status, purveyors of greater knowledge) is incorporated into our psyche very early in life. For example, one book reviewer suggested that while the Harry Potter novels appeal to both boys and girls, boys would have been less likely to read the series if the main character were a girl. Another noted that the author used only the initials J. K. along with her surname, Rowling, because there was some fear on the part of her publisher that if the author was known to be female, the book would be less likely to be read by boys.

The female concept of what constitutes appropriate female gender roles, then, has definitely expanded over the years; but it remains almost unchanged in terms of men's and women's biases regarding what constitutes the most desirable attributes in the mating game.

Male Gender

Until very recently, culture critics wrote more about changes in the female than the male gender role, apparently holding to the notion that masculinity was essentially ahistorical (a parallel with Freud's dictum that man is born, woman made). Nonetheless, over the past fifty years, a shift has occurred in the images of masculinity we most admire. The writer Neal Gabler uses movie heroes to make this point, drawing a distinction between midcentury heroes like the characters John Wayne played and the James Bond man. Gabler points out that Bond "emerged at almost exactly the same time as Hugh Hefner's *Playboy* magazine, which celebrated a hedonistic lifestyle very much like Bond's."[44] Unlike Wayne, Bond won praise not just for his victories over his foes but also for his ease in conquering women. This style of conquering women was imitated by any number of celebrities, particularly Hollywood stars, who flaunted their promiscuity and potency. Some eventually repented and converted—for example, Warren Beatty apparently underwent a metamorphosis in his fifties, after Madonna, with whom he was briefly partnered, made him look awkward if not foolish on one of her videos. But the stereotype of the swashbuckling, conquering male still prevails in celebrity culture.

Bond also exhibited what some would consider a feminine interest in appearance and style that would have been foreign to Wayne. As Gabler says, "operating in the postwar *Playboy* ethos, Bond didn't need to divide his true masculine self from his urbane exterior. He was sophisticated and feral, soft and hard, smooth and rough, modern and traditional, intimate and bold, the consumer and the producer all at the same time." Bond seemed to mediate comfortably between these two warring halves of contemporary manhood, enabling male viewers in the 1960s and 1970s "to identify with him in ways that they were increasingly unable to identify with more conventional, basically anti-hedonistic heroic types like the Wayne image."

The hedonism and the consumerism, emphasizing male beautification, that Gabler described have come to haunt men in the same way that the female equivalent haunts women, and have resulted in what some cultural analysts consider a decline in male self-regard. It is here that I see a crossover from the male homosexual world, a world that has influenced all our views of style and chic—not too surprisingly when we think of the important male homosexuals in fashion, hairdressing, and interior design. Then, too, it has become increasingly apparent that many gay men spend a lot of time and effort—at the gym and elsewhere—to maintain an attractive appearance. Not just the idea that thin is healthier but also the ideal of a taut body, already part of movie culture, swept the corridors of male power and has spread to a large segment of male heterosexual culture. Just compare photographs of our current crop of power brokers with those of an earlier generation. And let's be fair—the current crop look better.

This shift toward male beautification also reflects a shift in power. Women, who now have more power, often insist that their men shape up.

In *Stiffed*, Susan Faludi proposes that men, like women, are increasingly caught up in an "ornamental culture," by which she means that men are becoming more like women, not the other way around. In her view, men are also becoming disempowered. Men have "become soft: the modern man is more obsessed with his image than his job, which changes too frequently to be a firm basis of identity, and demeans its holder to boot."[45]

I've already suggested that gay men influenced Mae West's style, and she in turn contributed to the vogue of the blond bombshell. Gays are still setting the pace for ideals of beauty and sexuality for women, and also for heterosexual men. We now see men seeking some luxuries, in response to women and gays. And it should not be forgotten that lesbians were among the first to join the workforce at the turn of the twentieth century, though they were not identified as such. All the mutual influences and borrowings between male and female, straight and gay, have yet to be explored.

Each of us is willy-nilly forced into a dialectic of power. This is true in our early psychological development, as our will begins to emerge, counter to that of our parents; and it is equally true in our psychosexual development, as we negotiate the power struggles endemic to sexual development. We each develop a psychological profile somewhere on a power continuum, and gender is certainly a major influence on where we locate ourselves on that continuum. But our identification with either the weak or the strong is formed not just by our psychic history but by the social, cultural, and economic realities of our time.[46] No doubt the various psychological theories of the way women come to feel a loss of agency through early interpersonal relations and sexual development are to some degree pertinent. But these theories fail to address the way primary issues of power and hegemony, mediated through cultural beliefs about the natural order of things, affect our psychological and communal lives.

A truly credible theory of gender must go beyond Freud's emphasis on nature, nurture, and interpersonal relations, beyond his "ahistorical theory of man and society," to give full due to the world in which we live and its impact on our ideas about masculinity and femininity, male sexuality and female sexuality. We must also pay attention to the impact on one another of men and women, gays and straights. We tend to copy what we admire and envy.

It is not possible to theorize about female sexuality and femininity or male sexuality and masculinity on the basis of genital differences and early development alone, without considering power and hierarchy. A theory of power must examine not just how power is exercised but also how it envokes resistance among the disempowered. Were it otherwise, as suggested earlier, power could be extended indefinitely; we would all be subject to the most dominant. At first, the powerless attempt to prevent any exercise of power directed against them—or if not to prevent it, to resist submitting to it. Ultimately the powerless resist power through the articulation of a counterposition: it is just such a shift in the dialectic of power as regards men and women that we are currently observing. We should not be so reductionist as the evolutionary psychologists who invoke our genes as both an explanation of our behavior and a justification for a return to a recently overthrown status quo.

Our lingering gender stereotypes and accompanying value judgments—the positively sanctioned buccaneer businessman, the negatively sanctioned boldly professional woman—may be the last gasp of the old order, a final cultural outburst of nostalgia and backlash. Perhaps we shall soon see our culture as ready for a new order. But whatever the verdict, and despite our sometimes retrograde judgments of what is suitable for male and female behavior, the ongoing cultural revolutions offer clear evidence that attributions of power are subject to radical change. Even if the unconscious is timeless (as it may or may not be), our patterns of expressing sex and gender have changed as a result of gay liberation, feminism, the political pressures of various sexual minorities, the Pill, the separation of sex from procreation, and the work of sex researchers and psychoanalysts. With such further social and scientific changes as will undoubtedly take place, we should expect that the shaping and expression of our drives—which are in fact the fundamental *matériel* of the Freudian unconscious—may surface in ever new incarnations. Although unconscious impulses and wishes may sometimes emerge and swamp conscious ones, they in turn bear the imprint of the preconscious and conscious attitudes and beliefs that permeate an ever-changing *Zeitgeist*. The traffic between culture and psyche is always two-way, if not round-trip.

7

Sadomasochism: Interpersonal Power Corrupted by Aggression

*"To lie at the feet of an imperious mistress,
to obey her commands, to ask her forgiveness—this was for me
a sweet enjoyment."*

JEAN-JACQUES ROUSSEAU, *Confessions*

Thus far, I have given little attention to how aggression can contaminate power. Unlike assertion, aggression encompasses hostility and is accompanied by some transgression against its target. Aggression can sometimes be morally justified—for example, in war, though even in war there are limits to how far it can go before it becomes an outrage or a war crime.

Aggression is a component of power struggles and various abuses of power. It can also infect ongoing relationships, converting a dominant-submissive relationship into a sadomasochistic one. Sadomasochism is complicated because it can be embedded in separate but often overlapping spheres, the sexual and the relational. In a sexual situation, aggression in the form of controlled sadism or masochism can be experienced as pleasurable, but this is far less true of relational sadomasochism, particularly, say, for the wives of batterers.

In keeping with general psychiatric and psychoanalytic usage, I refer to *sadomasochism*, instead of *sadism* and *masochism*, to make the point that the purest sadism is generally laced with masochism and masochism with sadism. Sometimes, the same person may be masochistic in one relationship and sadistic in another. Consider Carl, a successful fortyish businessman, who splits his emotional life between a wife whom he oppresses and his secretary, Gloria, by whom he is enthralled and whom he placates moment to moment. When Gloria tells him that she is involved with a younger man—and one who works in a position subservient to her—Carl suffers, but his desire for her explodes. Whenever she is out of his sight, he begins to obsess about whether or not she is at that very moment sleeping with the other man. Carl has a dominant position in the business world, but in his psychic world he is under the spell of Gloria. In the deepest recesses of his mind, he appears to be reliving (and trying to revise) a relationship with his mother, in which her largely rejecting behavior toward him was punctuated with moments of intense intimacy structured around their conspiratorial alliance against his tyrannical father. While part of Carl plotted with his mother against his father, he also raged against her in his heart for what he believed was her lack of consistent love for him. This split in his feelings for his mother is relived in his two intimate relationships. He now wants to dominate and humiliate his wife just as he felt his mother dominated and humiliated him, while his subordination to Gloria echoes his abject longing for his mother's love, which he received only in brief moments.

At one end of the sadomasochist spectrum, sadism is not restricted to personal relationships but may take the form of rape or murder of a stranger, while, at the other end, masochism may disconnect from any personal relationship and degenerate into a variety of self-destructive behaviors. But my main focus here is on the way sadomasochism infects intimate relationships.

Let me begin by describing sadomasochism in the sexual realm, because it was there that the definitions of sadism and masochism originated. The sexologist Richard von Krafft-Ebing christened the erotic wish to inflict pain as *sadism*, adapting the term from the name of the Marquis de Sade, whose works are centered on what we now call sadomasochism. The word *masochism* is derived from the name of Leopold von Sacher-Masoch, whose novels, particularly *Venus in Furs*, provided brilliant descriptions of masochistic yearning.

Because sadism and masochism were first identified in sexual terms, it has become conventional to think of them as a source of pleasure. The sadist is said to derive sexual pleasure from inflicting pain, the masochist from receiving it. (Hence the well-worn joke: Masochist—"Beat me, beat me!" Sadist—"No.") But this is oversimplified. In enacted sexual fantasies, sadistic and masochistic pleasure can be obtained without actual pain. For example, merely playing the role of the humiliated or the humiliator may suffice. The basic pleasure of orgasmic release may sometimes be the farthest thing from the conscious mind of either participant. Still, it is useful to bear in mind that some people are very strongly motivated toward sadomasochistic sexual fantasies and enactments and seek them out again and again.

Over the past several decades, sadistic and masochistic fantasies and perhaps their enactments as well have been mainstreamed. Such fantasies and enactments may or may not be more common today than they once were, but they do seem to be more prevalent, more often portrayed in fiction and more openly discussed. This cultural trend extends to heterosexuals as well as gays and lesbians, but it first received public prominence in the open establishment in the 1970s of gay S&M leather bars. And nowhere were such establishments wider open than in San Francisco's South Market District, which according to writer Frank Browning "housed the world's largest collection of leather bars and S&M clubs."[1] As AIDS researchers began to explore the various expressions of homosexual activities, "they were stunned by matter-of-fact accounts of men whose nipples were attached to chains and stretched, whose testicles were twisted in leather thongs, whose mouths were gorged on the penis of one unknown man while another would plunge his fist and forearm so deeply into their bowels that he could feel on his fingers the contractions of the heart."[2] Of course, many of the S & M enactments that took place with such abandon in the 1970s drastically declined with the advent of AIDS in the gay population.

But sadomasochistic enactments are hardly the province of gays only. Browning tells of a CBS reporter who discovered while interviewing the owner of an S&M shop about gay sadomasochism that ninety percent of his clientele was heterosexual. The differences between straights and gays may have more to do with how public the practices are than in how prevalent they are. Organized groups of S&M heterosexuals and of lesbians have emerged over the past two decades. In the 1980s, the emergence of S&M lesbian groups led to an odd confrontation within feminism; S&M lesbian groups claiming that S&M sex was liberating came into open political conflict with the organized feminist stand against S&M pornography.[3]

While there are wide cultural swings during different eras in the degree to which sexual acts are suppressed or allowed expression, cultural critics have yet to explain the cultural background for the escalating public enactment of sadomasochistic sex. But we do not have to go far to find the historical origin of contemporary sadomasochist iconography. In her essay "Fascinating Fascism," written in 1974, Susan Sontag called attention to the way the insignia of fascism—leather, Nazi helmets, steel spike collars, caps, chains—had been recruited to sadomasochistic sexuality. Fascism was a radical, ultimately malevolent attempt to reconfigure power in the real world. Paradoxically, sadomasochists in the West have recruited its historical legacy to provide the shards with which to construct their dress-up fantasies in its own new key. Sontag notes that while "Sade had to make up his theater of punishment from scratch, improvising the decor and costumes and blasphemous rites [now] there is a master scenario available to everyone. The color is black, the material is leather, the seduction is beauty, the justification is honesty, the aim is ecstasy, the fantasy is death."[4] These props are utilized not only by S&M gays, but are also the regalia of choice of many bikers.

This S&M iconography made its way into the general culture in the 1970s principally by incorporating the conventions of hardcore pornography into high fashion, that featured black leather, studs, and dominatrix spike-heeled shoes and fashion photographs that suggested sadomasochistic activities. Shiny black leather has become ever more prominent as the costume of choice, as important as denim was to an earlier generation.

Closely related to this sadomasochistic strain in our current society is the "body modification" movement, which includes not only the now rampant tattooing and piercing crazes but also corsetry, branding, and scarring by knives. Body piercing first appeared in the gay community, but was then picked up by punk-rockers in New York and San Francisco, and was mainstreamed when it was adopted by major fashion models. Tattooing, on the other hand, has always been associated with the biker crowd. While some young practitioners may be merely conforming to a current fashion or trying to appear hip or "bad," the symbolism of body modifications is not lost on most of them. The imagery of body piercing symbolizes sexual slavery and sometimes gives a specifically masochistic pleasure all by itself. When one of my friends, a professor of psychology, asked a graduate student why she wore a lip ring, she responded without hesitation, "for the pleasure."

Many works of popular culture now invoke sadomasochism as a central theme rather than as a subsidiary one. In 1969, when Luis Buñuel's film *Belle de Jour* was released, it was considered shocking. (Interestingly, this film made a connection between childhood sexual abuse and masochism long before psychologists or psychoanalysts did.) While *Belle de Jour* still retains its brilliant cinematic qualities, its shock value is gone— any number of films and novels explicitly depict sadomasochistic sex and relationships. They include movies such as *Blue Velvet; Basic Instinct; The Cook, the Thief, His Mistress, and Her Lover,* the documentary *Crumb,* and novels such as A. M. Homes's *The End of Alice* and Susanna Moore's *In the Cut.*

Psychoanalysts have long observed that contemporary events, novels, and movies can give people access to their own suppressed fantasies and desires. If we harbor preconscious sadomasochistic fantasies and impulses—and nearly all of us do to some extent—our culture currently provides an abundance of imagery and content that can bring these fantasies to consciousness.[5] Many of us who are not active practitioners may be drawn to the S & M scene as voyeurs or fellow-travelers.

The increasing openness of S&M is connected, chronologically and politically, with a wave of liberation movements, including gay rights and the women's movement. (The civil rights movement was staid by comparison. Indeed, by making the image of the black slave unacceptable as a sexual icon, it removed one object of sadomasochistic fantasizing that had a long history.) The conservative columnist John Leo suggests that body modification represents a repudiation of Western norms and values.[6] He believes that the new "primitivism" is connected to a growing dissatisfaction with, and anger about, the impact of technology on the environment and a decay of communal values in public and private life. While plausible, such hypotheses are difficult to prove. But it may be that an erosion in family cohesiveness and community is making people increasingly anxious, frustrated, and even enraged. Some may seek to release their disturbing emotions through sadomasochistic fantasies or enactments—which are methods of taming isolation and of controlling their own angry impulses and the fear of aggression directed toward them. These fantasies may also become a way of communicating with one another—and they now have an outlet on the Internet.

Many gifted fantasizers intuitively understand that fantasy serves a psychological function. This is what Dominique Aury (pen name Pauline

Réage), the author of *Story of O*, is telling us when she writes about the fantasy life to which she retreated in her mind, before she actually wrote it out for the man she loved (and ultimately for the world): "I no doubt accepted my life with such patience . . . only because I was so certain of being able to find whenever I wanted that other, obscure life that is life's consolation, that other life unacknowledged and unshared."[7] She says of a series of sadomasochistic fantasies that were so violent they horrified many people: "All I know is that they were beneficent and protected me mysteriously." This is generally true; whatever form a fantasy takes, its intended effect, for the fantasizer, is "beneficent and protective."

Story of O, one of the most frankly and astonishingly sexual books of the century, served still another purpose. Aury first set it down in writing so that her lover could share it. Her strategy was to revive a waning love affair, to keep her lover's interest in her alive. As "Aury" explained to the writer John De St. Jorre: "What could I do? I couldn't paint, I couldn't write poetry. What could I do to make him sit up?" Her solution to this age-old dilemma has a touch of Scheherazade. As St. Jorre explains: "Because she knew he [her lover Paulhan] was an admirer of the Marquis de Sade and had written a learned introduction to his works, she began to draw upon her own sexual fantasies, which, she said, had begun during her lonely adolescence. The conjuncture of Paulhan's taste and her fantasies gave her the idea of writing something."[8]

Her seduction strategy worked on two levels. Paulhan encouraged her to publish *Story of O*, which was an enduring, international sensation, and he continued his affair with her until her death.

Masochistic fantasies and enactments are described by some of our most creative writers. Daphne Merkin touches on her fantasy life in "Dreaming of Hitler: A Memoir of Self-Hatred." She writes that during her adolescence her intermittent dreams about Hitler took place in a green glen:

> In the dreams I stood at the end of a long field of grass, and from the other end a man walks toward me. The man was dressed in a khaki uniform and tall, glossy black boots; his eyes were a piercing light-blue with tiny pupils and he sported a perky, abridged mustache. The man coming toward me could have been anyone, a father or a boyfriend, but he was recognizably none other than Adolf Hitler. Adolf Hitler was smiling at me![9]

Like a proper Queen Esther dream in which Esther saves the Jewish people through her seduction of Haman, Merkin convinces Hitler that he does not hate the Jews. But while she dreamed of Hitler paying attention to her, in her waking life her "father is permanently out of reach, a figure who mostly frightened me, a German Jew whom I would distrust, who was given to ear-splitting displays of temper. . . . Around my father I feel the helplessness of appeal; the attack dogs of his derisive impatience are barking inside me, straining at the leash, ready to jump if I make the wrong move."

Perceptive in her self-understanding, Merkin reports that her "grandiose fantasy of redeeming the man in the mustache and boots" has diminished, but she misses the wondrous sense of accomplishment it brought: "There I was, the same girl who feared her own father, reversing the tide of history, demonstrating powers of understanding and persuasion that were unguessed at in my observable existence."

Perhaps not surprisingly this same author has also written an essay entitled "Spanking: A Romance," in which she reveals that her fantasy preoccupation with S&M started early.[10] She searched in literature to find others who, like her, expended "a lot of energy in keeping his or her passion a secret," and she set up a mental category of famous people who were drawn to masochistic practices. Only in her mid-twenties did she find an "appropriate" partner, a man who had mastered some advanced sadistic skills (psychological rather than physical): "His wish to control me—to offer and then withdraw affection on an erratic and hurtful schedule of his own devising—coincided with my secret wish to be mastered, but it never occurred to him to spank me and I never asked." Some of his demands nonetheless allowed her to feel degraded; she experienced them as thrilling.

Only in her late twenties did she finally convey her wish to be spanked to another man, someone from a different world and therefore someone to whom she considered it safe to communicate her desire. In the beginning, she says, "the reality of spanking . . . was as good as the dream." She married this man, even though she already had complaints about him, including the spankings—they were either too hard or not hard enough. She says in an aside that she suspects that she wanted "to be spanked to death—transported out of sorrow into a state of numbness, of permanent unfeeling." This may be related to her intermittent depression, which she describes in another essay.[11]

But let us not lose track of the presumed beneficence, the essential safety of the sadomasochistic fantasy. The S&M practitioners Gloria Brame, William Brame, and Jon Jacobs argue in their book *Different Loving* that safety is essential in S&M encounters. Unlike the Marquis de Sade, who believed that the ultimate philosophical liberty was the freedom to violate and destroy, they contend that sadomasochism as practiced by consenting adults "largely abides by the credo 'Safe, Sane, and Consensual.'"[12] They argue that Sade is the wrong author to represent sadism, and that Leopold von Sacher-Masoch, Pauline Réage, and even Anne Rice (whom they view primarily as a writer of sadomasochistic erotica) fail to serve as appropriate models "for real relationships." Defending their version of sadomasochism, they insist that "most pornography dealing with bondage and sadomasochism depicts severely dehumanized portraits that are as irrelevant to the actual practice of D&S (dominance and submission) as a sleazy porno movie is to romantic love. The masturbatory spectacle is all. The emotional content nonexistent."[13]

By training and temperament, I consider even "safe, sane, and consensual" sadomasochistic sexual encounters potentially maleficent. That said, the authors of *Different Loving* provide testimony to the way sadomasochistic sexual relationships act to parse power. They offer shrewd insights into how we can use sexual scenarios to express (and contain) a variety of our power needs. It is the gratification of these power needs in joint or enacted fantasy that the authors claim constitutes "a fundamental form of erotic excitement, shared by equals, and often an intellectually enlightening experience:"[14]

> *My soul yearns to be able to let somebody else take control, to be able to not have to make the decisions, to not be concerned about what errors I'm going to make. . . . I think some of this goes back to twelve years of Catholic school: It's dirty to have sex. The Virgin Mary was the mother of Christ and she is the one we're supposed to look up to. [Having been] taught that sex is bad, I've wondered if perhaps the only way I can enjoy it is if I'm completely tied down and helpless. Because, if I'm helpless, I can't stop the person from doing that terrible sexual thing to me; I can't help it if I came, because I'm tied down and he made me come. (Slave V)[15]*

> *Submission is an alternate way of dealing with power, a way of exploring the nature of your own power, how to access it and turning*

it over or not. Choice *is the key. S/M is a tool for surrender. . . . You know, the more power you give away, the more power you must have! You can't give away what you don't have.* (M. Cbele)[16]

The authors say that in the culture of D&S, the sexual submissive is usually someone who exerts power in real life: "Which comes first is unknown: the submissive impulse, which may lead one to overcompensate in adulthood by pursuing high-powered careers, or stressful careers, which lead individuals to seek an outlet in submission. The archetypical submissive is said to be a top executive who longs to yield all responsibility during erotic play."[17] Yet they find that the need to escape responsibility is not restricted to high-powered executives: "Submission is a turning away from the social and a penetration into a sacrosanct internal space. This may be why many submissives compare their erotic experiences to religious or spiritual surrender. The surrender is a means of achieving a kind of freedom from the ego, a condition where one is completely trusting and undefensive."[18] Echoes of Dominique Aury. From this perspective, in a trusting relationship masochism allows one "to explore absolute powerlessness in a safe context, knowing that no actual harm will occur and that one will not be condemned or ridiculed."[19]

What kind of power do dominants seek in sexuality? The authors of *Different Loving* argue that "if submission is an escape from ego, dominance is the ultimate ego trip, a time when one exerts absolute control over another's reality and holds the key to his or her partner's pleasure."[20] They stress that what is particularly "electrifying" for dominants is to engage in sex with a masochist who is an equal in real life, especially if they can reduce such a person to "a condition of erotic helplessness."[21]

However, even those who believe that sadomasochistic sex is liberating, acknowledge that coercion can have a dark side if a dominant pushes a submissive to engage in activities he or she dreads. A dominant might, for example, compel her partner to accept increasing levels of painful stimulation. And some dominants punish submissives who "willfully" disobey; even if their intent is not to harm the submissive, it may cause the submissive pain or displeasure.

While purely sexual D&S's do not believe in punishment, it forms an intrinsic part of what Brame, Brame, and Jacobs call lifestyle relationships—more inclusive than sexual relationships only—where discipline may be one critical aspect of the dynamic. They suggest that "life style submissives often desire both the risk and the reality of punishment, because it reinforces the reality of the power relationship. Sometimes a submissive will purposefully misbehave—usually in playful ways—to incite the dominant to punish him or her."[22] "Life style relationship" means nothing more or less than two people who attempt to build a permanent union based on a shared S&M or D&S sexual script embedded within an overall relationship script. But the central script can become *the* all-important ingredient, thus leaving out certain aspects of what people commonly think of as a growth relationship.

While a significant number of people engage in consensual S&M, D&S, or B&D sexual role playing, many men seek gratification of this kind with call girls. Here the customer calls the shots, exercising power no matter what kind of sex he chooses. Still, call girls sometimes turn the tables, exerting their own power by "outing" their johns. In their book *You'll Never Make Love in This Town Again*, a group of Hollywood call girls go on record debunking the reputed sexual prowess of some leading male actors, who sometimes require extreme if not bizarre measures to achieve sexual release and who not infrequently request a sadomasochistic encounter.[23] A complication here is that whatever people proclaim about the merits of these practices, they often are embarrassed to disclose that they engage in them. But adding to the thrill of breaking a taboo, part of the spice of their encounters is the risk of disclosure—a wrinkle that in this instance got out of hand, wrecking the essential premise of safe play.

For some troubled men, there is a slippery slope from acting out S&M sexual fantasies with call girls to forcing sadistic sex on nonconsenting partners, up to and including sex murders. Many fiction and nonfiction books are about serial sex murderers, the extreme end of the spectrum of nonconsensual sexual sadists. (We should take note: the readership of these books is of such magnitude—just look at our best-seller lists—that we know the fantasies buried in the plotlines appeal to a wide readership, though the inner connection probably flies just under the radar of self-awareness for most of them.) Interestingly, the foil of the sexual murderer in these stories is often a cop who is sentimentally drawn to hookers.

The absolute living master of this fictional genre (stories of sex killings and sentimental cops) is James Elroy, author of *L.A. Confidential* and *The Black Dahlia*, which deal with the tripartite themes of sexual victims, sex killers, and victim-oriented cops. But nowhere has Elroy

written more compellingly about sex run amok than in *My Dark Places:*
An L.A. Crime Memoir, his brilliant and harrowing autobiography that
centers around his partnering with a homicide cop, Bill Stoner, to investigate the murder of his own mother some thirty years earlier, when Elroy
was ten years old.[24]

Elroy's memoir of self-discovery, a kind of enacted crime story-cum-
recherches temps perdu, throws eerie but uncannily accurate illumination
onto the darker recesses not only of the readers of the crime stories, but
also of the real-life victims and perpetrators, the people for whom S&M
and B&D never stay "safe" for very long.

Elroy was six years old when his parents separated. From then on he
had split his life between them, but his sympathies were with his father.
He had hated his mother from the time she had divorced his father, with
a hate that had made him "exclusively" his father's son.[25] After the split,
his mother started drinking more but didn't bring men home: "My father
figured she was shacking up on the weekends."

When the ten-year-old Elroy first learned that his mother, Geneva
Hilliker Elroy, had been murdered, during or after a sexual encounter with
an unknown man, he had just spent the weekend with his father. He cried
not out of grief for his mother but for the benefit of the cops: "I cried
tears all the way to L.A. I hated her. I hated El Monte [the town where
they lived]. Some unknown killer just bought me a brand-new beautiful
life."

After his mother was killed, Elroy began to live full-time with his
father, who was deteriorating badly. Elroy didn't like girls, but he liked
divorced mothers, preferably those who were pale-skinned and red-haired
like his own mother, though at the time he never consciously made the
connection to her.[26] He hated her and lusted for her. Without much
supervision, he refined what he called his "Crazy Man Act."[27] But it
wasn't just an act. Still pre-adolescent, he became a thief and a voyeur.
When he was eleven, his father gave him a book by Jack Webb, the star of
Dragnet on television. He was fascinated with "the saga of dead-end lives
up against authority. . . ."[28]

Webb's account of the Black Dahlia case, so called by a reporter
because the victim was dressed in black, sent Elroy "way off the deep
end." The killer had tortured and mutilated his victim, Betty Short, for
days. Looking back, Elroy says that Webb "didn't understand the killer's
intentions or know that his gynecological tampering defined the crime.

He didn't know that the killer was horribly afraid of women. He didn't know that he cut the Dahlia open to see what made women different from men."[29] Elroy instinctively understood the victim: "Betty sure wanted powerful things from men—but could not identify her needs. . . . She turned herself into a cliché that most men wanted to fuck and a few men wanted to kill."[30]

Elroy did not have to live too long with his father before coming to the conclusion that he had been better off with his mother. Obsessed with dead women, Elroy lived through a druggy, boozy adolescence, stealing, drinking, reading and fantasizing. He became what might charitably be described as a version of a juvenile delinquent. A lung infection and fear turned him sober.

Considering Elroy's painful and destructive adolescence and young adulthood, it is a minor miracle that he survived. Ironically, what saved him were his fantasies about dead women which eventually helped him become a major crime writer. Gradually he allowed himself to think about his mother and her murder.

By the time he teamed up with the investigator Bill Stoner to investigate his mother's death, Elroy already had a cult following as a crime writer. He had locked himself up for a year to write *The Black Dahlia*. "I lived with one dead woman and a dozen bad men. Betty Short [the victim] ruled me. I built her character from diverse strands of male desire and tried to portray the male world that sanctioned her death. I wrote the last page and wept. I dedicated the book to my mother. I knew I could link Jean [the name he called his mother by] and Betty and strike 24-carat gold. I financed my own book tour. I took the link public. I made *The Black Dahlia* a national best-seller."[31] His wife, Helen Kanode, persuaded him to pursue his obsession about his mother and her death.

Investigating his mother's murder with Stoner, Elroy concocted serial theories about his mother and her singular death and constantly revised them. One of his later theories was that she had not been killed resisting sex, but had been killed for demanding sex the second time around: she wanted more sex or male attention, and this led to her death. "I trusted my new theory. It made me feel this big wave of love for my mother. I was her son. I was hooked on more, as bad as she was. Gender bias in my time favored me. . . . She force-fed me the survivor's instinct she never developed herself. Her pain was greater than mine. It defined the gap between us."[32]

Elroy and Bill Stoner agreed that "Booze and dope and random sex gave you back a cheap version of power you set out to relinquish. . . ." The two men placed ads requesting clues to the killing and they received a number of replies. Six middle-age daughters told essentially the same story: their fathers were wife-beaters, abusers, took off with the rent money, and sought out underage women. The daughters had gone into therapy and defined themselves in therapeutic terms. To Elroy the women sounded smug, "entrenched and content in their victimhood."[33]

Here Elroy identifies something that is familiar to therapists. As I suggested earlier, the frequently encountered self-labeling as a "survivor," signaling triumph over victimhood of one sort or another, has emerged as one of the most important heroic scripts in our culture. Yet, the survivor script (excluding, of course, the life stories of actual survivors of concentration camps and other disasters) often conceals an underlying masochistic narrative—one of redemption through suffering, converting a tortured or sexually abused childhood into a heroic one.

Eventually, Elroy began to feel split between his current forty-seven-year-old self, investigating his mother's death and life, and the ten-year-old-boy whose memories he was exploring. However condescending Elroy sometimes sounds about therapy, his may be one of the all-time great self-analyses. In investigating his mother's murder, he reconstructed his own past. His childhood loyalties began to flip-flop. His father now appeared "more desperate and anxious to impress. . . . My father was a liar. My mother was a fabricator. . . . He brought my mother up and shot her down. . . . His stories were self-inflated and spiteful. He defamed my mother."[34]

As Elroy's memories grew stronger, he concluded that his father was a fundamentally weak man with a macho cover story. In his mother's mind, "All men were weak. . . . You could not control their weakness. . . . Disillusionment was enlightenment. . . . She saw me as her redemption. . . . She didn't want me to turn into my father. . . . She lived in two worlds. I marked the dividing line. She thought her dual-world scheme was sustainable. She miscalculated."[35]

While Elroy had viewed his mother as a drunk, a whore, and a hypocrite, he was able to retrieve the "good mother" part of her for himself. Her killer had become irrelevant: "He was dead or he wasn't. . . . He was only a directional sign. He forced me to extend myself and give my mother her full due. She was no less than my salvation."[36] As a result of this rehabilitation of his mother in his memory and in his feelings, perhaps Elroy made his peace. As a celebrator of dead women, he found a career and perhaps refound himself.

What Elroy describes is the non-vanilla side of sadomasochistic sex—sadism and masochism unanchored from the bonds of mutual consent or relationship. Too much aggression tilts the individual's internal balance in such a way that recreational sadism becomes deadly. If too much guilt and self-hatred are involved, masochism is not a sweet surrender; at best it is a game of Russian roulette. A journey to a deeper self-discovery, such as Elroy's, is, paradoxically, what is denied in safe S&M sexual play and is short-circuited, with deadly effect, in the true sexual predator. Elroy's life shows how the tortured powerlessness of a hateful childhood can and cannot be tamed in the fantasies of the bedroom. It is worth noting that Elroy was able to go beyond the partial redemptions of fantasizing and writing out his fantasies, to a more thorough-going confrontation with his past only after the success of his first books gave him the initial stake of real power that he needed to ante up to play this much higher-stakes game with himself.

IN THINKING ABOUT sexual sadomasochism, one does well to consider the extent to which issues of real power are effectively neutralized at the threshold of the encounter, because what happens then determines in large part whether what follows will be safe, sane, and consensual or whether it will be contaminated in a way that allows aggression and victimization to enter in. In parsing relational sadomasochism, it is important to evaluate whether the actual power balance between parties is sufficiently stable to tolerate conflict or the imbalance caused by the essentially gratuitous use of the relationship to express childhood grievances and frustrations. Sexual sadomasochism ranges from consensual submission and dominance to murder; analogously, relational sadomasochism ranges from sadomasochistically tinged relationships to virulent sadomasochistic interactions.

Here is an example of the "vanilla" end of the relational spectrum: Mrs. Danzig and her maid, Victoria, had a long-standing affectionate relationship, as good as one can expect between an employer and employee working at very close quarters. They had been together for fifteen years. But Victoria had moments when she resented being a maid, particularly if she was having trouble at home. She would then "forget" to do something or would watch television when Mrs. Danzig was out. For her part, Mrs. Danzig, who was sensitive to slights, sometimes turned the screws on Victoria if she felt Victoria was becoming slack or "uppity." On occasion, when Mrs. Danzig was frustrated with something that had gone wrong—the best vase broken or the dinner burned—she would lose her temper. This made her feel better, but twice, after such a blowup, Victoria had left her keys on the table and failed to come in the next day—the classic "in-your-face" defiant gesture of legitimately vexed or perennially disgruntled maids and housekeepers. Each time Mrs. Danzig had called Victoria and abjectly apologized.

Now, in the midst of wrapping Christmas presents, Victoria had mistakenly thrown out the instructions for an electronic game. Mrs. Danzig exploded; but when Victoria burst into tears, she knew she'd gone too far, became very apologetic, and tried to smooth things over—she gave Victoria an unusually substantial Christmas bonus and sent her home for the weekend. On Monday morning, however, she was surprised to find a message from Victoria on her answering machine, saying that she was not coming back.

Mrs. Danzig used her husband as peacemaker. She was still angry, though, and to save her pride told him that she would take Victoria back only if Victoria notified them by Saturday that she would return the following Monday. Saturday came and went. On Monday morning, the phone rang very early: it was Victoria, announcing her intention to return. Mrs. Danzig quickly calculated that if she gave in now, past the deadline, she would never be in control again. So she said to Victoria, "It sounds as if you're not really happy here. Maybe you want to think about it." Victoria, who had expected to be welcomed, was somewhat taken aback; she hesitated, saying she wasn't sure. Now Mrs. Danzig, trying to get Victoria to beg, said she considered their relationship over. But Victoria wasn't having any and ended their phone conversation.

At this point, neither one was willing to apologize, and they let their relationship die. As it turned out, both of them suffered because they found no substitutes for each other, but they were too proud to give in. This relationship was, of course, far more subtle than a straight-up sadomasochistic interaction, but each invoked latently sadistic measures to bolster her sense of control and self-esteem. Then they miscalculated.

In a true sadomasochistic relationship, sadism and masochism are more front and center, more pervasive. How does the sadist find a masochist, and vice versa? What is the prelude to an enduring sado-masochistic interaction? Some gesture must be offered and accepted for each party to recognize the other as available on "friendly" psychological terms. This recognition—through an action initiated by one person and endorsed by a second person—generally happens quickly, and the participants may not even be fully aware of it.

Darlene, an assistant buyer, was having an affair with Dan, an up-and-coming buyer eight years her senior. Before their affair began, Dan had told her that he was seeing someone else, but that it was an unhappy relationship because the other woman was tormented. In fact, he said he was afraid to leave her because she might harm herself. Nonetheless, he implied that he would leave eventually, and he could then approach Darlene honorably. When Darlene reacted sympathetically, he approached her without breaking off his other relationship.

One incident tells it all. About a year ago, Darlene went on a buying trip to Europe and brought home a special kind of tea for Dan. His girl-friend, Betty, perpetually fearful that Dan was unfaithful, suspected that the tea was from Darlene and insisted that he return it. This he did. Betty's insistence that Dan return the gift was a clue to Darlene that Betty was unsure of her ground. Darlene felt hopeful. The clue Darlene failed to pick up on was that there had been no need for Dan to tell her all this. Dan was recruiting Darlene as an ally and a sympathizer; he was stalling. He was still with Betty and not making a move to get out.

Darlene, whose personal background leads her to want to please, felt more hurt than angry, and didn't stop to consider the game Dan was playing. Her need to please and to control relationships in this way was at the heart of her response. Dan wasn't ready to give up Betty, but he didn't want to lose Darlene either. By returning the tea he was telling Darlene how bad Betty was, but he was not negotiating openly and honestly—he was dancing on a hot stove, trying to placate both women.

What predisposes someone to participate in sadomasochistic relationships? The psychoanalyst Marie-France Hirigoyen provides an astute analysis of how one person inducts another into a sadomasochistic relationship. A sadomasochistic relationship goes through two phases: (1) the seduction of the "victim" by the seducer and (2) the development of the sadomasochistic bond, emotional or physical.[37]

In what Hirigoyen calls the "seductive stalking period," the seducer—male, let us suppose—approaches his potential mark with apparent admiration of her, stressing his fascination with her and making her feel special.[38] The ideal victim—or "mark"—is somewhat depressed, and in the beginning, her exciting encounters with her seducer stimulate her to overcome a low-grade sadness. Flattered by the seducer, she warms up. Depressives, who may experience a sense of inner deadness, often look to the excitement of relationships to make them feel special, especially if the suitor or the situation is difficult or slightly dangerous. The seducer's admiration of his victim may or may not be authentic, but in either case it serves as the first step in a long-practiced "choreography" of induction into sadomasochism. The seducer gradually changes course and begins to destabilize his "victim" by withdrawing praise and becoming critical.[39]

As the victim loses self-confidence, her ability to oppose her oppressor is eroded. She capitulates to her partner to forestall abandonment. (Similarly, children sometimes submit to authoritarian, even brutal parents because this seems preferable to abandonment.) The seducer's assault is so finely timed and dosed that the spider traps the fly. The victim hopes desperately for the restitution of the time when she seemed to be the world to her lover. The abuser, for his part, tries to separate her from her friends and family, who might tell her the truth. Because the victim concedes authority to the abuser, she cannot defend herself.

If the victim should try to escape, the attacker experiences panic and explodes in fury. He disparages and insults her and insists that she remain quiet. But only rarely does he become physically abusive, because, despite appearances to the contrary, abusers are deeply dependent on their victims. Separation-anxious themselves, they feel they are being rejected if their partner asserts any independent will.

The abuser, generally narcissistic and filled with envy, targets women he views as important—for example, those who can take him into certain business or social circles. But instead of feeling grateful, he becomes even more envious and escalates his criticism. Despite an appearance of strength, an abusive narcissist has usually failed to achieve psychological stability, because of trauma and rejection in his own childhood. His own emptiness impels him to destroy any happiness he observes in others. Deprecating others, he elevates his own self-esteem. Thus he appears to do to his intimates what was done to him in his childhood.

The victim, not herself abusive, finds it almost impossible to imagine that anyone could be motivated by a wish to destroy her independence and pride. She believes that her partner's abuse must be a response to some hurt she has caused him, and she naively supposes that if she explains her motivations he will understand and apologize. To avoid flare-ups, she attempts to intuit and assuage his every need. But as she submits, he shifts into higher gear, and thus a vicious circle begins. Therapists generally see such victims only after they have begun to suffer from pervasive anxiety, depression, or stress-induced illnesses. But they also see abusers, who having pushed too far, may suddenly feel abandoned, threatened, or attacked.

For Hirigoyen, abusive relationships are a perversion of an ordinary balance of power; the narcissistic seduction draws the victim into a situation of dependency and of attachment. As she becomes dependent, her suggestibility increases and she is more ready to become submissive in response to any fear of rejection. The seducer has achieved emotional and intellectual control over her.

Perhaps more common than the conscious seducer—Hirogoyen's term for the abusive partner in a sadomasochistic relationship—are those who fear abandonment and are unaware of their own sadism. These are true relational sadomasochists. They sometimes act out their internal split—between sadist and masochist—in two simultaneous relationships.

Up to now I have used the masculine pronoun for the abuser, but there are women, too, who are abusers. Some years ago, I saw in psychoanalytic therapy a woman I will call Veronique. She entered treatment at the suggestion of her lover, Jonathan, a devotee of psychoanalysis. He believed that she was reluctant to leave her marriage to be with him out of a fear of intimacy, not because she felt guilty about her husband. Enthralled with Jonathan, Veronique complied with his request that she seek help. At the time, she was in her early forties; her son was almost an adult, her career in full flower. She was a high-functioning woman with a number of circumscribed sexual perversions and a history of angry outbursts directed at both her intimates and her employees. Still, in contrast to the emotional roller-coaster of her personal life, her therapy went very smoothly.

Veronique had been in therapy before, in her twenties. She had entered this earlier therapy at her husband's insistence and had experienced extremely painful memories of forlorn rejection while she lay on the couch—as well as rage at being there. At that time, she felt completely disorganized; often she would not get out of bed but would spend lazy mornings masturbating while floating sadomasochist reveries. She was drinking, refused to have sex with her husband, and could barely hold down a job. She indulged in potentially self-destructive behavior—for example, driving while drunk. She soon began to hate her therapy and despise her therapist. Throughout, she loathed being on the couch, but she never directly confronted her analyst. Instead, she acted out her hostility—missing sessions, arriving late, remaining silent, and seducing one of his patients. In retrospect, there is little doubt that she was acting out a hateful transference to her therapist, although at the time she felt judged rather than vengeful. The analyst finally ended the therapy, with the gloss that they were stalemated but that she was free to come back at any time.

Without the benefit of therapy, she still managed to evolve from a disorganized, fragmented, angry person into a more purposeful one. Through her enactment of a number of minor sadomasochistic perversions, she contained her rage in less ruinous kinds of acting out, and through sublimation she was able to turn some of her self-destructive behavior into a concern for the poor, the downtrodden, and the dysfunctional.[40]

By the time Veronique started treatment with me, her public persona bore little resemblance to the incapacitated young woman she had once been. With her husband's help, she had transformed herself into a power player in the world of magazines. She was known for her sharp tongue, her incisive intelligence, and her flawless memory for work-related details—though she never took a note.

But over time, some of her problems reemerged. In particular, she felt a growing discomfort with her husband and began a string of affairs. Despite her astonishing memory for her work, she had little ability to provide a coherent narrative of her life; her account of her adulthood was even less organized than her recall of her early years. Moreover, she had very little recall of themes from session to session. Only through painstaking work were we able to patch together a coherent life narrative.

Veronique had never consciously allowed herself to dwell on her anger, resentment, and envy. Yet she was far more subject to rage than she could acknowledge to herself. At work, she was notorious for temper tantrums, discourtesy, and dismissive, even hostile behavior. But she was out of touch with the emotional component of such behaviors—she thought the cause was simply her busy life and the demands of print journalism.

At home, her explosions were most often directed at her husband. Despite the stability he had brought her, the relationship had long since degenerated on her part into chronic resentment, which she rationalized as a response to his hostility. It never occurred to her that his anger might be a reaction to her abusive behavior. Consequently, she never saw herself as the perpetrator; she always felt like the injured party. (An honest reporter, she intellectually acknowledged that her husband, too, had long felt mistreated—even persecuted—by her. But emotionally she could not feel the merit of his reproaches.) Early in her treatment, her thoughts and associations centered on the struggle between her wish to leave her marriage and her fear of doing so.

As she disclosed more about herself, she began to see that her dependence on her husband stemmed from a damaged sense of self. Although she was perceived as a strong, "castrating" woman, she had always felt weak. She was an only daughter, the youngest of three children, and her parents had considered her awkward and ill equipped to cope with life. Retrospectively, her disorganization seems to have been the way she rebelled against her parents' rigid expectations. She fought back in the only way she sensed was possible—by disappointing them. While she caused them to suffer mightily, she unfortunately incorporated as her self-image the damaged self she presented to them.

Her high intelligence ultimately enabled her to do well academically and she found her way into a first-rate prestigious college—much to the distress of her parents, who wanted her at home and under their surveillance. Her decision to go away to college was the first evidence of her ability to separate from them. She fell in love with a man she saw as damaged, like herself, and with him she moved to New York City, where he went to business school and she took courses in art and literature.

After her boyfriend's graduation from business school, she broke up with him. She soon met and married her husband and began to work in publishing. In short order, her career took off, her success the result of her brilliance with language and her eye for new talent. But it also had something to do with her ability to attach herself to superachieving mentors, her "identity markers." Through association with them, she felt safe and whole, her self-esteem nourished by basking in their auras. She courted these mentors assiduously, using them to ignore her husband in the same way that she had used her passionate adolescent friendships to snub her parents. Through these highly idealized men, she found an avenue to what turned out to be a remarkable professional life. But she failed to internalize any sense of her own worth, all too readily crediting luck or her mentors. It was some years into her analysis before the downside of those relationships began to emerge—her sense of subservience and emotional surrender to these men.

Veronique was trapped in a dependent adaptation. She hated her husband and her mentors but used them as auxiliary batteries. Her ability to see herself as a separate person was compromised by her dependency and by fear.

Because she had seldom let herself experience her anger as such, her principal means of containing and exploring it, aside from contempt for her husband, was enacting perverse sexual fantasies with her lovers. Yet her anger might have been a more instructive compass for her to steer by, if she could have read it properly. Her need to immerse herself in a hostile, dependent relationship appears not to be a result of her parents' anger toward her, but of their vision of her as inadequate. The psychoanalyst Anna Ornstein, among others, has emphasized that sadomasochism is connected not only to a painful parental relationship and a compulsive repetition of that relationship later in life, but also to a self image "of a defective, denigrated self—inadequate, disgusting, castrated, undeserving and contemptible."[41]

Veronique's reluctance to see herself as angry served, in an illusory way, to protect those she depended on—her male mentors and me as her therapist. But it had another function. Her insistence on seeing herself as a good woman, not an angry one, served her wish to be different from her angry, destructive parents, to deny any psychological kinship with them. Her counteridentification to them was played out in her complete aversion to her parents' lifestyle, their political preferences and personal haughtiness. By denying that her parents lived in her, she symbolically killed them.

Veronique idealized key figures in her life to create a sanitized world, a world without rage. This was, in part, an impulse toward growth and thus part of the healing process. Though she needed to repeat past disappointments, she also had a wish to reopen the question of trust in the hope that her pessimistic expectations for a relationship would turn out to be wrong. Over time, as she came to understand her motivations, her relationships at work became more stable as the cycle of overidealization and deidealization diminished. But her tendency to idealize people continued in her relationships with her authors, where it was actually helpful.

Before our first meeting, Veronique had already idealized me. This was because of Jonathan's endorsement, and her idealized image survived her break with him. Thus her transference was, on the surface, dramatically opposed to the hateful transference in her earlier analysis. At the same time, she engaged in specific behaviors to limit her sense of dependency on me, symbolically limiting my control over her. For instance, she would look at her watch and end every session before I did in order to avoid feeling rejected by me.

My tolerance of her need to control me emboldened her to bring new material into the analysis, particularly the content of her perversions. This was important not only as such, but because it expanded the boundaries of trust, and allowed her to put aside her perceived need to be "good." She was able to show me her infantile, lascivious side. She came to see that other people were capable of integrating love, trust, and idealization into stable relationships—previously, she had conceived only of relationships like her own. Gradually, she was able to consolidate her own sense of strength while maintaining her ties to her previously idealized and now more realistically perceived mentors and to her husband and son.

Veronique's story demonstrates how someone can be motivated to enter into sadomasochistic relationships from both sides. Except for extreme cases, this is true of most sadomasochists most of the time, though typically one may have to get to know them very well to understand the masochistic identifications underlying their sadism and the sadistic streak laced through their masochism.

ORDINARILY, it is useful to distinguish sadomasochistic sexual enactment from sadomasochistic relationships. But of course they often overlap. Here perhaps I should spend a moment more on why and how sadomasochistic sexual enactments may not implicate sadomasochism in the overall relationship.

Technically, sadomasochistic sex typically involves unconscious psychological conflict and fantasies that provide pseudo solutions to a sexual conflict. That is, the individual cannot—for whatever reason—freely indulge in sexual passion within a romantic attachment. There is some taboo, some obstacle: a fear of being hurt, lessons learned as a child, an inhibition against showing desire or assertion. In a sense, the individual, confronting a sexual situation while deprived of the beneficent security of his or her secret fantasy, would be relatively powerless to act, if not frankly impotent. S&M and B&D provide fantasies of power (in which either oneself or one's partner may be imagined as the powerful one). Once a fantasy is enacted, it is freeing, making the conflict go away, at least for the moment. In this roundabout way, the fantasy uses the imagination to increase the scope of interpersonal power, though the solution is finally still make-believe, even if the man's erection or the woman's lubrication may be real.

Sadomasochistic relationships are different. They entail not fantasies of power so much as perversions of power. Relational sadomasochism does not facilitate play or gratification, and the only balance of power it achieves is corrupt. For some relational sadomasochists, their sense of autonomy requires cold domination of another, while mutuality seems possible only through submission. Sadomasochistic distortions are pathological versions of the normal conflict between mutuality and autonomy.

Sadomasochistic distortions in intimate relationships sometimes take the form of physical battering, a practice that differs from the colder abuse by malignant narcissists such as those Hirigoyen has described. Susan Faludi started her research on the psychology of men—incorrectly, she now thinks—by sitting in on a gathering of men who had been ordered by a court to explore why they were batterers. She says she made an unexamined, dubious assumption: that the crisis among American men was caused by something they were doing, unrelated to anything being done to them. But the men she came to know "had lost or were losing jobs, homes, cars, families," and she realized that they beat women because it gave them a feeling of being in power and restored their sense of being men. This kind of resolution was necessarily transient and served only to disguise the underlying problem—their powerlessness and the lack of control they felt.[42]

However, the psychology of battering extends beyond men's loss of prestige and power. When dominance becomes sadistic, or when submissiveness involves masochistic enslavement, the origins are not found exclusively in external stresses. Not all jobless men beat their wives. Sadomasochism must be understood in terms of individual psychology; it is a result of early life experiences and corrupted relationships.

Often, we can track sadomasochistic enactments from generation to generation as abused children identify with (or counteridentify with) the practices of their parents. Someone who participates in fairly extreme sadomasochistic interactions, in which suffering and humiliation are routinely sought or endured, has often suffered deprivation, trauma, or painful interactions with caregivers in early life. For some, the painful experiences of childhood are transmuted into a mode of attachment that is rationalized and even embraced as a sign of specialness. A girl who is spanked by her father may (unconsciously) construe this as an indication of his attachment to her and may therefore eroticize spanking. Alternatively, an abused child (whether the abuse is sexual or verbal) may unconsciously identify with the abuser. Whatever fantasies a child invokes to bolster self-esteem or counteract pain, these fantasies and the encoding of early relationships can become linked to fantasies of omnipotent dominance or of abject submission, which are later invoked as a means of reversing early trauma and gratifying early wishes. And just as submission may evolve into masochism, domination may evolve into sadism.

There is no absolute difference here between men and women. Both sexes appear equally vulnerable to masochistic and sadistic distortions of love. And both sexes are equally capable of seeking in another the dispositions they cannot face in themselves. One should not forget that what Freud first described and labeled as feminine masochism actually occurred in the fantasy life of men.

Most clinicians have had as many male patients as female patients who are tormented by masochistic submission in love. And there is ample evidence in literature of men's susceptibility (and attraction) to self-destruction in love. While male novelists have described the Pure Maiden, they have also described the Dark Lady, the powerful temptress who can lure a man to his death—she is a staple of male fantasy life.[43] The wish for humiliation or self-punishment also appears in men's fantasies as the big-breasted, high-booted, "phallic" woman with a whip. And a man drawn to the Dark Lady in fantasy often arranges to find her in the real world.

Just as there are as many masochistic urges in men as in women so, too, are there as many sadistic distortions in women as in men. Men and women, heterosexuals and homosexuals, are all capable of using intimate (and professional) relationships to gratify their unconscious longings for humiliation, self-punishment, or self-destruction—or their longing to dominate and abuse their partner.[44]

Those who are free of sadomasochistic distortions should not be too quick to judge those who embrace them—leaving aside, of course, sadistic killers. There are two reasons. First, our culture's fascination with serial killings and violent films suggests that many of us have sadomasochistic fantasies: if we do not create such fantasies ourselves, we nonetheless seem to be drawn to them as passive consumers. Second, and more important, it is apparent that S&M imagery and enactments often allow people to form relationships that might otherwise seem too threatening. While we may think of this solution as less than ideal, or as maladaptive, it does offer access to the world of relations—and that after all comprises a necessary, and sometimes the sweetest, part of our lives.

PART

Personal
Power

THREE

8

Agency: Authoring Our Own Life Stories

"With word and deed we insert ourselves into the human world, and this insertion is like a second birth."

HANNAH ARENDT, *The Human Condition*

Interpersonal power is power we exert in relationship to someone else, whether by domination and command, tears and entreaties, or compromise and cooperation. Personal power is power over oneself, or better yet, strength within ourselves; it is what is required if we are to insert ourselves into life as the active agent in our life story. To possess personal power is to be truly in possession of the self, to be able to use oneself as the instrument of one's own plans. When we possess it, we feel sure of ourselves; when we exercise it, we feel a kind of high. A rock climber quoted in Mihaly Csikszentmihalyi's book *Flow* captures the heart of this experience: "It's exhilarating to come closer and closer to self-discipline. You make your body go and everything hurts; then you look back in awe at the self, at what you've done. . . . It leads to ecstasy, to self-fulfillment. If you win these battles enough, that battle against yourself, at least for a moment, it becomes easier to win the battles in the world."[1]

To achieve wholeness, we must achieve some degree of control over ourselves and of our world. Yet we must not set the bar too high by aiming for absolute control or mastery; that would do little more than make our lives a frustrated, semi-enraged, self-blaming nightmare. A woman scammed out of two thousand dollars by a carpenter who insisted on advance payment and then skipped town found herself brooding about the experience. A psychiatrist friend told her to "think of it as slippage." He showed her how to think of slippage as a good thing: "It reminds us that we're not in control."[2] So she did, remembering all the times when she had lost time or money due to her own inattention, carelessness, or bad luck. So doing, she retrieved her sense of personal agency. We do well to remember that part of the so-called serenity prayer where one asks not only for "the courage to change the things I can change" but also for "the patience to accept the things I cannot change."

We begin our quest for control and mastery of ourselves and the external world in childhood. We do so in two important ways: by gradually acquiring skills and by forming a life plan in which we are the protagonist. To create this plan we begin to float a series of future-oriented fantasies that are really imaginative rehearsals for our future lives. I call them generative fantasies to distinguish them from simple wish-fulfilling daydreams. Every one of us embraces a number of these evolving, generative fantasies that are geared to future possibilities. They encompass our dreams of work, love, parenthood, achievement, adventure, fame, wealth, recognition, or adherence to a cause, among other aspirations. They are strung on a "wish thread," along which we shuttle back and forth, transforming childhood longings into possibilities for the here-and-now or the future.[3]

The research psychologist Daniel Levinson describes a similar process which he calls the formation of a life dream: "In everyday language, we say that someone 'succeeded beyond his wildest dreams' or that he 'dreamed a world he could never have.' These are neither night dreams nor casual daydreams." A 'dream' of this kind is more consciously intentional than a pure fantasy, but yet still not a fully thought-out life plan. It is a dream in the sense of Martin Luther King's historic 'I Have a Dream' speech, only it is personal." For Levinson, the evolution of the dream has consequences for adult development: "The Dream as a sense of self-in-the-adult-world is an imagined possibility that generates excitement and gives meaning to life."[4] Our generative fantasies and life dreams are the scripts around which we anchor our life stories. If they are to be effective, we must sometimes downgrade their heroic aspect in order to bring them to realization.

Here we must pause and take in the great paradox of personal power. If we are to have a real sense of our own agency, we must acquire a realistic, down-to-earth appraisal of ourselves, our skills, and our situation. If we are to act on our own behalf, we need to be grounded in reality. But this is only half the story. If we are truly to have a capacity to insert ourselves into life, we must also have a sense of what life might hold for us that goes beyond our present circumstances. We must have the capacity to imagine how things might be different, or, alternatively, how we might be different. Achieving and exercising personal power depends on a capacity for future-oriented fantasies and dreams. It also depends, whether or not we like to admit it, on having people who nurture and support our dreams along with our abilities. To begin with, though, we must achieve the rudiments of self-reliance and ultimately of agency.

Autonomy and Agency

We have an innate instinct to generate self-directed action, yet the way we express agency is almost inevitably connected in our development, and thus in our minds, to interpersonal relationships. This is because personal power arises out of what Hannah Arendt calls "a second birth" and what Judith Viorst refers to as "taking possession of ourselves"—both referring to our need to separate from our mother's embrace. We may learn to walk, talk, take baths and clean our rooms, play with our toys, and engage in sports no matter who our parents are; but the way they teach us, prohibit us, or encourage us, their own interests and personalities, and the way we identify with them are all factors that contribute to the ease or difficulty with which we attain self-determination. These same factors also play a considerable role in how much pleasure or abhorrence we bring to particular tasks.

Personal power and interpersonal power are interdependent, but they also retain a necessary degree of separation Put simply, we cannot insert ourselves effectively into the world, no matter how great our courage, unless we have first achieved a modicum of self-determination. No amount of interpersonal competence and comfort can compensate for our inner deficits. We can, however, use intimacy to mask our inabilities and to console us for the negative feelings that go with a lack in self-determination; in this way we can keep ourselves in the dark about our limitations. When the cozy dependency of a relationship is being used to cover over an inner lack of self-determination, that dependency is not usually apparent, either to the individual or to others, until it is threatened. Consider the apparently self-sufficient husband who falls apart when his wife gets sick, or the teenager who is the perfect student and model citizen until she leaves home to go to college.

Overcoming our infantile helplessness is a process that is roughed out in childhood and consolidated in the resolution of the power struggles of adolescence and early adulthood. The goal, of course, is the healthy development of a self-sufficient, self-reliant, independent adult. The most basic part of the process is achieving self-control, which involves skills in self-regulation and self-care, but ultimately, control comes to include the mastery of one or another part of the external world as well.[5] This developmental pathway can be fostered by parental encouragement, instruction, help, reassurance, and expressions of pleasure at the child's emerging power.

In the best-case scenario, parents support their children's growing independence. Ideally, when a child is small, the parents permit dependency, withdrawing their support bit by bit as the child learns to do for herself. As she begins to assert herself, her parents may even celebrate her efforts to forge an independent identity, restraining her only when there is a real danger. To do so, they must be fulfilled enough in their own right that they do not cling to their offspring out of their own needs. In the process, the child comes to possess something we call willpower, which is to self-control and self-esteem what the will-to-power is to the control of other people.

Not only are parents templates for the child to identify with, but the child will also use them, variously at different ages, as rivals and obstacles to be gotten around, or as people they can safely try their strength against. Siblings, too, serve valuable functions, being both object lessons in what to do or what not to do, depending on their fate; and they are also figures to differentiate from. As the scholar/writer Frank Sulloway has recently shown in great empirical detail, the tension between siblings is an important crucible of personality, particularly as younger siblings struggle to be different and thus are sometimes more open than firstborns to innovative ideas and life strategies. According to Sulloway, the relative weights of identification and of the counter-identification that go into shaping our own particular styles of self-care, self-control, and agency are crucially affected by birth order. Sulloway suggests that underlying identifications with parents are most evident in firstborns but for the later-borns are filtered in various ways through the ups and downs of sibling rivalry.[6]

Dependence on parents, an initially unthinking utter reliance on them as the only models children know, is obviously a major determinant of how they eventually come to understand and experience personal power. Serving as a counter-weight to their parents, children's own innate makeup and the influence of the peer group can encourage other styles of self-determination. Helen, for instance, remembers that her jealously overprotective mother dressed her every day and tied her shoes for her. One day at school, she saw that one of her laces had come undone, and it dawned on her that she had never ever tied her own laces. She was suddenly aware that everyone else of her age knew how to tie *their* laces and she was too humiliated to ask for help. Terrified, Helen sat down in a stairwell and struggled to perform this task for the very first time. Only when she saw another child approaching was she suddenly and miraculously able to tie the lace and avoid being humiliated in front of a classmate.

This traumatic but ultimately triumphant experience made Helen aware that her mother was different from most other mothers; what she sensed but could not yet articulate was that her mother was infantilizing her, unwittingly undermining her. Over time she began to insist on doing things for herself and was able to move out of her mother's constricting grip. Helen's fear of being shamed had motivated her to succeed—one example of the corrective effect of a peer relationship.

The weight of all these forces—parents, siblings, peers—work together to foster greater and greater steps toward autonomy, and most children, as they move toward adulthood, gradually rely on their own capacities as the main source of their security. But this desire to set your own course can be realized only after some basic skills have been mastered, beginning with self-control. As suggested in Chapter 1, this is extremely difficult because in early life, a child is biologically geared to seek pleasure, but limits must be learned. Self-control is rarely achieved without an internal struggle. The ever growing army of nutritionists, personal trainers, coaches, and gurus bear witness to the fact that problems of self-control continue to plague us into adulthood.

Our ability to master self-control as children has consequences for the future. The child psychiatrist Erna Furman tells us what should be intuitively obvious: there are "connecting links between a youngster's care of his body and belongings and the adult's ability to look after his health, home, and property. . . ."[7] Acknowledging that the know-how of mastery is necessary, she argues that "inner helpers, particularly self-esteem," enable us to use those tools. What this means is that we internalize both what our parents teach us and the degree of respect they have for us as individuals, and both are prerequisite to a capacity for true self-reliance. Paradoxically, while self-control is a prerequisite for the child to gradually disengage from her parents, it can develop only when some degree of identification with her parents has taken place and some actual support for her efforts, whether from parents or other interested parties, has been given.[8]

Adolescence is ordinarily the time when becoming self-reliant and independent assumes paramount importance. It is also the critical time when we begin to achieve a sense of autonomy and agency commensurate with adult capacities. The ultimate overthrow of parental authority begins with puberty. The school child generally achieves a modicum of self-reliance and develops a realistic perspective about her parents' limitations. But the upheavals of puberty will challenge this level of self-determination. Between the ages of eleven and fifteen, the child's personality seems to change in conjunction with the physiological and anatomical changes of puberty and the emergence of sexual desire. The analyst Joseph Noshpitz describes the altered circumstance of adolescence: "The acquisition of a mature body [is] a heady thing, a seductive, evocative experience that leads one to want to use that body, to do things with it. . . . Excitement, thrills, novelty—every kind of stimulating experience beckons it invitingly and the avid youngster responds."[9] The adolescent experiences a revival of feelings and issues concerning the body, its care, control, and uses, and also about its visibility and the shame and embarrassment connected to it, that were perhaps last encountered this intensely in the preschool and early school-age years. Adolescence plays us all a nasty trick—boys somewhat differently from girls—in that the physical changes of puberty coupled with resurgent levels of both energy and inhibition work to dislodge the autonomy that we have spent the latter years of childhood, roughly from ages eight to twelve, achieving. Then again, for the lucky few, for the natural athletes, the nascent beauties, the changes may bring new assets and sources of interpersonal power, but that is separate from the issue of self-control, which concerns us here.

Because assimilating the new body and the upsurge of sexual desires is so fraught with difficulty, fears of losing control are common during adolescence. Viorst notes that simultaneous inner and outer changes can forever fracture "our self-as-child identity, leaving us with a serious case of who-am-I, or what Erikson calls an identity crisis."[10] Althea Horner suggests that eating disorders develop at this time because adolescents are attempting to "gain omnipotent control over the body, its form and its impulses."[11]

Moreover, the reemergence of some variant of the Oedipal struggle often accompanies the onset of puberty. What is important to observe here is that the second Oedipus of adolescence is more than simply a revival of the first Oedipus of the late preschool years, though it is also that, as the child's soaring imagination begins to rework themes of rivalry and passionate longing that were first crystallized in the family romance. The Oedipus complex of early childhood is, as Erik Erikson observed, chiefly an affair of the imagination. And it is of an essentially limited imagination, the little boy imagining he will marry Mommy because she is the only married woman he knows. When the parents let the child be a child, the Oedipus remains an affair of the imagination and no more than that, a happy dream that tells the child he is entertaining big plans for himself.[12]

The revived Oedipus of adolescence can similarly be an affair of the imagination. But it can also be quite different. Parents who intrude into their children's lives at this stage do them no favor. Insofar as the mother sees her daughter as a real rival, or the father suddenly finds himself making his daughter into his little darling all over again, they are missing the boat entirely as parents. What the adolescent needs is support and encouragement in learning how to manage assertion and sexuality, not a triangular drama that raises the stakes by pulling the teenager back into the family constellation.[13]

Yet it is not uncommon for parents to be daunted by their children's burgeoning sexuality and attractiveness as their bodies emerge into adult form. It is uncommon for parents to admit as much to themselves, but the child is no longer so childlike and presents himself or herself to the parent as a much more serious rival and/or potent source of consternation born out of unwanted attraction. We can sometimes catch a glimpse of this in a movie or novel: in the first of the Lethal Weapon movies, policeman Danny Glover is surprised by his teenage daughter, played by an exceptionally lovely young actress, coming down the stairs in a very short prom dress, asking with her walk, "Daddy, how do I look?" Glover turns abruptly away, as though he had burned his eyes and makes a face to the camera that reveals his discomfort: a Daddy is not supposed to see what he just saw. The moment goes quickly, but it gets a big laugh—no doubt in unconscious recognition by the audience of similar feelings.

If an adolescent's assertiveness is met with serious intimidations from his rival parent, he will symbolically equate self-assertion with aggression and murderous violence, and as a consequence, he may come to fear retaliatory violence. The lifelong pattern may be set in which he inhibits assertion, not just out of fear but out of guilt as well. If the inhibition is symbolically extended to even benign acts of assertion, it can sometimes result in extreme passivity or anxiety.

Adolescents' identification of their own agency with that of an esteemed role model—often the same-sex parent—does not make them immune to conflict with their parents. Quite the contrary. At puberty and during adolescence, parents tend to become even harsher in their criticism because they are so often shocked at and fearful of their child's lurch into freedom. As a consequence, the adolescent's struggle to write his own life script frequently precipitates the revival of power struggles with his parents, making the overthrow of external authority seem more difficult and sometimes even hazardous.

There are several kinds of families and interactions that can impact negatively on the capacity for agency. Overcontrolling parents may produce either infantilized dependents or rebels. If the price of writing our own life script is our parents' anger, hurt, or withdrawal of love, we may forgo the right to an independent life, making do with the default roles left to us, living by the rules they impose on us, accepting the goodies they give us in exchange for forsaking what may seem like the overwhelming task of assuming command. Alternatively, we may enact a flat-out rebellion that leads to equally inauthentic choices, made simply to defy our parents.

In a good-enough adolescence and young adulthood, our parents will neither abandon nor engulf us, neither punish us nor make us feel guilty, as we differentiate and choose our own paths. Rather, they will gradually give us more and more control, supporting us as we separate and forge an independent identity, restraining us only when there is real danger. Of course, like parents of young children they themselves must be fulfilled enough not to control us but rather to help us to fly free. Even in the best circumstances there is some tension as adolescents and young adults move toward true agency. Parents may be ambivalent— happy to see their children grow to independence but incipiently aware that one of their own great projects, raising and guiding their children, is coming to a close.

Adolescents and young adults are particularly prone to battle with the fears about their capacity for independence and mastery, as the task to become independent outside the protection of the family becomes primary. If they have failed to internalize the capacity for self-control and self-reliance or to develop sound independent judgment, they enter a battle that can sometimes prove fatal if drugs or alcohol are invoked as a substitute for emancipation, independence, and mastery. More often, though, they work out their inner struggles in constructive ways—in goal-directed activities or in fantasy.

Adolescents' transition to full-fledged agency can be facilitated by an independent, strong figure with whom to identify. This may be a parent if we're lucky, but sometimes it is a mentor, a teacher, or an older sibling. Sometimes it is even someone we have only observed from afar or read about or seen in a movie. Adolescents can be remarkably resourceful in going outside the home for such modeling when they need to. One man who deplored his father's lifelong passivity consciously sought out and identified with the more active and assertive of his friends' fathers, and found among them a softball coach who helped make him a star athlete in high school, a gift he now honors by assuming the same role vis-à-vis adolescent boys in need of a mentor. Adolescents also transfer their dependency needs outside the family to friends, and soon enough, the peer group develops its own power hierarchy.

But if in ordinary development adolescence is the crucial time when self-mastery becomes consolidated, when fantasies and dreams of power begin to be inwardly coordinated with realistic self-appraisals and knowledge of limits, I would be wrong to leave the impression that this is a one-chance-and-out situation. If this development has not taken place in adolescence, then the late twenties may bring a quite dramatic change. And if not in the late twenties, then in the mid-thirties, or later still, in midlife proper, or sometimes even at retirement age. The point is that the opportunity is always there, although the right combination of inner and outer provocation, of altered circumstances coupled with new vision, may be hard to come by.

One way children and adolescents assert their independence from their parents is through their discovery that they can keep secrets. Secrets demarcate the inner life as something they may, if they choose, keep private. Also, secrets shared with friends make for strong bonds, elevating peers to conspirators in the lurch to freedom and deepening the feelings of intimacy. Increasing interdependence with peers helps children and adolescents diminish their dependency on their parents, and begin to create worlds of their own, which they imbue with increasingly greater importance. Secrets, something we can confine in our minds, make us feel more important. They also attune us to the pivotal role of our inner life, which encompasses among other things feelings and fantasies.

Mastery and Fantasy: Parallel Roads to Agency

At the same time that children and adolescents are developing self-control, and the rudiments of self-determination and self-reliance, they are also learning to master the external world—that is, learning how to manipulate their environment, to control their world to some degree. They do this in two ways: directly, by interacting with the real world; and vicariously, through the imagination.

Reality-based Modes of Mastery

In addition to their magical investment in make-believe control and power, children and adolescents develop power more realistically. They enter a world of peers, and they learn skills and games—they play cards or ball, study piano or ballet, or play the drums in a school orchestra. They also learn how to manage their time, how to share in household chores, and how to balance homework with the Internet or television. Television and the movies and the knowledge they acquire from the outside world open them to ever-expanding possibilities.

While some adolescents and young adults aspire to master objects, be they yo-yos or Frisbees or pottery wheels, others strive to demonstrate physical prowess—running track, snowboarding down a mountain, playing pool or darts. Still others care for or train animals. The care and feeding of a pet can be a very satisfactory way to establish a sense of control and mastery.

Sarah, a young woman I know, decided at age twenty that it was time to leave her parents' house. A previous excursion into independence eighteen months earlier had ended disastrously when she found herself confronted with the loneliness of solitary life, the formlessness of too many days spent in her own company with nothing to give them structure or rhythm. This time, with an almost prescient sense of her own needs, she got a dog along with an apartment. Lizzie proved to be not only a loving companion who could assuage her loneliness, but what I would call a transitional object in the domain of power. Sarah now felt responsible for the physical and emotional needs of another creature. Taking Lizzie to the vet for her sequence of shots, housebreaking and training her, walking her three times a day, tending to her illnesses, learning the particulars of *her* dog's habits and tastes—all these provided Sarah with a sense of mastery and therefore of personal power, enabling her to make a real maturational leap.

Such interactions with animals are a common feature of growing up. Susanna Rodell wrote in the *New York Times* that "as a child I felt terrorized by the world. But on my horse I was invincible." She said that riding "gave [her] the chance to test [her] physical courage, to take risks, to get respect, to exert [her] will over something bigger than [herself]."[14] These are also themes developed in the novel and movie *The Horse Whisperer*. Much of the story's appeal is in its ability to portray the redemptive potential of our bonds with animals. Prepubescent Grace's relationship with her horse, Pilgrim, allows her to escape the world of her parents, "a complicated world where dominance and compliance were never quite what they seemed," and to enter a world where she could eventually decipher and negotiate the rules of power. It was Pilgrim's spirit that attracted her. When she first saw him in Kentucky "he didn't let her touch him, just sniffed her hand, brushing it lightly with his whiskers. Then he tossed his head like some haughty prince and ran off flagging his long tail, his coat glistening in the sunlight, polished ebony."[15] While *The Horse Whisperer* is a novel that explores the complicated patterns of powerlessness and power as they play out in all the main characters, the description of Pilgrim's meaning to Grace is at the novel's center. Pilgrim gives Grace a world of her own and allows her to inure herself against the complexities of her life. This is what many adolescents and young adults need—a world of their own, a safe context where they can experiment with and master the devices of autonomy.

Many children and adolescents also begin to work, often at home, but often, of course, baby-sitting, mowing lawns, delivering groceries, and so on, to make their own money. On the one hand, these activities provide a sense of competence, and, on the other, they ensure enough money to buy things they want for themselves without being solely dependent on their parents. Adolescents also begin to run marathons, climb hitherto unbreachable mountains and rock faces, and do power-spinning or Pilates at the gym. Some of this is about mastering the world, some about mastering themselves.

From Make-Believe to Autonomy: Generative Fantasies and Life Dreams

At the same time that children and adolescents are performing in the real world, they are also floating fantasies and dreams about what will come, some of which are fanciful, some rehearsals for the future. They begin to practice or rehearse mastery not just in their everyday lives but also in their imaginative lives, quite apart from any Oedipal narratives. Their longing for power is readily apparent in the fantasies, games, and stories that appeal to them. From early childhood on, they begin to try on power scripts in their creative play: "I want to be a mommy, a daddy, a fireman, a cop, a doctor, a scientist, a writer." Sometimes these fantasies predict future choices. But whether or not children literally pursue their childish dreams, these dreams are part of the process of learning that they *have* choices and that their failure to make them becomes in itself a choice by default.

The Pokémon craze revealed young children's budding desire to possess power in the form of control and mastery. Embedded in the Pokémon stories and movies is an underlying fantasy that children have control of one or more of the Pikachus, bizarrely gifted animal-like creatures, who use their magical powers on their behalf. By owning a Pikachu doll, children de facto become Pikachu Masters, giving them the fantasy of accessing power in the world. At least in their imaginations, children are no longer completely in thrall to their parents but have vicarious access to the Pikachus' power.

Children also begin to fantasize alternative lives for themselves. Freud showed how the longing for parental authority invariably undergoes an internal metamorphosis early in childhood, in the form of the "family romance fantasy." In this fantasy, a child constructs an imaginary mother and father who are the "real" parents. Children daydream, for example, that they have been adopted or abducted from their "real" parents, who are generally infinitely superior to the everyday parents with whom the children unhappily find themselves. The children believe that the fanta-

sized parents would love them fully and perfectly in a way that would satisfy all their desires.

The family romance fantasy has at least two sources: children may be
angry at their parents for what seem to be unjust restrictions, or they may
become disillusioned when they realize that their parents are not all-
powerful. Either way the issue is power. Withdrawing idealization from
their unsatisfactory parents and transferring it to the longed-for parents of
their imagination, children create a set of fantasied parents—generally,
though not inevitably, noble, rich, or famous—who not only love them
unconditionally but who are powerful in the external world and can have a
significant impact on it. Thus, the child develops a built-in escape clause
that allows his issues of control to be moved outside the immediate relationship with his parents, and into the wider world. It is as early as this that
our imaginative life begins to play a major role in our real-life adaptations.

At the same time, the family romance acts to strengthen the child's
own sense of self. Bruno Bettelheim argues that the family romance is
essential to the development of personal authority, insofar as the transformation of the good mother into an evil stepmother is an impetus to
develop a separate self. He may overstate this, however, because there is
certainly an instinctual component to the quest for autonomy.[16] But he
correctly emphasizes that a major impetus for the family romance is the
need to "develop initiative and self-determination."[17]

An example of the family romance fantasy can be found in the Harry
Potter novels, which bears out Bettelheim's insight that such fantasies
promote a sense of self-determination and personal power. Harry is an
orphan whose mother and Wizard father were killed by an archwizard, the
villain Voldemort, when Harry was just a baby. As a consequence, Harry
was sent to live with an aunt and uncle, the Durstleys, who are Muggles—
they have no magical powers and hate and fear Wizards. They dote on
their own son, Dudley, and are ashamed of Harry's Wizard blood. Harry is
a kind of male Cinderella, relegated to a tiny closet at the foot of the
stairs, systematically deprived while Dudley is overindulged. One day,
Harry gets to tag along to Dudley's birthday celebration, but Dudley and
his friend get huge ice cream cones, while Harry only gets only a cheap
lemon ice pop.

Harry suffers through ten miserable years of neglect and abuse before
the Wizards send for him. Hagrid, a giant, accompanies him to the Hog-

warts School of Witchcraft and Wizardry, a magic world parallel to the world of the Muggles but invisible to them. At Hogwarts, Harry discovers his magical powers; he will ultimately become the instrument for undoing a conspiracy against the good Wizards, masterminded by Voldemort. The plots of the Potter novels—all based on the idea that even the magical world is divided into forces of good and evil—catapult Harry out of any straightforward family romance fantasy into an ideological war between the forces of good and the forces of evil, each organized around a shared belief system and mission. (Here, early in our lives are the rudiments of our search for causes and belief systems.)

Adolescents also use make-believe to experiment with power. In the fantasy game Dungeons and Dragons (a craze in the 1980s), the players tried to increase their various assigned powers by digging up magic talismans as the game proceeded. To this ostensible objective was added the further challenge of using your wits to figure out how to cope with each new confrontation, whether dragons or sorcerers. Presiding over the drama, like some absent-yet-present parent figure was the "game master," the nonplaying player whose job was to organize the adventure but remain on the sidelines while it unfolded. This was the real power position if you will, available to the teenager willing to renounce his own desire to play and to fantasize.

Adolescents may also experience vicarious mastery through television shows and popular literature. Teenage girls often become enchanted with witches and witchcraft, for example, through movies like *Practical Magic* (based on a novel by Alice Hoffman), which is about sister witches. Witches have been featured in several television series, such as *Sabrina the Teenage Witch*, *Buffy the Vampire Slayer*, and *Charmed*. The Hallowell sisters in *Charmed* have special powers: Pru can move objects telekinetically, Piper can momentarily freeze time, and Phoebe can foresee the immediate future. Magazines and books present witch-related subjects such as astrology, herbal cures, and color therapy. One bookstore in Manhattan devoted twenty-one feet of shelf space to "Magical Studies." Some observers suggest that witchcraft appeals to many feminists because it features female deities.[18]

Andrés I. Pérez y Mena, an assistant professor of anthropology at Long Island University in Brooklyn, believes that witches appeal mostly to middle-class female teenagers, suburban or rural (rather than urban). He theorizes that these girls "have few distractions and even less control over their lives and practice sorcery to exert power over their existence."[19] Such interests are not an adequate substitute for changes in behavior or for social action, of course, but they may be a harbinger of a desire to achieve power in reality, not just in fantasy. Phyllis Curott, a lawyer who describes herself as a witch priestess, says that a witch is attractive because she "stands outside the notion of acceptable behavior—she challenges the power structure, she's dangerous, she's angry."[20] Thus she offers a possibility of power realignment to teenage girls, and to grown women.[21]

For boys, a widespread form of vicarious mastery is found in their hero worship of superathletes. An example is Michael Jordan, who is not only a brilliantly gifted basketball star, but a leader with the ability to pull in his team, almost single-handedly bring them from behind, and win in very unlikely circumstances. Jordan is also an advertising icon and the sneakers and other products he endorses allow his admirers to own a symbolic piece of him. (There is a kind of unconscious identification at play, similar to the identification we make with fictional characters.) Of course, there are some teenagers (at least there were a few years ago), who would argue that Magic Johnson was a better player because he made the players around him better, indeed, made them into perennial winners. He only took the last shot if he had to. Then there is Derek Jeter, the soft-spoken, smooth fielding Yankee short stop, who has the uncanny knack of somehow always being at the right place at the right time. He is also—ask any adolescent girl in Manhattan—oh so cute. But Alex Rodriguez, equally good in the field and only a little less cute, hits for more power. My point is that as adolescence proceeds, the image of the superstar becomes more differentiated and the youngster begins to choose heros who have particular traits that match his own inclinations. The endless arguments over who is a better ball player—and why—that are so endlessly rehearsed that middle-aged men over beer can still recite the main points from memory serve an important function for the young. They are a vehicle for gradually differentiating our dreams of who it would be worthwhile to be like, all of this under the safe cover of seeming to talk objectively.

Concomitant with changes in our behavior and relationships, we toy with fantasies that conjure up both realistic and grandiose dreams. Fantasies of omnipotence can be a defense measure against internal conflict and even fragmentation. Though the reality checks that proliferate in adolescence often diminish the grandiosity of childhood, it is not yet time for grandiosity to disappear altogether. Reluctant to give up fantasies of glory, the typical adolescent may, however, temper them. The psychologist Eric Klinger quotes an anonymous student: "I was one of the top tennis players in the US but was not ranked or anything. I just played for the fun of it and could beat about anybody. I lived in a big house in the mountains with my own private tennis court beside it. I played tournaments now and then to earn money to live on, but I didn't have everyone all after me to be in the papers and play for any teams. I kept going over certain plays in my mind and how good I was."[22] This might be considered a typical fantasy of late adolescence, in that it has been deliberately downgraded in certain ways to keep alive the imaginative possibility that it might still come true.

Many fantasies of early adolescence are so grandiose that they cannot be sustained. Sooner or later, teenagers invariably notice the discrepancy between their fantasy life and what is realistically available, given their own resources and talents. The psychologist Jerome Singer believes that the pain of late adolescence arises in part when the discrepancy between what is wished for and what is possible becomes apparent and many "dream balloons are likely to be punctured."[23] No surprise, then, that from adolescence to middle adulthood, reveries come to center on increasingly realistic plans for work and other achievements.

Many fantasies are related to a career or furtherance of one or another cause. For example, a woman whose mother's erratic behavior tormented her during childhood and adolescence recognized that her mother was psychologically disabled. For a long time, the daughter hoped she could help repair their relationship and make restitution to her mother for the things missing in her life. This never happened, but her rescue fantasy fuels many of her feminist activities. What she could not do for her mother she tries to do for women in general. Another woman, whose father died when she was entering adolescence, watched her mother deteriorate, unprepared to cope with supporting herself. Up to that point this daughter had always imagined herself as a pampered wife, like her mother, but now she became interested in a television show about a woman lawyer and began to see a different kind of life for herself.

Fantasies of repair or restitution are quite common in adolescence. Sometimes they involve self-sacrifice for the good of others, which is especially attractive because it requires control over one's own desires. A dream of doing good often entails self-purification and the suppression of "forbidden" or threatening fantasies, often sexual. (That is, sometimes we use one fantasy to suppress another one.) Our fantasies have various roots. For adolescents and young adults, fantasies are often motivated by a rebellion against their parents' materialism and self-interest. Some fantasies focus not on a happy future but rather on the possibility of failure, loss, or disaster. These fantasies are warnings; they range from self-blame for erroneous judgments to fear of the loss of loved ones to a dread that one will fall prey to cruelty, misfortune, or even madness. The fantasy that one will simply not live very long, which is a fear fantasy rather than a wish fantasy, may memorialize a trauma from early life or dramatize the fact that one does not yet have a life plan. All these fantasies continue their subterranean existence well into adulthood.

Some of us seldom create our own fantasies but still participate in the world of fantasy as consumers rather than producers. Reading fiction is satisfying, in part, as Freud observed, because it puts "us in a position where we can enjoy our own daydreams without self-reproach or shame."[24] Our own fantasy may make us feel ashamed or guilty, or may simply seem too grandiose, but a similar fantasy in the work of an author, a filmmaker, or another artist can be enjoyed and even modified to suit our needs and plans. The creator becomes our secret collaborator, giving voice to our longings.

One of my patients, Mr. Kenney, became fascinated, as an adolescent, with several fictional characters—in particular, Horatio Hornblower, C. S. Forester's eighteenth-century British naval hero.[25] Hornblower is an intelligent and courageous leader, adored by his men, feared by his adversaries; but he is also an overly sensitive man, plagued by self-recrimination and doubt, uncertain with women.

Mr. Kenney would recount Hornblower's passions and fears with great emotion. Hornblower was conquering the world at the same time as he seemed to fear the shadows of his own insecurity. Like Hornblower, Mr. Kenney feared women almost as much as he fretted about his own inadequacy. So he was able to identify with the feelings of his fictional hero, connecting himself with every crest of his career, every trough of his ego. These were stories about Mr. Kenney's feelings about his own life— especially the corporate world that he had come to loathe even as he had risen in it. He had designed and implemented some of the best-known marketing campaigns in the United States, yet he was afraid someone would ask him a question at a board meeting. The similarity between him and Hornblower was so great that a friend who had read one of the novels said, "I thought I was reading about you. *You are* Horatio Hornblower."

Since his adolescence, Hornblower had been important to Mr. Kenney because they were awkward in the same ways and because Hornblower had succeeded nonetheless. The "borrowed" Hornblower fantasies gave him the hope that his limitations need not impede him, since similar limitations had not impeded Hornblower. Fantasies, then—whether we create our own or borrow them—give us direction, hope, and solace in the pursuit of our dreams.

What I call generative fantasies and what Levinson calls "the Dream" tend to crystallize in adolescence or early adulthood. Some of these fantasies are real-life aspirations that we bring to fruition on our own or with the support of a teacher, a parent, or a mentor. The lucky adolescent and young adult will find a slightly older person to act as a cheerleader and mentor or both; some young people seem to know intuitively how to recruit a mentor, even in the form of a fictional character. A mentor serves many functions: moral compass, coach, enthusiast, older friend, adviser, and someone who can sort out conflicts. In essence, a mentor does for a budding adult what a good enough parent does for a child—encouraging growth by having faith in the adolescent/young adult and endorsing his or her hopes and dreams.[26] It is difficult to have a dream and keep to it in any case; to do so entirely on one's own is virtually impossible. And while "mentoring" has become a fashionable topic among successful young people, who seem to feel they have additional "quality time" to bestow on someone, the fact is that a mentor relationship is elusive, hard to plan ahead of time. Still, almost everyone who is truly successful can, if asked, readily identify one or two mentors who were crucial earlier, whether in late adolescence or in adulthood.

Failures in the Acquisition of Autonomy and Agency

Anxiety and dependency are the towering enemies of autonomy and agency. What predisposes us to fear-driven adaptations, dependency, passivity, or obsessiveness—symptoms of a failure of autonomy? By and large, these predispositions are already apparent in childhood. A child may be afraid to go to school alone or get on the bus even though her peers are doing so. If her parents fail to encourage her independence or do not address her anxiety, she may develop a school phobia, may be frightened of spending a night at a friend's house, may be too timid to learn to ride a bike or ice-skate, may be unable to go on a Ferris wheel. Gradually, these symptoms separate her from her peers, and she drops off the path of increasing independence and activities. Her fears also attach to her school work, to her examinations, and act to limit her dreams of what she can become. She retreats into a kind of morbid dependency on her parents. In other children, fear may be more specific. One child, for instance, may do very well in school but fear all sports involving physical contact. Another may be adept at anything physical but may become anxious over an intellectual task.

In some children, anxiety appears to be hardwired; but in others, it is clearly learned. If parents fear for a child's very survival, the child will likely become dependent. Sometimes a child's dependency is caused by clinging parents—dependency is at the heart of the parental bond, and the child will sacrifice independence to remain close to the parents. If all this precludes activities with peers, the child will miss out on the spurt of growth so often attendant on the camaraderie of shared adventures.

Anxiety can also be engendered by constant criticism or disparagement of the child's first attempts at independence. It may also be a result of trauma—illness, an accident, or the loss of a caregiver. One woman's anxiety began in her early years, when she was hospitalized for a ruptured appendix. Thereafter, her parents treated her as a child who might be lost if they did not constantly keep their eyes on her. Through their oversolicitousness, she was socialized into an abject dependence. Her first awareness of her disability came when she felt invisible in social interactions; she realized that while she might appear to participate, she was experiencing herself as an observer.

Our tendency to idealize our parents or surrogate parents, to see them as the energy source from which we derive vicarious power, can persist far beyond childhood. If our parents foster dependency, we may fail to exert our will. Then, being loved—not self-reliance—becomes the prerequisite for our sense of wholeness. (Alternatively, we may be caught in a downward spiral of adolescent rebellion.) If children fail to develop a sense of personal power, they will be susceptible to recurrent separation anxiety. They may also rely excessively on others as a source of strength. And they may give up the goal of personal power, regressing to a wish for a distorted form of interpersonal power: wholesale dependency, sometimes camou-flaged as romantic love in which submissiveness and ingratiation, rather than mutuality and interdependence, are paramount. Then, dependency and love may become symbolically interchangeable.

Parents may inhibit their children in many ways—by declaring an activity dangerous (for example, climbing trees or playing stickball) or bad (for example, disagreeing with one's parents or masturbating). Unfortu-nately, such inhibitions do not always remain confined to the orginal con-text but tend to spread to other areas. This is true of nonsexual and sexual inhibitions. Thus, an inhibition might begin with injunctions against masturbation, but the resulting frustration alters the child's self-image and impairs the child's ability to make choices or to become the author of his or her own life story. The original idea, "I cannot do *that*," becomes broader—"I cannot *do*," referring to assertion of any kind. Similarly, if an inhibition begins with self-assertion, it often overflows into sex. A renun-ciation of assertion in any behavioral area reverberates elsewhere.

Later in life, failure of autonomy is evident in an inability to control and regulate gratification. A man is unable to stop smoking even when his doctor tells him he has emphysema. A fat woman says she hates being fat but cannot stop eating. Sometimes, of course, our need to feel that we are in control over our own bodies can go over the edge and become hyper-control, and then we may find ourselves in the realm of anorexia. An anorexic has what would be for most of us an amazing ability to control her eating, even to the point of starvation. However, the other side of the coin is that she cannot easily reverse the process, and may not be able to force herself to eat enough to stay alive. Such problems are generally entwined with dependency problems.

Caroline, an intelligent and creative young adult, functions best in structured situations. Although she was relatively symptom-free in col-lege, after graduation she was unable to choose a career. She eventually found a job, but it is not commensurate with her capacities and offers her no future. Not only is Caroline stymied in charting her own life course (a failure of agency), but she also suffers and struggles with issues of self-control—she has bulimia. Her binges of gorging and vomiting relieve the free-floating anxiety she often experiences when alone, but each binge lowers her self-esteem even more, and in the long run increases her anxi-ety and undermines her self-control.

Caroline disguises her inability to form a life plan by signing on to others' projects. She can act, and be assertive, on behalf of her friends' interests and causes, though not on her own behalf. If she's involved with a boyfriend, she's deferential and takes the blame for whatever goes wrong, taking a submissive, almost masochistic, position. Her overeating and bulimia seem to be part of these dynamics. Her passivity suggests an identification with her mother, who was overcontrolled by *her* father.

We may fail in self-care, autonomy, or mastery when we identify with parents who were impaired in the same way. Not only identification with a parent who lacks personal discipline but also rejection of a parent who is obsessive about self-maintenance may skew our sense of proportion. Some overweight women had a mother who was committed to appearance and beauty and valued little else. The daughter's extra pounds are sometimes a reproach to the mother for being too narcissistic to pay attention to her child.

Failures in self-determination lead to extreme dependency and are a frequent reason that young patients enter therapy. A markedly dependent twenty-four-year-old woman undergoing psychoanalysis for agoraphobia (anxiety in open spaces) at the insistence of her increasingly frustrated parents plaintively announced to her analyst early in treatment: "I am a very simple girl and would be content to lie on your couch forever." While the first part of the statement was an accurate assessment of her current adaptation, the second revealed her unconscious purpose in coming for treatment. Not surprisingly, her dreams had a predominant pattern, expressing the hope that the therapist would offer magical gratification. The following dream was typical:

> She was in the dining room of her therapist's home. The table was bountifully stocked with food. The therapist sat down at one end of the table, the therapist's spouse at the other end. Then she sat down with their two children and felt herself one of them. She awoke pleased and happy.[27]

It is hard to imagine a more primary dependency than this. The wish is undisguised and fulfilled. The food in such dreams is a symbol that harks back to one of the earliest gratifications of a need, the relief of hunger.

Another patient used essentially the same symbol, but with a different twist. Sooner or later, all patients realize that the therapist will not fulfill their magical expectations. When this happens, they feel deprived and respond with anger. In this case, a young man had just been presented with his first bill. Until then, the patient's pattern was to recite his troubles almost ritualistically and wait expectantly for the therapist to provide a solution. The bill provoked the following dream:

> He walked into a restaurant and sat down at a table. The waitress was a dull, stupid-looking woman. The patient ordered a seven-course dinner. The waitress brought the food and put it on the table. The patient began to eat, but he had no sooner put the fork to his mouth than the waitress suddenly, with one swipe, cleaned all the food off the table and slapped down the bill. The patient was furious and protested he hadn't eaten yet, but the waitress wouldn't listen and insisted that he pay.

In his associations, the patient identified the dull, stupid-looking waitress as the therapist. He complained that he was being asked to pay for services not yet rendered—that is, the complete resolution of all his problems. He was unconsciously enraged at the therapist for not gratifying his magical expectation that his difficulties would vanish with no effort of his own. In effect, the patient had renounced reliance on his own mastery and instead sought dependency in which all responsibility would be shouldered by the parent-substitute, the therapist.

The dependency fantasies in these two dreams literally make use of food as the substitute for maternal sustenance. For many patients, another symbolic solution to the problem of frustrated dependency is to symbolize sustenance in pseudosexual terms, using either the breast or the penis as a source of dependent gratification. Thus their problems can be disguised as sexual desire, in which a longing for a woman and her breast or for a man and his penis become symbols of dependent security and power.[28]

Dependency can be quite subtle. A woman can be very active in the world, with a full schedule of work, occasions, and "quality time" with her children, yet remain deeply troubled by a sense of impotence, of life passing her by, of never truly being herself. How can this be? When we look closely, we find that her activity is always contingent on getting the "green light" from someone else. Similarly, a man can go the gym five days a week—if he has somebody to go with him. A woman can bake world-class pastries—if her husband makes a point of asking her to do so. He can go to the moon and back at work—if this is what the boss wants. And so forth. Sometimes, you can hear this need for a green light in someone's conversation; he or she has developed a knack of raising a topic, but then waiting for the other person to take a position before weighing in with his own view. In therapy, the ball is always in the therapist's court: the patient will return a shot but will never serve. This may not be apparent at first, if the patient is adept at reading subtle interpersonal clues: he or she seems to initiate topics but has actually decided, preconsciously, that this is what the therapist wants to hear about.

Ongoing dependency produces a need for constant reassurance from our intimates. People who have difficulty "hatching," whether because of their own nature or because of excessive parental discipline or control that discourages independence, will remain vulnerable to anxiety. Their powerlessness and learned passivity produce a feeling of weakness that can be countered only by reassurances from their friends or an "identity marker"—a person whose friendship allows them to feel important. (This represents a perversion of the mentee/mentor relationship, evident, for example, when a middle-aged academic still needs to introduce himself as the former student of a famous scholar.)

Sometimes the identity marker turns out to be a celebrity with whom an individual has had no more than a passing sexual relationship. A beautiful young woman hospitalized in the old psychiatric unit at Bellevue once told me that her mark of distinction was that she was intermittently called on to perform oral sex on a well-known athlete. Psychologically frail to start with, she elaborated this actual but tenuous relationship into an extended romantic fantasy in which the athlete married her and, as a couple, they socialized with his ex-wife, also a celebrity, and her new husband. This fantasy gave her the double boost of socializing with two celebrities; it also incorporated an Oedipal resolution, since the athlete and his former wife were considerably older than she was.

Any apparent disapproval or disengagement on the part of an identity marker can precipitate a collapse or crisis; the individual feels weak and powerless and experiences intense anxiety. The actual threat may be very slight—an omission, perhaps, rather than a direct act (for example, not receiving an invitation to a prestigious annual dinner after having been invited in previous years).

Any impairment of agency and autonomy is detrimental to the personality as a whole. Carl, a man in his late thirties who looks at least a decade younger, still thinks of himself as a boy, dresses like a teenager, and remains emotionally dependent on his aging parents. Although he visits them only three or four times a year, he is in constant contact with them by telephone and consciously takes great care never to say anything that might offend or displease them. Their control over him is financial. They are wealthy, and they have always told him, as an only child, he will eventually inherit all their money and that some of it is already in trust for him, though he has not been allowed to touch it. No matter how old he is, they still think he is unable to manage money on his own. This is just one aspect of the systematic way they have undercut any belief he might have had that he was able to make independent judgments. Originally, Carl tried to gain his parents' good opinion through submissiveness. But then he turned the tables on them by refusing to work. This has terrified them and forced them to continue supporting him, giving him the gratification of seeing himself as a rebel, and disguising the fact that he is as dependent as ever.

A common reaction to impaired agency and autonomy is an attempt to develop power in one arena to compensate for powerlessness in another area. Some of us respond in "weak" ways, turning to alcohol, drugs, food, or sex; some try to extract validation from others. We seek reassurance from friends, revive an activity or interest in which we once succeeded, or soothe ourselves with shopping (spending money is a symbol of power). If we fail to establish a sufficient sense of mastery, we may revert to daydreams of power in the form of domination over others or, vicariously, in a preoccupation with the rich, the famous, and the powerful.

There are also those who react against their own sense of paralysis through defiance, antisocial behavior, and self-destruction. Here I want to underline the risk of becoming destructive. If, as Rollo May insisted, powerlessness leads most readily to violence, then humiliation must be the trigger. And a person who is not in command of himself or herself, who is not a self-directed agent, is likely to encounter humiliation at every turn.

Paradoxically, however, our very limitations sometimes become the spine on which we come to hang our professional success. One man used his submissiveness and dependency to achieve success in a cutthroat industry. With him, I first came to appreciate the psychological importance of internalized conversations—conversations with others that we run in our mind, supplying the lines for both participants. Unlike most patients, he reported what happened to him almost exclusively in terms of "he said, she said." It didn't dawn on me for a long time that this form of communication mirrored the content of his thoughts; his stream of consciousness was based on conversations—remembered conversations, rehearsals for future ones, or conversations he never intended to have but used to clarify his ideas. Unlike most of us, he always gave the best lines to the other person. His very real business acumen resulted from his almost supernatural ability to intuit the needs of his immediate superiors, the result of his intimate knowledge of the thinking processes of the other that was rehearsed so often in his head.

These conversations, whether replays from the past or rehearsals for the future, served a multitude of functions. The conversations he remembered having with his grandfather, for example, served as a guide to good behavior. His grandfather's advice, suggestions, and prohibitions, rather than being internalized in his own voice, remained in his mind in his grandfather's voice. His grandfather had been the dominant figure of his childhood, particularly because he felt that he had never lived up to his parents' expectations and recognized that they considered him inferior, intellectually and physically, to his sister and brother. Though his mother was at times verbally abusive and his father sometimes physically transgressive if he ignored their injunctions, he still loved them. But their disapproval made him wary with women—fearful that they would find him less than interesting. This had interfered with his forming a deep love relationship with any woman with but one exception. The one exception, however, boded well for his future growth, because the woman he married was no slave to others' opinions but a free spirit. His choice was the first sign that he respected rebellion and that he longed to break away from his family.

His idealization of his grandfather was projected onto his bosses, whose expectations, as I noted above, he usually figured out in advance through his internalized conversations. This gift, neurotic in origin and sometimes constricting him personally, served him well professionally, and he was promoted to jobs with more and more responsibility. When he had risen high enough that it became essential for him to make independent judgments, he felt a crisis of confidence, acutely aware that all his decisions had previously been filtered through the make-believe conversations he had in anticipation of any meeting with a boss or even a colleague. But he weathered this crisis, too. His is an apparently paradoxical course of development in which submission and the ceding of authority to someone else indirectly led to his expertise, to preeminence in his field, and ultimately to an internalized sense of independence and agency.

I BEGAN THIS CHAPTER by quoting Hanna Arendt, who said, in effect, that one needs the will to insert oneself into the human world in word and deed. This requires courage, but also more than that. For where the roots of personal power, of agency and autonomy, have withered, the courage to take steps against the person we hold responsible can become transformed into vengeful fantasy or worse, impotent destructiveness, whether directed against the self or another. This may be how the stunning, unprovoked, incomprehensible violence we read about in newspaper headlines first gets hatched in an individual's mind. Consider the following headline story, which was once well known, and its most surprising denouement.

In 1959, at the trial of Burton Pugach, a lawyer then in his thirties, Linda Riss, a secretary in her twenties, testified that she had tried to break up their relationship after discovering that Pugach was married. In response, he threatened to have her "blinded by acid" if she refused to marry him after he got a divorce. Evidence showed that he then hired an accomplice who threw lye in her face. He was convicted of maiming and other crimes.[29]

Shortly after his release from prison fourteen years later, Pugach married Miss Riss, prompting a considerable number of headlines. But the story did not end there.

In 1996 Pugach, still married to Linda Riss, was charged with threatening to kill another woman after she broke off a five-year affair with him. His wife testified that he was a "wonderful, caring husband." He was acquitted of criminal charges and convicted only of noncriminal harassment. In an interview in the winter of 2000, Pugach said that from then on there would be no more women and no more trouble. His wife, then sixty-three, looked back on the saga almost wistfully: "It was melodrama, but now it's sort of dull, like anyone else's life. We are now like an old married couple." She sounded nostalgic, even though the lye had destroyed her vision in one eye and had damaged the other so badly that eventually she was completely blind.

In summing up the story of his life, Pugach said he "regrets every day for what I did to my wife . . ." but claimed that extenuating circumstances, professional setbacks, and alcoholism had left him unable to cope with their breakup. What is strikingly telling about his closing remark to the interviewer is the metaphor with which he summed up his situation: "Since my release from prison, I've had complete acceptance from this community. No one would throw this in my face."

This metaphor, given the violent act he chose, seems bizarrely appropriate to capture how he feels—how every psychologically impotent person feels—in response to criticism or confrontation. To him, criticism is having something thrown in his face, and this is likely a clue to the way he felt in early life—blamed, chastised, criticized, humiliated. It is surely not coincidental that he chose to hire an accomplice to throw lye in the face of someone he believed rejected him, as a mode of restoring his own personal sense of agency. His story is reminiscent of a number of recent cases in which fired employees seek retribution on bosses and fellow workers through shooting sprees at their former place of employment. Having a job taken away from them meant losing the very thing that made them feel functional and made them feel they were in charge of their lives.

The story of the now "dull" Pugach-Riss couple is remarkable, of course, because Pugach appears to have found his true love match in the long-suffering Linda Riss, whose dependency, it seems, has outweighed her instinct for self-preservation, let alone self-assertion. In a relationship such as this, where the ordinary resources of personal power were so strikingly absent, love is truly blind.

Finally, I want to make the point that personal power does not depend on talent, gifts, or achievement in the world, though it certainly can be enhanced by them. Indeed, personal power often appears in a gritty response to adversity, as though a latent life force is awakened. For example, our strength can first emerge when we face a serious medical problem. We sometimes encounter people who have indeed been crippled since childhood, figuratively as well as perhaps literally, people whose disabilities have caused them to succumb to their parents' oversolicitousness, or overprotectiveness or, in a different scenario, to the wounded narcissistic rage of parents who can not bear to have a "defective" child. But just as often, we encounter people who have been impelled to greater independence and self-reliance by an early disability. Alfred Adler, the originator of the idea of an "inferiority complex" (if not the exact phrase), made a special point of this, emphasizing that some people learn to compensate for their difficulties and may even develop special talents as a result. Adler was equally perceptive in describing the neurotic variant of this process, in which early disability gives rise to demands for special treatment—invariably accompanied by episodes of defensiveness and outright hostility when these demands are not met.

Many of us first find the upper register of our strength in times of acute trouble. Extreme circumstances reveal just how important it is to us to maintain some command of the situation. For example, definitively learning whether we do or do not have a specific illness may cut anxiety even if the outcome is negative. A study from The Center for the Biopsychosocial Study of AIDS at the University of Miami found that patients who tested positive for HIV (sero-positive) "display clinical levels of anxiety, intrusive thoughts and avoidant responses during the week of sero-status notification. These measures returned to their initial non-clinical baseline levels within five weeks after notification in both the sero-positive and sero-negative groups."[30] By and large, we can cope with bad news because it allows us to focus on a plan of action, whereas uncertainty increases anxiety.

Similarly, gene testing for breast cancer in women with a family history of the disease provides information that allows them to make informed decisions. Angela, a woman in the genetic testing program at Memorial Sloan-Kettering, had a constant round of mammograms, sonograms, MRIs, breast exams, and biopsies for more than twenty years because there was a history of breast and ovarian cancer in her family. Her family history and the medical tests were thrust on her by fate. From the outside one might not see how mastery or personal power might be involved. Then gene testing became available.

Being tested and found negative is obviously a relief. But, to repeat, being found positive, while clearly not the desired outcome, gives the individual a chance to exert some control. Angela originally chose to be tested because she discovered there was a chance she could be negative— one of her relatives had turned out to be negative. When she was told on the phone to come in for the results, she knew the news would not be good; otherwise they would have told her on the phone. Angela did test positive. Nonetheless, she felt empowered because she "knew what she was looking for." After careful deliberation, she decided on a bilateral mastectomy, believing that it was the right decision even though she as yet had no disease. Her choice gave her the time to talk to different surgeons and to determine who she thought was the best. As it turned out, on microscopic examination postsurgery, the doctors discovered that she had an intraductal carcinoma; it was in the earliest stage, so the intervention was effective. "I feel I made all the right decisions for all the right reasons and as a result I sleep very well at night," Angela said. "I believe genetic testing saved my life."[31] For Angela, the basics of personal power were there all along, but the crisis only brought them out. This is what autonomy and agency are all about.

9

Men, Women, and Personal Power

"A man of about thirty starts as a youthful, somewhat unformed individual, whom we expect to make powerful use of the possibilities opened up to him by analysis. A woman of the same age, however, often frightens us by her psychical rigidity and unchangeability. . . . There are no paths open to further development; it is as though the whole process had already run its course and remains thenceforward insusceptible to influence—as though, indeed, the difficult development of femininity had exhausted the possibilities of the person concerned."

SIGMUND FREUD, *"Femininity"*

Regardless of gender, we all face the same basic life tasks and challenges. We each must establish an independent identity; develop and manage our relationships; develop our capacity for self-assertion, self-determination, and autonomy; find a means of support; seek pleasure and creative outlets; establish meaning in our lives; and face and come to terms with loss and death. But we will each approach and cope with these shared human challenges in different ways. That said, some of the approaches differ because of gender.

Men and women seem to have their own set of psychological vulnerabilities and strengths, though there is a great deal of individual variation. At each stage of life, men and women experience different pressures and expectations from themselves, their families, and society. Consequently, to some degree men and women will seek different paths to power and will experience different psychological and role conflicts in relation to issues of power.

Sigmund Freud, brilliant though he was, was as biased about women as his contemporaries. He believed that masculine personality traits were the norm. Women, he suggested, "retreated" into their feminine personality traits when they discovered at a very early age that they could not be the men they "naturally" wanted to be. His explanation of female psychology was based on what he called "penis envy." His theory was that as soon as a little girl discovered that she had no penis and could never hope to have one, she felt shocked, deprived, inferior, and angry. To resolve this conflict she normally began to retreat into a submissive, passive, masochistic, childish personality. She then began to form dependent attachments to men and in so doing found some kind of substitute for her own missing penis.

Freud believed that penis envy rendered a girl powerless, not only in terms of her childhood experiences but in ways that would affect her future. While Freud believed that this pattern was normal, inevitable, unchangeable, quintessentially female, and appropriate and desirable for all women, he made an exception for his female disciples, whose "unresolved masculinity complexes"—so he believed—allowed them to excel.

Only much later would psychoanalysts and other theorists realize that Freud's view of female psychology was mired in nineteenth-century cultural attitudes toward women and that his psychological explanation was far from adequate. Traditional male interpretations of female psychology (Freud's included) involve projecting male psychology onto female psychology. Men's insistence on penis envy as central to women's psychology is in part a projection of their own feelings toward stronger and more powerful men.[1] In fact, men seem more interested in penis size than women are and susceptible to envy—to worrying about the size of their penis in comparison with other men's penises. As I have written elsewhere, penis envy and not just castration anxiety is pivotal in the mental life of men.

When women had few approved avenues for self-assertion outside the nursery and the kitchen, when they had little authority over the course of their lives, when they faced cultural admonitions against their sexuality, many felt shortchanged by life, to say the least. It is not difficult to see how women came to experience psychological distress, probably leading to the so-called "nervous afflictions" that were once so common.

History, it turns out, is the great leveler of grand theories, whether historical, sociological, or psychoanalytical. The changes over the past century in the way contemporary men and women seek power showed that some of Freud's formulations about gender and gender roles were wrong. Women have made good use of their new opportunities, and their residual envy of men, such as it may be, can scarcely be considered anatomical.

Men and women have the same aspirations to power, though in different arenas and to different degrees. Both sexes express power through sexuality and by forming intimate, loving relationships. Most want children, and parenthood confers power in two ways: not only through identification with the powerful parents of one's own childhood but also through the transcendence of reproduction, the projection of some trace of one's self into the future. But women remain the major caregivers, and men still maintain more freedom to exercise self-determination and agency in choosing their life work and in undertaking a variety of esteem-building adventures.

Until the middle of the twentieth century men possessed access to much more clear-cut and socially sanctioned pathways for expressing personal power than did women. This difference can be attributed in large part to different childhood experiences and cultural directives. Gender has implications for power, with men and women living to some degree in separate realities. The major difference still hinges on the relative values the two sexes place on agency and attachment. Men are more apt to favor autonomy and agency—in exaggerated form, what the psychologist Lynne Layton calls defensive autonomy—over attachment and dependency. Women favor connectedness. However, it should be noted that some women now come close to the predominantly male model of autonomy, and sometimes to defensive autonomy as well.

While men's concepts of masculinity have only recently begun to change, women's concepts of femininity were on a wacky, liberating ride for much of the twentieth century. Women's liberation, however, has not been all of a piece. Its two strands, as described by the writer and film critic Molly Haskell, have different ramifications: one promoting personal freedom, the other professional freedom. According to Haskell, "flappers . . . represented one strand, the life style side of the coin: claiming the right to drink and smoke and party alongside men, challenge the double standard. But just as today's sex-and-the-city girly-girl babes look askance at the *Ms.* magazine generation that paved the way, so the flappers distanced themselves from their more earnest beneficiaries, the down-in-the-trenches suffragist-maiden aunts as they saw them—who had cut their political teeth in the Woman's Christian Temperance Union with all its Puritanical overtones. . . . Female characters as portrayed in films prior to a wave of movie censorship in 1934 were still more interested in men than votes, in love than jobs, and for all their sexual gallantry, for all the fun they had and the tunes they called, when the party was over and the music stopped, they looked a little older than the men . . . and it was still a man's world."[2] The integration of these two sides of liberation—personal behavior and professional access—has been decisive for the changes in how women now regard themselves, though it is still hard for women to put together the full package, particularly if children are involved. But to the degree that liberation has been effected, it has brought about profound consequences—both positive and negative—for women and men.

Women

One might claim that we are witnessing a gender revolution in progress, that is, a revolution in the roles prescribed for women and men, but primarily for women. The women's movement advocated a radical shift in the ideal feminine role. Traditionally, a woman thought of herself as what Simone de Beauvoir called the "other," achieving fulfillment vicariously through her nurturance of husband and children.[3] Now, fulfillment is seen in terms of the self and sought through personal gratification (including sexual pleasure) and autonomous achievement; consequently, both personal freedom and work have assumed increasing significance for women.

For every person, the sense of self as female or as male becomes the scaffolding around which personality develops and behavior takes shape. Studies now show that little girls and little boys go their separate psychological ways even before they are old enough to recognize that they have different sexual organs. The male brain and the female brain develop somewhat differently after a certain point in fetal life, and this apparently leads to some differences in behavior, including males' greater aggressiveness. Nonetheless, most of what society considers masculine or feminine patterns are acquired, not inborn.

More important than her genes or hormones to the little girl's developing identity is her situation in the family and in society. The process of developing a feminine way of being begins in her earliest relationships within her family. Her parents and the larger culture directly or indirectly teach her about what emotions, behaviors, reactions, and ambitions are considered ideal for girls and what kinds of activities and rewards are available to her as a female. She also becomes well aware of what will be denied her. Meanwhile, the little girl begins to identify herself as female and to imitate her mother. Over time her sense of femininity is also shaped by her relationships with her father and her siblings.

As she gets older, a girl learns still more from the culture at large, including her peer group, about what constitutes normal, appropriate, approved, and rewarded behavior and roles for girls and women. By the time she's out of adolescence, the young woman has formed an ideal of femininity which she will try to live up to and against which she will measure herself. However, in a time of changing mores, such as ours, cultural values may well have changed by the time a girl reaches adulthood. This presents a conflict for some women today: outwardly they may espouse a new femininity, but inwardly they may be influenced as much or more by the feminine ideal with which they grew up.

Traditionally, women learned to value relationships, love, and intimacy as the validation of their femininity, whereas men proved their masculinity through autonomy, work, and achievement. While men, too, seek love and family, and women increasingly endeavor to make contributions in the workplace, each gender still tends to have its own central psychological mission. A man may not feel comfortable in his relationships until he has established a niche in the working world. A woman who has not found love, marriage, and motherhood may feel she has fallen short of the prescriptions of femininity, despite real accomplishments in her career.

For some women, the overriding importance of succeeding as a wife, lover, and mother may make them psychologically vulnerable to certain social factors—among them the relative shortage of men. Wars, men's earlier mortality, and homosexuality have combined to make men a comparatively scarce commodity for women, especially as they age. Adding to this, men in our culture tend to find older women less desirable. The writer Susan Sontag has dubbed this phenomenon the "double standard of aging." As a result, women have a higher risk than men of being alone, and sometimes that risk is enough to make them give up their dedication to a career.

Motherhood, traditionally the defining career for women, is still one way for a woman to assert her power in identification with her own mother—and for many women it is the greatest glory. But some women do not want to have children, and even ardent mothers-to-be have fears and ambivalence about pregnancy and childbirth.

A distinction is often made between labor and work, with labor being less valuable. Compared to work, labor is considered unskilled, consisting of activities like hauling and lugging, pushing and pulling. Perhaps it is no accident that the birth process is called labor, not work. Yet the choice of words is quite striking, given that work is usually said to involve a product—and a baby would seem to be quite a product indeed.

Although a woman might be the angel of the household, hers is also the body that labors to bring forth children. From one perspective, childbirth is a labor of love, but it is also daunting. As the science writer Natalie Angier puts it: "For mothers that will be expected to suckle and care for the young, the antecedent to the arrival of dependent newborns—that is giving birth—is a feat of almost cataclysmic stress. This is true for mammals generally. . . . Yet the role of birth as the crucible for bonding is nowhere better exemplified than it is among woman."[4] Angier points out that unlike other mammals, the human female requires outside help with the birth process, and therefore women want the support and companionship of others, often being terrified at the thought of giving birth alone. (Interestingly, only when delivering babies became the prerogative of the general practitioner or the obstetrician, generally male at the time, rather than of the sister, mother, or midwife did the process of helping birth babies become work.)

No matter how independent a woman may be, pregnancy makes her vulnerable. Giving birth and raising children have shaped women's lives to such a degree that until recently women were limited in comparison with men in the range of strategies they might invoke for achieving personal power.

In the middle 1970s the poet and essayist Adrienne Rich wrote of "motherhood in bondage," arguing that while we "speak of women as 'non mothers' or 'childless;' we do not speak of 'non fathers' or 'childless men.' . . . In trying to distinguish the two strands: *motherhood as experi-*

ence, one possible and profound experience for women, and *motherhood as enforced identity and its political institution,* I myself only slowly began to grasp the centrality of the institution. . . . Under that institution, all women are seen primarily as mothers; all mothers are expected to experience motherhood unambivalently and in accordance with patriarchal values, and the 'nonmothering' woman is seen as deviant."[5]

It should not escape us that Rich is talking about power. She has observed: "The right to have or not have children; the right to have both children and selfhood not dependent on them; these are still being fought for, and this fight threatens every part of the patriarchal system. . . . The myth that motherhood is 'private and personal' is the deadliest myth we have to destroy. . . . The institution of motherhood—which is maintained by the law, by patriarchal technology and religion, by all forms of education . . . has, by the most savage of ironies, alienated women from our bodies by incarcerating us in them."[6] For Rich, women's struggle for self-determination is being fought out in the domain of their female body. She is not warning women against becoming mothers; her aim is "to release the creation and sustenance of life into the same realm of decision, struggle, surprise, imagination, and conscious intelligence, as any other difficult, but freely chosen, work."[7] Rich may be using the word *work* deliberately (or perhaps unconsciously) to imbue pregnancy and delivery with the dignity and self-determination that work, in contrast to labor, connotes.

Historically, women have been constricted in many other ways as well. Until recently, women were involved in conflicts over the very ownership of their bodies. As late as the nineteenth century and the first half of the twentieth, women were expected to respond to their husbands' sexual advances, no matter what they themselves felt. Many women resorted to headaches and psychosomatic illnesses as a way of controlling their own sexuality. (This was an effective tactic but relied on the powers of the weak.) When reliable methods of birth control became available, a troubling question for women was who was empowered to decide about whether or not to use them. A similar question arises over abortion. (While it may be unnecessary to say so, let me emphasize that not all women agree on the answers to these questions.)

According to the social critic and psychoanalyst Juliet Mitchell, "sexuality, which supposedly unites the couple, disrupts the kingdom if uncontrolled; it, too, must be contained and organized. Woman becomes, in her nineteenth century designation, 'the sex.' Hers is the sphere of reproduction. . . . To put the matter in a more generalizing fashion: men enter into the class-dominated structures of history while women (as women, whatever their actual work in production) remain defined by kinship patterns of organization."[8]

Women's emergence from biology and into culture had begun—though in fits and starts—well before the women's movement of the 1970s. Elaine Showalter writes that by the late nineteenth century, the traditional patterns of gender behavior and relationship were undergoing change: "As early as the 1880s, relationships between mothers and daughters became strained as daughters pressed for education, work, mobility, sexual autonomy, and power outside the female sphere."[9] In short, women have been seeking self-determination and a greater degree of agency for well over a century. Even today, combining pregnancy and motherhood with a career makes paths to personal power more circuitous for women than for men.

Far more women work today, including those with small children. While many of them work out of necessity and may still subscribe to more traditional values, many have internalized the work ethic of middle-class men—the overt expression of ambition and the desire "to go the distance" professionally.

Even so, one still hears the remark, "So and so is really successful for a woman." And, indeed, statistics continue to show that women do not reach the upper echelons as easily as men. For example, Laurie J. Flynn reported in the New York Times the results of a survey indicating that although working women have made substantial headway in Silicon Valley, high tech remains a man's world: "Slightly more than half the women surveyed said they worked in high-technology jobs . . . [But] of those women who work in technology, 45 percent agreed they had to 'Fit into a masculine work place' to advance, compared with only 23 percent of the women in the survey who did not work in technology jobs. And 28 percent of women who work in technology said that gender was a significant barrier to advancement, compared with 15 percent in non-technology jobs."[10]

When the barrier to success is external, one is dealing with sexism and the solution is political. But when such obstacles exist, they must also be dealt with by the individual woman, and she must be able to recognize when a problem, however much it has been internalized, is based in external reality. A black professional once told me that the most significant event in his therapy was his analyst's remark that he was suffering from discrimination and not from paranoia. Comparable clarifications spare women the burden of internalizing responsibility for all failures and attributing them to personal deficits—a pronounced tendency for many women. At the same time the woman must be alert to personal psychological problems that may lie hidden behind the invocation of prejudice, even when prejudice is present in reality.

When external barriers are internalized, the problem goes beyond the cultural and becomes psychological; and the solution requires individual change. Women increasingly seek psychotherapy to help them in their search for autonomy and self-realization, which they believe will come through professional or creative achievement. Therapists working with these women are beginning to encounter many work-related inhibitions, which are caused in part by role conflicts, ambition without clear goals, fear of failure, fear of deviance, and fear of success.[11]

Role Conflicts and Role Strain[12]

Role conflicts are best understood in the context of the significant shifts that have taken place among the urban and suburban middle class as a result of the sexual revolution, the women's movement, and the crisis of the family. This triad has both positive and negative implications for all areas of women's lives, critically affecting role expectations and values and pushing women toward work and professional commitments.

Although at its inception the women's movement was grounded in demands for economic and political equality for women, it has progressively focused on liberation from role stereotypes as well. At the same time, there is considerable social alarm over what has been called a crisis of the family. Increasing divorce rates, ambivalence toward parenting, and differences in values between generations have been cited as evidence that the nuclear family is declining. More and more women, fearing that their role as wife may not be permanent, believe that at some point they will be called on to support themselves and possibly their children, and that they therefore require some focal point other than marriage. To put it simply, personal relations are considered unsafe because they do not promise stability. Many women acknowledge that the impetus to work comes at least partially from this fear of not achieving any long-lasting and gratifying relationship.

Thus, feminism can be seen, in part as an adaptive response to threats to women's security from the presumed disintegration of the family—although it may also rationalize further attenuation of family bonds. Consequently, many women have come to consolidate their identity through work, and their professional identity may provide them with sufficient self-esteem to explore other facets of life. Success at work may be a prelude to a greater capacity for love, just as newfound sexual energy may be a prelude to increased self-esteem in other areas. At the same time, though, these shifts are problematic for many women.

Many women are caught in the crosscurrents of change. Despite the dramatic shift in cultural values, old and new values coexist. Lacking absolutes, women are subjected to role conflicts. The realistic difficulties of combining motherhood and a commitment to work cannot be overestimated. For women, the years from age twenty-five to thirty-five are critical for both childrearing and laying the groundwork for a successful career. Working mothers express guilt over neglect of their maternal duties simultaneously with anger at their children for distracting them from their professional commitments. And of course when a woman comes home from work she may still have the problem of putting dinner on the table.

Women suffer, then, from what is euphemistically called role strain—the problems inherent in managing separate and sometimes conflicting roles. But this term does not adequately describe the level of stress working mothers experience—the chronic fatigue, the anxiety, the sense of always being behind, the near panic. This remains true even if a man participates in the tasks of running the house and the family, because the woman, by and large, keeps her role as what I call the "psychological parent."

The psychological parent is the one who takes responsibility for dealing with all the details of childrearing—knowing where the children are, how they are to be transported, who takes over if the child-care arrangement falls apart, and so on. Although fathers may perform some of the tasks of child care, many fathers are better able than mothers to put the child out of their minds and concentrate on their other work. Fathers rarely think of themselves as being "in two places at once," while it is precisely this feeling that causes intense inner strife for many mothers.

(However, this may now be changing among some men in their thirties or younger.)

Even those rare women who seem to put work and motherhood together with relative ease testify to the strain—whether it is recurrent exhaustion, self-neglect in terms of exercise or appearance, or most commonly, a lack of private time, solitude, and the leisure to think one's own thoughts. Those who aspire to creativity may be hardest hit.

Women who seek self-fulfillment through professional achievement as the route to personal power are often literally caught between two worlds—without the guarantees or protections of the traditional world and without role models or the psychological skills required for success in the new world.

Issues of Ambition

Many more girls than ever before are permitted and encouraged to have aspirations related to work. And many young women, like men, are avidly pursuing careers. But this is not true of all girls, and many women who are trying to actively pursue career goals grew up dreaming passive dreams. Some women have fantasized about being famous ever since they were girls. Women in their forties and older probably fantasized about being movie stars; younger women often dream of being rock stars. In either case, the fantasy often turns on the event of being discovered. Few of these women take realistic steps to achieve expertise in acting or singing, but even so, they are disappointed when nothing happens. Fantasies of achievement without effort mirror the career trajectories of the few successful role models most women know about: princesses in fairy tales and movie stars. In these stories, one is rewarded for innate gifts like beauty, not for skills acquired through practice.

Ambition coupled with passivity can be understood as a problem inherent in female psychology or as a problem resulting from socialization. A few psychoanalytic theorists still believe that the coupling of narcissism with passivity is intrinsic to women, implicit in female psychosexual development. But while passivity or narcissism may indeed be important in some individual cases, using these concepts to explain such a widespread phenomenon disregards the long reach of women's experience in the first two-thirds of the twentieth century, when ambition and the desire to work were discouraged as inappropriate.

Marietta Tree, though distinguished from most women of her generation by her illustrious Peabody roots, might be thought of as emblematic of a transitional generation. Born in 1917, Tree, like most of her generation, believed that a woman had only one route to power. Early in her life, she became well aware of the power of her beauty in attracting men, and through her birth into an advantaged class, she knew she would have access to powerful men. According to her biographer, Caroline Seebohm, by the time Marietta was twenty-one, she had explicitly proclaimed to a circle of friends, "I intend to get power through connection with a man."[13] She married advantageously, more than once. Ronald Tree, her second husband, was enormously rich, but their marriage was far from perfect; he was bisexual if not homosexual. When he chose to be buried next to his longtime butler, Marietta wryly remarked that there was no room left for her in the cemetery. She had already taken Adlai Stevenson as a lover perhaps in response to her complicated marriage to Tree. At the time, Stevenson was the American ambassador to the United Nations. In 1961, he recommended that Tree be appointed the U.S. Representative to the UN's Human Rights Commission of the United Nations. Tree, who was originally uninterested in political and economic power for women, had no qualms about exercising the kind of power that was available to her—the power of beauty and charm—as a springboard to achievement. Given a real position she acquitted herself with distinction throughout her professional life.

Dawn Steele, born in 1946, roughly thirty years after Marietta Tree, had more opportunity to direct her own career trajectory, eventually becoming Chairman of Columbia Studios in 1987, the first woman to head a major Hollywood movie studio. Her career began after she ran out of money in college, and took a job answering phones at *Penthouse* magazine. She noticed that just before an amaryllis plant blooms, it looks a lot like a penis, and she marketed this bawdy perception. This was the 1960s, the heyday of sexual liberation, and her idea launched a fad of placing an amaryllis at the head of the bed. She went on to Paramount and, with the advocacy of a number of men, became a producer, with such films as *Flashdance* to her credit. Her stellar career was still enough of an anomaly for a woman that she did not exactly embrace sisterhood; she admitted that she felt "threatened by other women in those early years. . . . I was so busy climbing up the ladder, staying above the water. If there was only room for one woman in a room, I wanted to be her. I'm not proud of it. I certainly don't feel that way now. It was an absolute evolution for me."[14] Unlike most successful women of earlier generations, she did not stay exclusively male-identified.

Nora Ephron, who was given her first job as a director by Dawn Steele, says: "Dawn certainly wasn't the first woman to become powerful in Hollywood, but she was the first woman to understand that part of her responsibility was to make sure that eventually there were lots of other powerful women. She hired women as executives, women as producers and directors, women as marketing people." She was hurt by her reputation for being tough, hard, and mean, although tough, hard, mean men were not subjected to the same criticism. But unlike most successful women of earlier generations (and some contemporary women), Steele moved from an exclusively male-identified self-image to seeing herself as a feminist, who took it upon herself to promote women.

In their careers, women must strike a balance between their need for self-assertion and agency, on the one hand, and for connection, on the other. A full-out push for power in the external world, whether it is climbing an academic or a corporate ladder, may distance women from the intimate world. Knowing that the demands of an extremely strong personal ambition may damage the quest for interpersonal stability, many women have sacrificed their ambitions in order to preserve their intimate ties. They privilege interpersonal power over personal power.

Even without long-standing ambitions, some women may feel impelled to pursue a career—to protect themselves economically, to find intellectual stimulation, or to make themselves more interesting. The creative imperative, the goal of autonomy, of becoming oneself, while admirable goals, are sometimes more easily wished for than achieved. Such an imperative creates especially poignant problems for those women without specific ambitions or passionate interests, who may underestimate the difficulties of finding a direction and pushing the envelope. This is particularly evident when we realize how many successful careers can, in fact, be traced to embryonic interests going back to childhood. Yet many women, from childhood on, focus primarily on interpersonal relations and the acquisition of social skills; this is evident from the books they read, from their preferences in conversation, and from their boredom with impersonal information. Some girls born in the 1980s still prefer a script similar to Marietta Tree's. When they grow up and, perhaps, feel betrayed by the empty promises of a traditional marriage, they may expect a magical liberation through work—once again being passive. Too often, this brings a deeper sense of failure, as they internalize blame for yet another disappointment.

Fear of Failure

Fear of failure is associated with low self-esteem and shame connected to a previous failure, which inhibits achievement-oriented behavior. A woman's low self-esteem sometimes comes from an unconscious identification with a maternal figure who was seen to be either passive or relatively inept in the world outside the family. While mothers may be revered, they, like women in general, are generally not given the same status as men. Whatever its origins, fear of failure becomes self-reinforcing because it precludes the trial and error necessary to develop skills, confidence, and self-esteem. It may be true then, in some metaphorical sense, that wars are won on the playing fields of Eton. Fear of failure is not always conscious and frequently goes unnoticed; in the workplace, inhibitions are often seen as lack of motivation or commitment to more feminine pursuits.

Even when women do succeed at their work, they may not internalize their success in a way that would build self-esteem and confidence. Instead, success is attributed to something external: good luck, a good connection, someone else's encouragement and help. Also, a woman's success may be attributed to her social skills and to key relationships rather than to any real competence. Consequently, some women function imaginatively and competently in auxiliary roles but feel unwilling or unqualified to take the initiative and act on their own behalf.

Fear of Deviance

Until recently, women's jobs have been of relatively low status; high-achieving women were somewhat rare before the 1980s. Fear of success has been interpreted in different ways, but it has been suggested that some women fear that were they to become successful they would fail to be chosen by a man.[15] Fear of deviance can be understood as a special kind of fear of success, to be distinguished from the fear of success that is usually described as a result of a specific neurotic conflict. The threat of social ostracism, particularly by men, is especially potent when we consider that women are socialized so that success is defined primarily as desirability to males and ultimately as marriage—external expectations that are internalized in the ego ideal. Fear of the consequences of deviance sometimes limits success. However, over the past ten to twenty years some of the strictures girls and women once felt have diminished and women are moving ahead full throttle, as evidenced by current medical and law school enrollments and many men are now attracted to high-power women.

A few decades ago, an affinity was often noted between successful career women and male homosexuals, sometimes based on their shared "deviance." Career women and homosexual men had stepped outside conventional boundaries, and nonconformity or rebellion was often part of their self-identity. When they were successful, they shared the pleasure of "beating the system." The affinity still exists, but more now perhaps because of shared interests and the appeal of friendship with the opposite sex without the complications of sex and romantic love.

Special Problems of Successful Women

Women are often afraid to "go public," and this may manifest itself as fear of public speaking and public exposure. Putting oneself forward is sometimes experienced as sexual, not simply assertive, because competition among women is traditionally sexual—the goal of which is to be noticed by men. One woman said that she felt most comfortable speaking publicly when she was pregnant—pregnancy was proof of her femininity. Other women have felt more free to express themselves during pregnancy, and some feel this in midlife. This may be due to an unconscious sense that pregnancy or middle age is a biological safeguard against sexual exhibitionism. (Men, too, may fear public speaking, but the dynamics are different, centering on issues of competition and inhibition of assertion. But of course, women can have this problem, too.)

Women may tend to personalize work situations, a pattern that stems from the overriding emphasis placed on affiliative ties in female psychological life. Some quite successful women may still fail to distinguish their personal career trajectories as separate from that of the boss they work for. Such women, as a consequence, do not consider switching firms when it is appropriate, feel overanxious at times of transition, and hesitate to leave a mentor. Some merge their goals entirely with those of their company.

Sometimes, women also misunderstand power. Far from having a defective superego, as Freud suggested, some women are compelled to speak truth to power, whatever the circumstances. For example, a successful woman might disagree with her boss or mentor in an open meeting and will be surprised at how ferocious his response is. Some of these women have been rewarded, particularly by their fathers, for being sassy, outspoken, and scrupulously honest, and, to some degree, these very attributes, having helped distinguish them early in their careers, are very hard to discard. Moreover some women continue to confuse their relationship to a powerful person with holding power in their own right. Or they confuse status with power. Here again, a focus on personal affiliations obscures the reality of power.

Self-evaluations by women at all levels of achievement are filled with the sense of fraudulence and a fear of exposure. The roots of this fear may be found in the way women are taught to please, to ingratiate themselves, to make people comfortable, even if it means denying their own feelings. In sexual life, this can be seen in the still existing (though diminishing) practice of faking orgasm—*Sex and the City* notwithstanding. Faking orgasm is based on deference to the male, the need for his approval, and the shame of presumed sexual inadequacy. Above all, it is motivated by fear of losing a male sexual partner. If a woman fears that she is a fraud in the workplace, this may be understood as a tendency to dissemble or ingratiate in order to gain approval and, thus, as related to an overriding need for love. Constant pressure to be ingratiating leads to a feeling of inauthenticity, which emerges in different ways—for example in the fears of successful women that their "fraudulence" is about to be found out and exposed. Faking orgasm is *not* the source of these other fears and behaviors, but they are symbolically linked. "Faking it" often has a prominent place in the imagination, even among women who achieve orgasm easily.

What is prominent in the psychological life of many women is not penis envy but fear of loss of love, which belongs with a cluster of traits frequently observed in women in our culture: dependency, fear of independence, fear of abandonment and of being alone, and unrelenting longing for a love relationship with a man. These characteristics do not derive from early development, as so many of the first generation of psychoanalysis supposed. They originate rather in the fear of being a single woman, which in turn is a response to prevailing social attitudes toward women who are still unmarried when they have reached a certain age. Self-preservation then becomes linked symbolically to female-male bonding, which emerges as a preoccupation with finding a partner.

Job and Family

The major unsolved problem for many contemporary women is the integration of work with family life. This problem takes three major forms. The first is that a woman must deal with her guilt over discarding the ideals of her mother and the sense that she may be abandoning her children. The second problem that she must come to terms with is over not being able to be full-out at work—unable to work late or on weekends, for example. But the biggest problem facing most working women, whether they are working to support their family or to fulfill their wishes for self-actualization, is figuring out how to manage the dual responsibilities of job and family. This unsettling situation is often compounded by real concerns over who will look after the children.

Priorities may be changing. The emphasis on the woman as a person and on self-fulfillment outside the roles of wife and mother did not come about simply from the women's movement or from the "me" generation. It was and is a natural outcome of economic conditions and the fact that many married women must work to maintain the family's standard of living. Today, even women who adhere to the values of dedicated motherhood and do not self-identify as feminists may well have to support themselves and their children at some point in their lives, because of divorce, death, or economic pressures. This knowledge, whether conscious or unconscious, subtly changes women's plans, survival strategies, and values.

One more factor—the implications of which have not yet been confronted—is the effect of knowing that old people are no longer necessarily cared for by their grown children. The expectation that one's last days may be spent in an old-age home or retirement community may erode the absolute commitment to provide for one's children, no matter what degree of selflessness is involved. If an intense attachment to one's mother has gone out of fashion, this may turn out to have consequences for mothers' unconditional love of and commitment to their children. As one woman patient in her fifties put it, hers is the last generation to be bound by duty to both parents and children, and she has no expectation that she in turn will receive comparable consideration from her children.

The increase in the number of women working, whatever its causes, has shifted our perception of family obligations and mutual interests. Sheila Rothman has suggested that it is no longer assumed that what benefits a woman—for example, working—automatically benefits her husband and children. In fact, it is sometimes feared that what benefits husband and children depletes the woman. Even so, most mothers are still devoted to their children's interests. They have yet to abandon their commitment to mothering, but they face the problems inherent in mothering and working at the same time—a prime example of the complexities of role proliferation.

Men

Men must find their way in a hierarchical situation at work where they will be judged every day in every way. Since most of what is written about the world of work refers to the middle and upper classes, we generally focus on how men negotiate power to climb the ladder. The quotation from Freud introducing this chapter strikingly refers to the middle or upper classes, disregarding any class distinctions in order to universalize differences between males and females. While many generalizations are apt when comparing the two sexes, some of these are trumped by class.

The fact is that the same problems do not apply across all classes. *The Honeymooners*, starring Jackie Gleason—a classic television sitcom of the 1960s—addresses issues of power among working-class men. *The Honeymooners' Companion* gives us the plot synopsis of each episode: "Ralph is a fat, jealous, conclusion-jumping, bigmouthed bus driver with an ego that is dwarfed only by his waistline. He has a wife who alternately battles and babies him; a friend who is a constant source of companionship, aggravation, and sewer jokes, and a walk-up tenement 'castle' on Chauncey Street in Brooklyn of which he has persuaded himself that he is the 'king' to offset his pawn/jester status in the outside world. In his leisure time, he bowls, plays pool, rails about male supremacy, and dresses up like a Raccoon. Because he is poor and has always been poor (and because his wife is forced to share his poverty) he tries too hard to get rich overnight. Ironically, his crazy harebrained schemes, though doomed to failure, seem to assure him that he is edging ever closer to success."[16] His is the plight of the ordinary man, even to this day, alleviated only somewhat with the boom times that moved many blue collar workers into white collar jobs.

In any serious consideration about paths to power, several variables must be included—not only gender but also class and race. One reason men choose (or need) to be dominant at home is to compensate for their powerlessness in the world. Most men, not just women, live much of their lives in a subordinate position, particularly in the workplace. Men's harshness to women is often more extreme among minority groups or lower economic groups, in which men have relatively low status in the world and thus have an intense need to restore their sense of power at home. This need to assert power underlies the exuberant, macho dress and swagger of many working-class men. But lower or lower-middle-class men are also celebrated as sexually charismatic or as major heroes; for example, Stanley Kowalski as played by Marlon Brando in A *Streetcar Named Desire* or Bruce Willis in *Die Hard*.

Historians, sociologists, and others have begun to look at the impact of the women's movement on male roles and have studied the fears engendered in men of all classes by the changing balance of power between men and women. These changes precede the women's movement. According to the sociologist Michael A. Messner: "The transformation of the United States from a largely farm and small business economy to urban, industrial capitalism both bolstered and undermined the social basis of men's power over women."[17] Because of the change in ownership of individual businesses and farms, fewer men worked for themselves; most worked for wages. To the degree that men controlled earnings there was a new foundation for masculine power and prestige. But because men worked outside the home, they spent less time with their children. As a consequence, women became more responsible for the socialization of boys not only at school but at home. By the end of the nineteenth century, the mother's power in relationship to her children was surpassing the father's power: "women were teaching boys to be men."[18] Moreover, the man, though he might now have more prestige, sometimes had less security than men had when jobs and ownership were passed from father to son on farms and in small businesses.

The very factors that took men off the farms served to catalyze the creation of a new woman, who repudiated the cult of true womanhood and threatened men as never before. Messner points out that while she may have been a far cry from today's new woman, she could and did find work, wanted the right to vote, increasingly sought to live apart without a male head of household supervising her, and claimed a right to higher education. In the early twentieth century, she began to seek the new forms of entertainment available as part of urban nightlife, now accompanied by other women and no longer dependent on being escorted by men. The balance of power had previously tipped strongly toward men, especially when violence and fighting were pervasive; but during the period of industrialization and modernization, which was "more rule-governed and 'civilized,'" the balance began to tilt toward women.

Women's quest for control of their bodies posed another threat to men, as did increasingly open homosexuality. Messner, whose special interest is the history of sports, observes that "the modern institution of sport was shaped during the time when women were challenging existing gender relations and helps to explain the particular forms that sport eventually took."[19] In his view, British men responded to the threat from women by instituting combat sports such as boxing and rugby. In America, bare-knuckle prizefighting was a "solution" to the "rise" of women, part of a masculine backlash in the late nineteenth century against the threat of an incipient feminism.[20]

For Messner, "Modern sport is a 'gendered institution,' . . . a social institution constructed by men, largely as a response to a crisis of gender relations in the late nineteenth and early twentieth centuries."[21] These men created the Boy Scouts of America and sports as bastions of masculinity. Sports became mobilized to define a gender grid that differentiated men from women and high status men from lower-status men. Messner suggests that a culturally dominant conception of masculinity was being forged which was legitimated within and through sports: "Sports bonds men, at least symbolically, as a separate and superior group to women."[22]

The Balance of Power between Men and Women

Undoubtedly, women's gains at work have threatened men's security. Undoubtedly, too, the current intense interest in masculinity and masculine identity is a reaction to feminist critiques of male power and privilege, and to women's entry into what had been regarded as male safe houses—clubs, certain industries, and so on. Moreover, as women have claimed their own sexuality they have made more sexual demands on men. Men's responses have been far from uniform and are in fact quite complicated. Many men felt positively about the women's movement of the 1970s, but some disregarded it and others responded with anger. There has been a mixture of acceptance, guilt, denial, support, and a rearguard refusal to acknowledge change, but on the whole, progress has been steady—and has caused dislocations for both men and women.

One response (perhaps unexpected) was the fear aroused in men, and their invocation of older models of masculinity in order to design a "new man." As R. W. Connell, a sociologist and historian, suggests, "the idea of 'men's issues' created as a mirror image of 'women's issues' of the 1970s, soon turned into a defense of men's interests against women's. By the late 1970s, a number of 'men's rights' groups had formed to oppose women in divorce and custody cases."[23] In 1990, the poet Robert Bly launched a mythological reinvention of maleness to heal wounded masculinity. This movement was based on his best-selling book, *Iron John: A Book about Men*. Bly proposed that men needed to be initiated into manliness by other men and had to celebrate lost archetypes, which Bly derived from the brothers Grimm, invoking the Warrior, the King, the Magician, and the Wild Man.

Connell suggests that Bly's work became influential in "a period of deepening political conservatism, but also a period when the feminist critique of masculinity has powerfully affected the group of men (white, middle-class, heterosexual North Americans) from which Bly's adherents were recruited." Bly urged those men to stop feeling guilty about their privileges and to celebrate masculinity, essentially "to secede from women." Connell argues that Bly's cult of the virile warrior echoed the familiar rhetoric of American self-reliance, worked up by the ascendant right wing into a public celebration of aggressive individualism: "The entrepreneur, the competitor, the self-made man, are proclaimed the reigning heroes of American culture." Yet, as Connell points out, this image has very little to do with the real life of most men. The inherent contradictions between aggressive individualism—a mainstay of eighteenth- and nineteenth-century America—and the contemporary social order, in which most men work in hierarchical organizations, could not be genuinely resolved by a mystic cult of masculinity.[24] Bly's influence has diminished, but earlier his popularity may be understood as an emotional response to changes in the balance of power between the sexes, and also between classes.

The decline of men is the subject—and title—of a book by the sociobiologist Lionel Tiger, and of a discussion between Tiger and the feminist writer Barbara Ehrenreich, moderated by Colin Harris and published in *Harper's* magazine.[25] Harris asked Tiger: "You're worried about men, that they are under pressure—societally, occupationally, sexually—even as women are enjoying a long overdue ascension. . . . What's happening?"

Tiger, surprisingly, attributes men's crisis to the birth control pill. He believes that whereas the social problems of the early twentieth century were Marxist in nature, those at the end, including gay rights, single motherhood, and abortion were Darwinian—related more to a change in the way we control our biological destinies than to economics or class. He argues that "the introduction of the pill a generation ago yielded two counterintuitive results—more single mothers and more abortions. Paternity uncertainty has had a far more volatile impact than anyone would have predicted." Ehrenreich interprets the same facts differently, suggesting, instead, that men are leaving families because they want to. She believes that they resent supporting women "who don't earn their keep" and that the "whole quasi-Freudian psychology in which manhood was defined as holding a job, being married, and supporting your wife [was already] beginning to crumble in the Fifties and Sixties."

Tiger and Ehrenreich agree that power between the sexes is on a seesaw—that is, that empowerment for women has resulted in diminished power for men. Let me suggest that the change in this seesaw may work in another way as well: as men become less self-reliant and more dependent on the corporations for which they work, their loss of independence, power, and prestige may induce women to seek personal power because they fear that they can no longer rely on their men.

Tiger and Ehrenreich's debate emphasizes that our culture is in flux and that gender roles and sexual behavior are changing dramatically, even as the pundits disagree about why. Ehrenreich challenges what she sees as Tiger's concept of gender and evolution—that "the males are the hunters (their path to personal prowess and power) and the females just wait around for them to bring the meat home. . . . By creating this mythical view of our past . . . you made it impossible for anybody to talk interestingly about prehistory for a long, long time." Ehrenreich proposes instead a hypothetical era before "man the hunter" in which men and women cooperated communally. The argument boils down to what Tiger and Ehrenreich believe are the biological limits of human nature. Tiger, having created the term "male-bonding," is accused by Ehrenreich of dismissing bonding of *all people* as their core quality.

While the Tiger-Ehrenreich dialogue is informative and thought-provoking, they share the same bias: both privilege biology, and biology in the form of what ethologists call a closed program—a kind of reflexive action incapable of modification.[26] As a result, they both seem to neglect a major characteristic of humans: our capacity for adaptation and change, a fundamental source of our power. If an animal can learn through conditioning, it must be because of an "open program." Insofar as human beings possess highly developed exploratory behavior, the genetic program of all or nearly all of our behavioral patterns must be to the highest degree open programs. The logic of this is that one "explores" to learn useful things about objects, environment, and people so that *later* one can respond to them in useful ways. If the program were closed, the useful response would happen right away; there would be no "time" to explore.

Men, Women, and Achievement

According to one review of twenty-seven studies on the intensity of the psychological wish for power in the business world, male and female managers have the same aspirations.[27] In fourteen of the studies men scored higher in the need for power; in thirteen studies women scored higher. Upper-level managers of both sexes expressed the need for power twice as often as lower-level managers.

In one study, qualitative differences were found in the way the two sexes conceptualized power: "Men tend to experience power through assertive behavior—having power *over* another. Women tend to experience power by building up their resources in order to have more to give to others—having power *to* support, protect or enable another."[28] This is a good example of how different strategies of interpersonal power get applied to the goal of personal power.

But how was this finding established? Two psychologists, Ruth Jacobson and David McClelland, administered the Thematic Apperception Test (TAT) to a group of approximately 400 male and female entry-level managers. They studied responses "to pictures that were selected to gauge motivation to achieve power." Their responses, both male and female, clustered around three themes: "resourceful power," used to help, support, inspire, or protect another; "reactive power," used in an assertive or aggressive act against someone, especially someone in authority; and "powerlessness."[29]

This research was followed up eight to thirteen years later to see whether the tests predicted advancement, and the findings were as follows:

> Seventy-six percent of women who became upper-level managers had previously scored high in resourceful-power imagery, compared to thirty-two percent of upper-level men and only fourteen percent of lower-level women.[30]

The women who became upper-level managers were twice as likely as men to have seen power in terms of helping, supporting, inspiring, or protecting others. However, the approach women take at work may have more to do with their fear that a more dominant style would be badly received than with any natural tendency to be nurturant.

> Seventy-nine percent of men who eventually became upper-level managers had scored high in reactive-power imagery, compared to a mere ten percent of upper-level women, and thirty-three percent of lower-level men.

Thus the men who became upper-level managers were nearly eight times as likely as women to see power in terms of assertion and aggression. (Not surprisingly, another study found that "women are more effective as democratic leaders while men are more effective in hierarchical structures.")[31]

The majority of both men and women who became upper-level managers seldom experienced feelings of powerlessness:

> Only four percent of upper-level men and seven percent of upper-level women had scored high on powerlessness, compared to fifty-two percent and fifty-six percent of lower-level men and women, respectively.[32]

While men and women use different strategies in their quest for power, both can, of course, be successful. Yet something still holds many women back. The psychiatrist Linda Austin makes the important observation that single women are more likely to be successful than married women. In *Who's Who* women are "four times more likely than equally distinguished men to be unmarried, and successful married women are three times more likely to be childless than equally accomplished men."[33] In a survey of 650 men and women from New Jersey, designed to learn how women understood their progress toward achieving equal opportunity, the political scientist Roberta Siegel found that "housework commanded an extraordinary amount of their attention."[34] Women responded to this with resentment, coupled with passive resignation. It appears to be women's dual responsibility—in the home and in the workplace—that impedes their capacity to be full-out in their jobs. Interestingly, working women did not blame their male colleagues for their plight, but they did blame their husbands.

CHANGES IN the cultural unconscious—shared fantasies and narratives, beliefs and ideas that we hold out of conscious awareness—can probably take hold only over the course of several generations.[35] Differences in the way the male psyche and the female psyche are organized can easily be inferred from the novels and films each sex favors. Women are still drawn more to love stories (stories about intimacy and bonding); men are drawn more to tales of adventure (stories about derring-do and personal power). Some women feel diminished if they stand alone without a man at their side. Men feel diminished if they lose their place in the world of work. What this suggests is that a woman's status depends on her being married and a man's status depends on his perch in the world of work. (However, it is frequently noted that widows adapt more easily than widowers; this suggests that women can function on their own as well as or better than men.)

Given women's ambitions and all the very real changes in women's lives, what still holds women back from a run for the roses? Our lingering gender stereotypes persist, as do the value judgments with which we rationalize them. Our ideas have yet to catch up with the changes that are taking place in the everyday lives of men and women. We may be seeing our culture's lingering gender-think in the recent ascent of Hillary Clinton. Just as she was becoming the most humiliated wife in the history of the world, she was being promoted to celebrity icon, glamorized on the cover of *Vogue*. The culture hadn't been quite ready for a female co-President when the Clintons came to power and it rejected her as part of the two-for-the-price-of-one that her husband said we were getting, but it loved her when she did a stand-by-your-man number. (This suggests that we may be more forgiving of successful women after they have taken a tumble.) Perhaps we will soon see if the culture is ready for a new order. But whatever the verdict, and despite our sometimes regressive judgments of what is suitable male and female behavior, the ongoing cultural revolution offers clear evidence that attributions of power are subject to radical change.

10

Work and Power

*"Because thou has harkened unto the voice of thy wife and hast
eaten of the tree of which I commanded thee, saying, Thou shalt
not eat of it, cursed is the ground for thy sake; in sorrow shalt
thou eat of it all the days of thy life. . . . In the sweat of thy face
shalt thou eat bread till thou return unto the ground; for out of
it wast thou taken; for dust thou art, and unto dust shalt thou
return."*

GENESIS 3:17–19

Work may have begun as the pun-
ishment for our forebears' transgression in The Garden of Eden, but, in
countries like our own, it has become much more than a way of earning
our bread. Whereas in the nineteenth century the monied class priori-
tized leisure over work, our work is now the primary way many of us self-
identify and one of the predominant ways we achieve personal power. The
psychoanalyst W. W. Meissner believes that work has become a cardinal
virtue: "Society tends to cast a jaundiced eye on anyone who does not
earn his keep—whether in the form of the wealthy playboy or social gad-
fly, who seems to do little else than seek self-gratification and self-
amusement, or in the form of a welfare recipient, who spends too much
time accepting government checks and too little time seeking gainful
employment."[1]

Freud believed that love and work were the two poles of our development. Both become measures of our worth, of our self-regard. Some of
us derive our sense of personal power primarily from our work because
it is there that we acquire the personal qualities and assets (the self-
discipline, the approaches to problem solving, and the financial means)

which are needed to realize our various dreams. I have previously quoted Daniel Levinson to the effect that for many of us work *is* the dream.[2] The dream gets refined as we modulate fantasy through the lens of reality. To the degree that we are successful in living out our ambitions and life dreams about work, even in toned-down versions, we experience pleasure and pride, and our sense of personal power increases.

Many of us come to experience work as a veritable celebration of our agency. Our sense of power derives not only from the fulfillment of a dream or ambition, but also from the pleasure of mastery we attain in our specific fields. Doctors must know the human body, its maladies and cures; pharmacologists must know their drugs; mechanics their engines; hairdressers the hair; sailors the patterns of the wind; and businesspeople must know the marketplace and be able to balance supply and demand. We often find pleasure in both the process and the product of our work. Those who look after other people—teachers, dentists, doctors, the clergy—may find their work particularly gratifying. Workers who have some independence and some connection to their product enjoy their work and are proud of what they produce. Take a ride with a carpenter and as you pass by each house where he has worked he will point out the additions he has built, the fences he has put up, the decks he has added in the backyard. Talk to someone in construction and he will tell you which great skyscraper, which underpass, which tunnel or bridge he has been associated with.

Work is connected to power in still another way. I have already shown how personal power and interpersonal power often get bundled together, and this is especially true in our work lives. Success at work is often dependent on establishing, maintaining, and managing relationships with our subordinates, peers, competitors, clients, suppliers, or customers. The interpersonal skills we call on for our work are necessarily somewhat different from those we utilize in our intimate life. In work, what matters is getting the job done, and this frequently requires the ability to cooperate and compromise. Work relationships are generally more instrumental, less intimate than personal relationships but they are nonetheless gratifying. And deep friendships, and sometimes love affairs, develop at work.

Finally, our work positions us in a social hierarchy. The prestige and recognition accorded to different jobs depends on current social attitudes. For example, public school teachers are not as highly regarded now as they were in years past, and a pharmacist can be more important in a small town than in a big city. In large companies, our status depends, in part, on where we fall in the organizational hierarchy, and this generally carries over into our position in the social world. In the United States, our work plays a major role not only in the way we self-identify but in the way others see us. Upon meeting someone for the first time, the opening conversational gambit is often "What do you do?" When I first went to Europe many years ago, I soon discovered that Europeans considered this an impolite way to open a conversation—even though Europe is still much more class conscious than the United States. Perhaps in Europe one's class is obvious and it counts more than work in establishing one's position in society. As a consequence, the kind of work one does is less important in conferring status there than it is here.

How we choose our work is as varied as the choices at which we eventually arrive. Those of us who are lucky have already developed generative fantasies or life dreams about our work by the time we reach adolescence or early adulthood. These fantasies and dreams have many sources: they may be based on identifications or counteridentifications with parents or other adults who are important to us. We may identify with neighbors, friends, relatives, or characters from books or movies. A teacher, minister, or the parent of a friend may intervene to guide us, or serve as models. Some young men and women become policemen because their fathers and grandfathers before them were policemen, just as we see others whose fathers and grandfathers were doctors choose medical school. Some are born into business families where a secure position appears to await them. A few of us have talents which are of such magnitude that not to pursue their development would be almost criminal, whether those gifts are musical, mathematical, or athletic. Certainly among the historically disadvantaged classes, breakout depends on the possession of such a talent, hence the emphasis on and avid interest in sports and music in some minority communities.

Absent a life dream, our choice of vocation or profession depends on a complicated mix of innate skills, interests, talents, exposure, intelligence, shrewdness, and imagination; also involved are social background, educational opportunities; initiative or dependency; or just being in the right place at the right time and the reverse, plain bad luck. A choice can be serendipitous. One boy's absentee father showed up at his sixteenth birthday party and gave him a few shares of stock, which he followed with great interest. Although the stocks turned out to be worthless, the boy's passion had been aroused and he eventually went into investment banking. (We might guess that the young man's interest in stocks served to make him feel connected to his absentee father.) Since vocational opportunities now depend to such a large degree on education, many young people enter college in the hope that they will discover there what they want to do. A decisive event for me was reading Freud's *Civilization and Its Discontents* in my second year at college. Freud's pessimistic tone spoke to me, and I decided to become a psychoanalyst, which meant going to medical school. Of course, it was also during a decade when the cultural influence of psychoanalysis was at its height. Many of us pick up on what's in the air, what's exciting at the moment, and what confers status. In recent years, the popularity of business and the financial world has outdistanced that of traditional interests such as law and medicine. For those who enter the financial world, some are happy with the pursuit of profit and the excitement generated in doing deals, but others complain about being locked into golden handcuffs. With a drop in the markets, business school applications are down.

For teenagers, who may have limited financial resources and few connections, the Army is a major training ground for discipline, selfhood, and a vocation, which often combine to produce a feeling of inner strength. Some companies, such as UPS, love ex-Army men since the work they need done requires both staying within a command structure, never deviating from procedures, and being able and willing to work very hard in return for profit-sharing options. Other companies positively shy away from military personnel feeling that they lack initiative and creativity. One cannot help but note, however, that President Eisenhower had a previous military career, as does our current Secretary of State.

How we subsequently conduct ourselves in our working lives is the product not only of our dreams, desires, and talent but also of personality traits such as perseverance, initiative, vision, and the pleasure or displeasure we experience at work.

The Gratifications of Work

For most of us, the degree of command and control we exert in our work and the respect we receive for it determine how much satisfaction and gratification we derive and how much pleasure the experience accords us.

Much of the personal power we experience at work can be traced to our position in the work hierarchy, as demonstrated in the research of Mihaly Csikszentmihalyi. Csikszentmihalyi defines flow as the mental state accompanying the process of total involvement with life. It is normally correlated with "optimal experience"—a time when people report intense concentration and deep enjoyment. Csikszentmihalyi was surprised to discover that people reported more flow situations when they were at work than when they were at leisure. He observed that people actually work about three-quarters of the time they are at their jobs; the other quarter is spent daydreaming, gossiping, or conducting personal business. It was during the times they were actually working that people reported a high flow. Still, his subjects did not regard work as an optimal experience; they preferred leisure. Csikszentmihalyi considered this finding paradoxical: "On the one hand, our subjects usually report that they have had some of their most positive experiences while on the job. From this response it would follow that they would wish to be working, that their motivation on the job would be high. Instead, even when they feel good, people generally say that they would prefer not to be working, that their motivation on the job is low. The converse is also true: when supposedly enjoying their hard-earned leisure, people generally report surprisingly low moods; yet they keep on wishing for more leisure."[3]

Csikszentmihalyi and his team had not expected these findings. Because the results were counterintuitive, they considered several possible explanations. First, they suggested, people may be conditioned to think of work as a constraint, "an infringement of their freedom, and therefore something to be avoided as much as possible."[4] Alternatively, they suggested, that while there is considerable flow at work, "people cannot stand high levels of challenge for long periods of time. They need to recover at home, to turn into couch potatoes for a few hours each day even though they don't enjoy it."

Perhaps, too, Csikszentmihalyi suggested, "the problem seems to lie more in the modern worker's relation to his job, with the way he perceives his goals in relation to it. When we feel that we are investing attention in a task against our will, it is as if our psychic energy is being wasted. Instead of helping us reach our own goals, we are called upon to make someone else's come true. The time channeled into such a task is perceived as time subtracted from the total available for our life. Many people consider their jobs as something they have to do, a burden imposed from the outside, an effort that takes life away from the ledger of their existence. So even if the momentary on-the-job experience might be positive, they tend to discount it because it does not contribute to their own long-range goals." I favor this last explanation. Workers do not feel they are steering the boat or driving the car; they are not picking the destination. Because they work at someone else's behest, they do not control their own day-to-day activities.

Csikszentmihalyi's observations are important. Freedom from external demands allows employees (at whatever level) to feel self-directed and provides an internal space for self-will, for self-determination. If we cannot find autonomy on the job, we naturally seek it all the more avidly in our free time—even if we are simply looking for the freedom to do nothing. This may be why a husband is likely to be resentful when his wife insists on help with the children and household chores as soon as he comes home—thus denying him his cherished moment of freedom. It is also the reason career women who are simultaneously running a home feel so drained, so cut off from their inner lives and their own desires. They feel powerless despite their success; their dual script owns them, and they do not have the freedom to improvise as they go.

Not too surprisingly, Csikszentmihalyi's studies of managers and supervisors reported significantly higher experiences of flow at work (sixty-four percent) than did clerical workers (fifty-one percent) and blue-collar workers (forty-seven percent). The obverse was true when he looked at flow during leisure. blue-collar workers reported more flow during leisure (twenty percent) than clerical workers (sixteen percent) or managers (fifteen percent). Conversely, blue-collar workers reported more apathy at work than managers did (twenty-three percent versus eleven percent), while managers reported more apathy during leisure than blue-collar workers did (sixty-one percent versus forty-six percent). These findings are consonant with our culture's emphasis on independence and self-sufficiency as among our highest values.

If we think of Csikszentmihalyi's findings in terms of power, it seems clear that being relatively low in a hierarchy at work detracts from the pleasures of mastery. Even if the pleasures of the actual work are real and may be experienced as flow, they are counteracted by an undercurrent of resentment when people feel that their actions are in the service of their superiors. (A perhaps farfetched analogy: a woman has an orgasm in a sexual encounter she would have preferred to skip. The pleasure, however real, is blighted by a grating undercurrent of subordination and shame that spoils the experience.)

Employees at any level become demoralized when they feel that their autonomy is diminished by the requirement that their sole purpose is to fulfill other people's expectations. From this it appears that gratifications at work are correlated with the level of independence we command. This insight leads some managers to favor cooperative governance rather than a top-down organizational chart—to give an illusion (and sometimes, partially, the reality) of participatory decision making. Suggestion boxes, for instance, are intended not only as a source of potentially good ideas but also as a way of letting employees feel they are a part of a team. A more potent device is through profit sharing. And an even more potent device—more significant than money—is to give line workers control and authority over the line. This last option has almost always increased workers' morale and productivity and would seem to be a win-win approach. But by empowering the line workers or their representatives (the foremen) this device also disempowers the lowest level of managers, who now have nothing to supervise. One could always let them go, of course, but that would remove the bottom tier of the salary pyramid, potentially undercutting the entire salary structure right up the line. Thus, what works in one obvious way does not work in another way, and this can be a serious conflict in hierarchies. It is the line workers who ultimately pay by having their autonomy perhaps irrationally curtailed compared with what it could and should be if productivity were the only goal.

Of course, there are exceptions to Csikszentmihalyi's findings. For example, patriotism in wartime makes jobs feel more significant; rather than flying solo and competing against one another, we feel interdependent, engaged in a common cause and standing shoulder-to-shoulder against an external enemy. During the golden age of labor unions, the struggle between workers and the owners provided workers with a purpose in life and a concomitant sense of agency. Workers shared in the power of the unions and were part of a brotherhood. John Kenneth Galbraith observes just how effective the trade unions were: "[they] . . . set the limits to the power of the wealthy, thus serving as a good example of the dialectic of power, that is, its tendency to provoke an opposite and countervailing exercise of power."[5]

Herman Guttman, historian and theoretician of the working class in the United States, emphasizes how the unions limited the power of the wealthy owners through their victories in securing unemployment compensation, welfare benefits, medical care, and retirement funds.[6] These benefits freed the workers from any day-to-day abject dependency on the companies for which they worked. As a consequence of their political victories, the workers felt proud and purposeful. But, ironically, as Guttman demonstrates, their very success took some of the purposefulness out of the activities of the unions, and permitted some of their membership to disengage. Moreover, as the children of the working class rose to middle-class status, the strength of organized labor began to diminish.

Ultimately, we derive a sense of pride and power from our work only when we retain some measure of autonomy, are immersed in the process of work, or feel a sense of pride and power as part of a team, an important political force or of a national effort. For today's factory workers, the loss of pride in their position is twofold. First, there is no longer as much pride in belonging to the union, because it is less powerful in economic life and in the imaginative life of the culture. Moreover, blue-collar workers have lost a sense of security as corporations downsize, close headquarters, or move from one city to another. These circumstances weaken not only the pride, but also the security of blue-collar workers, many of whom fear for their livelihood.

The writer and journalist Michael Lewis writes about the difference between today's work force and the gray-flannel-suit-culture of the 1950s—the era of the Organization Man. Lewis observes that a small but growing number of people have begun to describe their jobs differently, emphasizing what they do rather than their affiliation with what their organization does: "Here were the prosperous children of the great American economic boom, an amorphous, unpinned-downable labor force. They were not full-time employees of big companies, just temps. But there was now sufficient glory in being a temp—rather than a full-time employee with hours and a boss—that a temp was no longer a temp. He was, in new-economy parlance, a free agent."[7] The greater degree of control we have over our own work life, the greater degree of self-reliance and personal power we experience, even if the job itself is far from ideal. Lewis cautions, however, that only about 12 million (according to the Bureau of Labor Statistics), are "workers with alternative arrangements." He mentions these free agents, he says, "not because they are exactly typical but because they point to something that is: a general drift away from old-fashioned corporate order and a tendency toward individualism in work life, especially among those who tend to invent new lifestyles for everyone else—Wall Street, Hollywood and now Silicon Valley." Lewis's observations resonate with Csikszentmihalyi's findings—many of us dislike feeling subordinate at work. Our job satisfaction is tied to our sense of self-determination. We yearn in our hearts for independence (or alternatively for guaranteed dependency), though the majority of us will not probably find either. The fear, distrust, and uncertainty so many of us feel about work as well as our feelings that we are no more than cogs in the machine erodes the power and pleasure we might otherwise take in our jobs.

Pleasure and Power in Different Kinds of Work

We may work as managers, employees, part-time help, small business owners (mom and pops), entrepreneurs, freelancers, or domestics. Different kinds of work require different skills and provide different kinds of gratifications.

Entrepreneurs

It may be our longing for independence that makes entrepreneurship one of our culture's favorite images of freedom, power, and success. Like the more recently arrived "temp" who works on his own and may even work at home, the entrepreneur remains an important icon. Entrepreneurs flourish everywhere, but our country's relative youthfulness and its expansion westward in the nineteenth century fostered entrepreneurs in many areas. While some entrepreneurs have come from families that go back several generations, our culture has been mobile and open enough to provide entrepreneurial opportunities for immigrants as well. We've had the oil wildcatters, the cigar store-to-communications magnates, and the pushcart-to-department store families. Perhaps dearest to our hearts have been the Hollywood studio impresarios, some of whom started as impoverished immigrants from Eastern Europe.[8]

For an entrepreneur, "job description" and personality are closely entwined. Ideally, entrepreneurs get the big picture before everyone else.

Henry Luce, the founder of *Time* magazine (named in honor of time, which he deemed our most precious commodity), believed his own insatiability for the news would be shared by other people—as did Ted Turner who founded CNN. Entrepreneurs are usually concerned with actualizing new ideas and inventing new kinds of business or doing deals. They differ from managers, who are primarily involved in operating a business. Unlike the manager's desire for stability and ordered growth, the entrepreneur sees a new possibility, a segué to a new focus, or a niche that needs to be filled. An entrepreneur is best viewed as an impresario, a kind of producer or director, who gets the show on the road but then lets someone else keep an eye on it. It is not only his originality, but also the power of his enthusiasm and his charisma that so often closes the deal. Entrepreneurship is an ideal role in which we can enact our fantasies of living by our wits, prospering by our initiative, and dazzling our associates. (My definition excludes many of the classic categories of entrepreneur—for example, the owner-proprietor of a small business whose primary purpose is to insure a steady living.)

Innovative entrepreneurs sometimes like to see themselves as the cutting edge of social change. Often, though, the entrepreneur's motivation has been interpreted narrowly as a wish for profit. The economist Joseph Schumpeter emphasized the entrepreneur's importance to technical progress; but Schumpeter nonetheless believed it was the possibility of making a profit that prompted businessmen to seek more efficient methods and to risk introducing them.[9]

Psychologically, however, entrepreneurs may be motivated as much by the ongoing excitement of risk-taking and negotiation, of achieving command and control, as by the possibility of profit. They are sometimes motivated as much by the promise of action as by the opportunity to make their mark on the world or to make a profit. Their motivation is well expressed in a quote attributed to Andrew Carnegie: "It is the *pursuit* of wealth that enlivens life; the dead game, the fish caught, becomes offensive in an hour."[10] Most entrepreneurs live for the ongoing game, the fish not yet caught, for the interpersonal maneuvers and coups that give birth to business ventures. Their need for action is such that many of them reenact cycles of boom and bust, never consolidating when they are up, never giving up when they are down. This is almost inevitable, given their psychological propensity for taking risks and for action.

Ingenuity, that archetypal American quality, is at the heart of the nation's romance with the entrepreneur. Many entrepreneurs are authentically creative, coming up with new ideas and detecting a change in the wind. In addition, they generally share a keen ability to turn interpersonal encounters to their own ends. They often exert their influence through persuasion and manipulation, mediated through charm and enthusiasm—a nonsexual kind of seduction. Entrepreneurs must be sufficiently enthusiastic about their projects to ignite a fire in others. This fire illuminates their self-image and stabilizes their sense of self.

New York City is, of course, a center for all kinds of entrepreneurs, but perhaps those most closely associated with the city and its changing contours are its real estate magnates. Gordon, who grew up poor, relates the serendipitous process by which he found his calling—a calling made possible only because he possessed the requisite gifts.

> I probably am now, in my life, at the height of power and it didn't come because of an effort or a consciousness to get there. Slowly, over the last ten years, I just went from day to day doing deals and getting involved in civic and industry type things and schools and all these other things, kind of like, it grew. I remember that Tevye in *Fiddler on the Roof* sings "If I were a rich man"—remember that song? He says, when you're rich, people believe anything you tell them. They think you're very wise. I think it's true at a workman's level. Working people will look up to their bosses and figure anything they say is the gospel. But at the level that I live my life, this is not true. You have to prove yourself every time you do something. Now, it's by deed, it's not by position.
>
>   I never thought of myself as smart, but I had command of friends from early on. When I was just a youngster—I'm talking seven, eight, nine, ten years old, the whole society of boys that I hung out with always revolved around me. I set the tone for what we were going to do, when we were going to do it. I never thought about it. I mean I wasn't the strongest kid, so it wasn't a bullying kind of thing. It was a mental exercise, or mental exercises. As I grew older, that continually happened to me. [Here he is talking about the "automatic deference" that charisma commands, and how early it is evident.]

It started out, not from having so much self-confidence, because I don't think that's what I had; I think it was just the reverse. I think that it was a way of overcoming my inferiority feeling as a child. Because my mother never gave me a feeling that I was a smart kid—just the contrary. When I was in about the fourth grade, she got called to school. She never went to school, she never looked at my report cards, she never looked at anything. I was holding her hand, and the teacher, Mrs. Walsh, said, "I want to skip him a year in school." And my mother said, "Why would you want to do that?" She said, "Well, because he's advanced beyond the fourth grade and we've got to put him in the sixth grade." And my mother said, "He's not so smart. Why would you want to do a thing like that?" So I'm standing here listening to this, and the two of them are having a quiet argument over me. The teacher says, "Yes, he is," and my mother says, "No, he's not." And she storms out of the school. She wouldn't give me permission to skip. So I didn't skip until the seventh grade—I went from the seventh to the ninth grade. But it must have seeped into my subconscious; after all, if your mother thinks you're dumb, you have to be dumb! How can you be smart if your mother thinks you're dumb?

So, I think that this played for me very, very heavy. And when I went to high school, then I mingled with these really smart kids. I thought I was in a group of smart kids [in grade school], and all of a sudden I see smart kids in Bronx High School of Science that are beyond anything I ever knew. It wasn't hard to have a kind of inferiority complex again. I mean I did pretty well. You know, I ran about an 85 percent or 87 percent average in that school, and that was like ten points added to your grades for any college that you went to. However, there were so many kids that were geniuses in that school. But not all of them ended up being successful, and not all of them looked like they were going to be successful in life. I continued to be the leader of my group of friends. [Being smart helps even if you don't know you are smart. He gets into a school that is very hard to get into, yet denies that he is traveling on his intelligence. But being smart is not enough.]

After high school, I went into the army, and decided not to get killed. It was 1950. The Korean War was at its height. There were huge casualties. It was right after the Inchon invasion. After being in the army for two or three weeks, I did very well on my exams there—the test scores—and I was in Fort Hood, Texas, and I decided that I was not going to go to Korea. So I went out looking for a job in the army. I'm a twenty-one-year-old kid. I mean, when I think back about the balls that I had to do this! I put on my class A uniform on a Saturday, and I'm still in basic training. I went around to every personnel office asking for the officer in charge. I'm at the lowest level in the Army you can be, because I got drafted. I kept asking if they needed help, like a job. Finally I walk into one guy's office, a young guy—couldn't have been more than twenty-seven or twenty-eight years old. It's Saturday morning and he's working like a dog. He was an enlisted officer reserve, who got called back, and he was pissed.

I told him I wanted to work there. "Why?" he said. "Because I can do anything." So he calls over to my battalion and gets my records and says, "OK, I'm convinced." He transferred me out of my unit into his office, starting there Monday morning. I worked in that office and I did the things I'm good at. I reorganized the place, and then I got promoted after four months to the day, from private to Pfc to corporal and then to sergeant in four days. He wanted me to run the office, and the only way he could do that was he had to get me a sergeant's rank. [Not only is Gordon smart, but he is also proactive, understanding that he has a shot at changing circumstances, controlling his destiny.]

The drive and the fire are going on continually, from being a little boy all the way through school and high school and in the army. [Here he finally acknowledges his drive.] I get discharged, and I've got to figure out what I'm going to do with my life. I was friendly with a guy in the New York state legislature, and he was teaching at this law school, and I went to see him. I asked him what I should do with my life. He said I could do whatever I wanted to do, and my other friend said I should become a lawyer. That's what I did—I decided to go to law school.

I went to this one law school because it had a night school and because my friend said, "You're going to get on Law Review." To get admitted to law school was beyond my expectations. [He makes Law Review and segués into real estate through a friend in the business.]

I realized that it was very easy to outfox most people. I didn't make a concerted decision on how to negotiate. It's such a combination of factors, including the old inferiority stuff that rose every once and a while, and now my renewed confidence in my intellect and my ability to see things that some other people couldn't see both in deals and in people. At the negotiating table, I never tried to show the other guy that I was smarter than him. The objective was only to make the deal. That far outshone whether they thought that I was smart or not. After a while, deal after deal after deal and you build a string of successes and get involved in so many outside projects that the reputation just grows with it. . . . If you're doing it intuitively, then your whole personality and intellect come into play, responding more or less to the circumstances. If you try to plan it or plot it, it's very easy to make mistakes. [This is his intuition or instinct for "getting" what the guy on the other side of the table wants or needs.]

I think of myself as having achieved power. But in a very soft, subtle way. I mean, I'm a leader in an industry that is one of the most powerful industries in the United States. I'm on maybe fifteen different boards, civic and educational boards. I've dealt with my life, going from situation to situation without having a game plan, so to speak, and without thinking of what I was doing as an achievement, but just going on to the next thing.

Mr. Gordon conveys some of the mental quirks and habits of mind that work for many entrepreneurs. In part, he relies on how to "outfox" someone else. This kind of shrewdness is not necessarily correlated with a high IQ, but relies on an intuitive reading of the other person, and the ability to improvise on the spot. This gift may be close to what Elias Canetti had in mind when he said that, "These are days when no one should rely unduly on his 'competence.' Strength lies in improvisation."[11] Not all entrepreneurs have the same gifts, but all of them do have a particular kind of intelligence that enables them to see and seize the opportunity, a personality that is by no means risk averse, and a kind of psychological savvy that immediately understands interpersonal nuance—

a keen grasp of what someone else wants and needs. They also have a sense of how pieces of reality can be fitted together to create a differently designed product or deal, a slightly different angle, or a sense of how different the near future can be from the present. For many of them, the pleasure is as much in the action as in the profit.

Corporate Life

Managers at all levels—from the CEO down—are by and large a different breed from entrepreneurs. Responsible for first defining and then meeting the goals of the corporation in which they function, successful managers must be able to crystallize the company's goals, to draw the big picture and get "their" people committed. Therefore, interpersonal concerns— how to influence or control those below you and above you—are paramount. Some of the most practical insights into effective leadership come not from psychologists but from people who've been there, done that. This is evident in a story the management consultant and psychoanalyst Abraham Zaleznick tells of Professor Douglas McGregor. McGregor had spent most of his career at M.I.T. teaching theories of group behavior and leadership. He specifically proposed that managers avoid a top-down hierarchical approach. To put his theories to the test, he took on the presidency of Antioch College, where he remained for six years.

Zaleznick quotes from McGregor's essay, "On Leadership," which he wrote toward the end of his stint at Antioch.

> Before coming to Antioch, I had observed and worked with top executives as an advisor in a number of organizations. I thought I knew how they felt about their responsibilities and what led them to behave as they did. I even thought I could create a role for myself that would enable me to avoid some of the difficulties they encountered . . . I believed, for example, that a leader could operate successfully as a kind of advisor to his organization.
>
> I thought I could avoid being a "boss." Unconsciously, I suspect, I hoped to avoid the unpleasant necessity of making difficult decisions, of taking responsibility for one course of action among many uncertain alternatives, of making mistakes and taking the consequences. I thought that maybe I could operate so that every-

one would like me—that "good human relations" would eliminate all discord and disappointment. I could not have been more wrong.[12]

For an expert in the field, this is a stunning—and admirable—insight and admission. Zaleznick concludes: "Understanding that unused power undermines the authority structure overcomes the tendency to give way to one's own passive wishes. But it is not simply the desire to use power that supports the authority structure. . . . The initiatives a chief executive presents must make sense, even create a sense of excitement, to gain the enthusiastic support of subordinates. Passivity in the chief executive can take many forms. One form is leading with process rather than substance."[13]

The writer Michael Korda surely would not endorse McGregor's qualms about being the top dog in a hierarchy. In his book on power in the corporate world (which he now claims was written tongue in cheek), Korda sets out strategies of confrontation and persuasion, and explains how to use the emblems of power in order to actualize power. Such emblems include having the best office, an ample expense account, easy access to the senior person in the business, and a car and driver. They are not only power's rewards and validation, but insignia that announce to someone across the desk the potential power that can be brought to bear. Essentially, Korda suggests that, even if real power is largely illusory, one can invoke the insignia of power in order to to manipulate others.[14]

Most experts on management take a position somewhere between McGregor's original position (play the role of advisor rather than that of boss) and Korda's position—let them know who has the power. For the management consultant John O. Whitney, the manager not only sets the goals and strategies, but must also take charge of the chain of relationships in his company.[15] As soon as the manager assumes a new position, he must quickly identify who will support him full-out and who will take a wait-and-see attitude. He should assume that those who thought his job was or should be theirs will be his natural enemies. Whitney astutely observes that the in-house person most responsible for choosing an outside person seldom if ever feels fully repaid. While a new CEO who is promoted from within knows the cast of characters better than any outsider, he may already have problems simply by having won over his competitors. Whether chosen from within or recruited from without, the new manager cannot hesitate to fire anyone who is either incompetent or subversive. Nor should he count on his kindliness to co-opt someone who is dead set against him. (Ignorance of this pitfall may be a special problem for women.) Whitney stresses the importance of putting together a group of loyalists and working to guarantee their longtime loyalty. He also emphasizes that the manager, by virtue of the power of his position, necessarily is the target of distorted perceptions of him. Such perceptions may be projections that have nothing to do with him but may nonetheless lead to overblown expectations of what he can do.[16]

The manager must be able to control his employees without creating enmity. Smart managers learn to do this without appearing to be authoritarian; when dealing with their people they make their point clear enough, but leave enough "wiggle room," to permit the subordinate to save face. Direction and suggestions are presented in such a way that the recipient does not feel criticized: even if he's done something wrong, he must be given a respectable out. The manager needs to command his people's loyalty yet needs to have enough information so that he can chart the business's course and sometimes change it. One time-honored means for achieving these ends, not without its own dangers, is to put rivals in adjacent positions in the flowchart. This way, any disagreement is sure to be kicked upstairs, ensuring a flow of critical information, and the possibility that the two will develop loyalty to each other and conspire against the boss is effectively undercut. Casey Stengel, the legendary baseball manager for both the Yankees and the Mets, advanced a related version of this strategy. On any team of twenty-five players, Stengel argued there are five who love you, five who hate you, and fifteen players who have not made up their minds. The secret to being a successful manager, Stengel advised, is to keep the five who hate you away from the fifteen who have not yet made up their minds.

In different industries, bosses and managers reward—and thereby control—their employees in different currencies. For example, if you work for a newspaper, the editor can give you a special perk or withhold it—put you on page 1 or page 3, above the fold or below it, give you a particularly hot overseas assignment or a particularly quiet local one. In the press, perks are more in the coin of opportunity or tokens of prestige rather than in the coin of money. On Wall Street, because the goal is simply to make money, the incentive system is more straightforwardly financial. In the newspaper business, because your reputation is the payoff, people are generally even more competitive than they are in an investment house where, because the goal is to make money in which the whole company shares, people are more cooperative and there's more of a system of mentors. Particularly with the rise of the analyst as an important figure within the financial industry in the past ten years—previously it had been the salesman or the manager—someone who runs a group relies a great deal on the analyst and may well reach out to mentor him. Thus as the investment world has evolved, being mentored has also become one of the incentives.[17]

In other kinds of industries, too, the incentives are primarily money. But as several management consultants suggest, money alone does not ensure loyalty, and generally fails to generate enthusiasm. Employees, particularly those at the managerial level, want some piece of action above and beyond profits; they want a problem to think through and to which they can respond creatively. (This observation confirms Csikszentmihalyi's contention that employees are more gratified when they are a part of the game plan, not just part of the muscle.)

Most managers have superiors of their own. Whatever their titles, they know that their life belongs to the company store. They are routinely expected to take their jobs home with them. Indeed, as the social critic Harvey Swados noted long ago, the pay differential between lower-level management and skilled labor is less than one might imagine, if one simply assumes that the manager is being paid for an extra twenty hours or so a week, the time he spends worrying about the job at home. Even when on holiday, a manager, far more than a regular employee, may be asked to come into the office or to check in by phone. If he wants to keep his status, the manager has less freedom than an ordinary employee simply to take a sick day or a personal day. Insecure managers may be so sensitive to the managers above them that they may tread even more lightly than necessary. But some lower-rung managers, prodded by their insecurities, may seek proof of importance by demanding to do things their own way—which generally turns out to be a mistake.

Relationships in the workplace have changed over the past several decades due to the significant transformations in how work is organized. Today, companies are focused on establishing brand loyalty from their customers, but the bond between company and employee is in decline—

and in many industries is now informed by the sole criteria of how much it would cost the company to train a replacement. Without feeling a sense of security or prestige at work, employees at many levels no longer have the pleasure or privilege of identifying with the company. The emotional toll of these changes affects not only the employees, but the employer as well. Many executives who are responsible for discharging long serving and loyal employees pay an emotional price for their actions. These are often decent men, caught up in a system that equates their value almost exclusively with their ability to produce improved bottom line figures. One way out of this dilemma which would not satisfy an employer of real conscience, but which is the rule nowadays in many industries, is to simply shirk the responsibility of doing the downsizing oneself and hire outside consultants to do the job instead. One's position in corporations appears to be less secure today then it once was as human resource managers come in and with the warmest sensitivity quietly give the ax to a pre-set fraction of employees.

Solo Flights: Professionals and Other Self-Employed Workers

For many years the self-employed—for example, lawyers, doctors, and single proprietors of small stores—seemed to be the backbone of our society. These professions and occupations offered a great deal of personal fulfillment and pleasure. Not only were they doing well by doing good; they were doing good within a well-defined community that acknowledged their help and expertise. Stressed and stretched as they might be, they controlled their own work life—or at least had the illusion of doing so. And they usually made enough money to be able to live comfortably in the middle or upper middle class. Moreover, they had warm personal relations with their clients or patients. Thus it was that many immigrants saw a future for their children, steering their education toward preparation for one of the professions or encouraging them to become store owners—that is, to seek independence and therefore to be able to control the trajectory of their work lives.

Yet the status of these independent workers—that they can even be thought of as "workers" represents a change in perception—has declined significantly in recent years. Single store owners—whether druggists or owners of furniture, office supply, or hardware stores—are finding it increasingly hard to stay in business against competition from huge chains. Doctors, too, have seen their profession change, as governmental regulations have affected their practices, and they are now consumed with justifying lab tests, filling out forms, and keeping track of third-party payment. Moreover, doctors and lawyers have found that their incomes are dwarfed in comparison with those of people in business and finance. Some enjoy their work sufficiently that they are willing to accept this decline in both independence and income. But the long-term results of this erosion of some of the perks of the profession are yet to be determined. Of course, the major perk that is lost is the control over one's own work life.

Distortions in the Arena of Work

In addition to outside social forces that diminish the power we should ideally realize through work, there are psychological conflicts that undercut our ability to engage fully in our work or to take pleasure in it. Some people, out of grandiosity or a need to force their parents, spouse, or relatives to look after them, either decline to look for work or fail to find sufficient pleasure or pride in their work to motivate them to stay on the job. They may quit or manage to get fired. (But the bottom line is that if they do not build a résumé, their situation gets worse, not better, as the years pass.) Others suffer from inhibitions that prevent them from pursuing even modest aspirations, and from seeking even simple jobs. These inhibitions may be the result of depression, phobic anxiety of the outside world, or of grandiosity—nothing is good enough. They may be a product of a power struggle with parents in which offspring feel justified in remaining dependent and demanding reparations.

Still others suffer from classic success phobias. By and large, success phobias originate in a competitive struggle with a parent—usually the same-sex parent—in which the child fears that if his success exceeds that of his parents, it will bring retaliation or abandonment. Success is equated with danger. The success phobia can be understood as the result of an Oedipus complex that has gone awry. Others feel so cheated by the circumstances of their lives that they seek restitution through alcoholism (escape) or criminal behavior (revenge).

At the other extreme, the potential for authentic power garnered through gratifying work gets contaminated by monomania or extreme ambition. There are those whose whole mental life is consumed with business. One of my first analytic teachers told me of a patient of his, a successful furrier who seemed to have no access to his own inner mental life. The analyst thought that inquiring about his patient's dreams might remedy the situation. But the furrier resolutely dreamt only of furry little creatures jumping a fence. The analyst tried to derive some symbolic meaning from these repetitious dreams, but finally concluded that the furrier was just checking out the best pelts. This kind of obsessive preoccupation devolves into such mononotous devotion to a particular pursuit that an individual has thoughts of little else.

Those who obsessively seek financial, business, or political power seldom wonder about the source of their motivation. Their desires seem to them transparent, self-evident. Who wouldn't share them? Extreme ambition—to be a phenomenally successful entrepreneur, a CEO, a military commander, or president of his country—often has its origin in the deepest recesses of his mind, far outside an individual's awareness. Perhaps a lust for power is a way of fulfilling the dreams of an ambitious father (as would be suggested by the almost identical aspirations of all the sons of Joseph Kennedy). Or ambition may be rooted in displaced sibling rivalry, the need to remedy early life weakness, a longing to rescue a parent whose own life is hopeless, or the dream of winning the heart of the princess. Whatever the reason, there are some among us who aspire to be leaders. Some may be motivated by the desire to help others through their leadership, but some want to control others and use them for their own ends.

Hans Morgenthau drew an astute analogy between perversions of political power and perversions of interpersonal power: "There is then in the great political masters a demoniac and frantic striving for ever more power—as there is in the misguided lovers, the Don Juans who mistake sex for love, a limitless and ever unsatiated compulsion toward more and more experience of sex—which will be satisfied only when the last living man has been subjected to the master's will."[18] It is this very insatiability for power that leads to ultimate defeat. A lust for power incites resistance. Those so afflicted often lead very stunted lives, since both their real-life and imaginative activities have been drafted full time in the search for more and more power. Sometimes the all-consuming lust for power is not so much the cause of a stunted emotional life but its result: those who despair of ever establishing intimate ties with their fellows opt instead to establish absolute command over them, substituting perverted personal power for human connections.

THE PSYCHOANALYST Erna Furman makes an important comparison between work and play: "The pleasures and satisfactions derived from work and play do differ, but they also share an important characteristic. They never provide direct gratification of bodily needs such as hunger or elimination, or of impulses, sexual and aggressive."[19] Such pleasure as we derive from work are more connected to our self-esteem and even to our narcissism. Our mastery of work helps us to define ourselves, and, in the best of circumstances, adds to our sense of worth. While we may work out of necessity, work becomes part of the way we evaluate ourselves and therefore an important part of our self-regard. Perhaps the genius of humankind is to make a pleasure out of necessity. The psychological, intellectual, or physical stretch we feel when we are full-out at work contributes mightily to that pleasure.

11

The Power of Creativity

"Whereas the scientist is pointed toward discovering order in the external world, the artist . . . toward creating order within. . . . both types of creativity are . . . motivated by a 'divine discontent' which is part of man's biological endowment."

ANTHONY STORR, "Psychoanalysis and Creativity"

For many people, creativity and power seem to have little to do with one another—power being regarded as heavy and dark, creativity as inspiring and uplifting. Yet drive and discipline are as essential to creativity as they are to the success of any other ambitious pursuit. In fact, we often use the adjective *powerful* to describe an artist's work. And creative people often feel a rush of adrenaline and power when their work is going well.

Creativity, the capacity for self-expression and originality, comprises all the arts: music and poetry, art and dance, design and architecture, all kinds of writing, business, and also intellectual and scientific disciplines like mathematics and physics. Tapping into our creativity, whether our capacity is modest or vast, allows us to achieve "flow"—a timeless, out-of-body oneness with whatever we are doing, a feeling of transcendence. (Yeats said it best: "How can we know the dancer from the dance?") A watercolorist who captures the light over a lake in late afternoon has this sense of flow. So, too, does the poet who finds a just metaphor for lost love, a critic who suddenly sees links between two writers who are superficially quite different, or the psychotherapist who, reviewing case notes, has an epiphany about the meaning of a patient's dream.

Creativity exists in a wide range of pursuits and at many levels of accomplishments. In our status-conscious world, we too often restrict the word *creative* to renowned intellectual and artistic geniuses. But many of us partake to some degree in the pleasures of creating. One woman I know is not only a brilliant pianist but an extraordinary and inventive cook—though she has a heavy hand with butter. Another woman designs and knits baby blankets for all the newborns within her purview. Some people have an uncanny eye for placing furniture in a room, others a flair for color. Some women who need a jump start to get their creative juices flowing turn to Martha Stewart, and it is part of *her* creativity to cater to our need for a little creative tutoring. And, of course, being genuinely funny is one of the most appreciated creative gifts. To partake of any of these creative experiences is to feel a special kind of gratification, an inner sense of pleasure and power.

The psychoanalyst Anthony Storr quotes Rosemund Harding to the effect that "In the man or woman of genius there are always present great technical skill and originality. The technical skill is usually built up from childhood. The future poet scribbles verses as a child, the future artist begins to draw as soon as he can hold a pencil."[1] Storr points out that even artists who begin their creative careers in midlife showed some precocity as children. Of George Eliot he writes, "Although 'Scenes from Clerical Life' did not appear in *Blackwood's Magazine* until the novelist was thirty-eight, it is known that she wrote both fiction and verse in childhood."[2] He notes that Picasso drew before he spoke and that the first sound he made was "piz," short for *lápiz*, a pencil. By age four Mozart was composing, and at that age Béla Bartók could play forty songs from his memory using one finger.

Just as fascinating is the failure of some child prodigies to develop into creative people of the highest order. Storr cites people "who are musically endowed in the kind of way which would be invaluable in a composer, but who are not impelled to write music. Such people can translate a tune in their head into notes on paper with a facility which is the envy of those who lack this gift. They can often read music fluently, transpose with ease; emend or arrange the composition of others, and interpret with sensitivity. In other words, they seem to possess the skills which are necessary to musical composition (a combination of gifts which seems rather uncommon) but lack the compulsion of originality."[3] Storr also observes that only about one out of ten child prodigies will go on to become an adult virtuoso. In trying to understand creativity, we have to consider two factors beyond talent: motivation and access to the deeper sources of creativity.

If we are to achieve the upper reaches of creativity, our talent must be animated by energy from deep within. Many people know that Freud considered the unconscious the source of our innermost desires; fewer people know about the broader unconscious, which encompasses problem solving and creativity. Yet all of us communicate with this unconscious to a lesser or greater extent. I discovered it for myself at a time when I was fascinated with riddles and puzzles, long before I knew anything about the Freudian unconscious. Solving the puzzle that I am about to describe would be very low on any scale of creativity, but the process gave me an indelible insight into how problem solving often occurs. I had been presented with a puzzle which runs as follows:

> You are lost on an island inhabited by two kinds of people, half of them congenital truth tellers, half congenital liars. You come to a fork in the road, and there is a man from whom you must learn which road leads to the castle that is your destination. You must devise a question such that the answer will lead you in the right direction no matter whether the man is a congenital liar or a congenital truth teller.

This is not the most difficult of puzzles, but the truth is that I struggled with it several days without being able to arrive at a solution. This was especially humiliating because I was vain enough to think I was pretty good at solving puzzles. Frustrated, I decided, by a conscious act of will, not to waste any more time, and I put the whole matter out of my head— or so I thought. A week later, much to my surprise, I woke up with the answer as my first waking thought. The mental work of solving the problem had gone on out of consciousness.

While the solution to the riddle is of little consequence, for the record, here is my solution: "Sir, if you were the opposite of what you are, how would you direct me to the castle? Do I take the road to the right or the road to the left?" The truth teller would of necessity give me the wrong instructions. But the liar, instructed to answer as a truth teller, would necessarily respond as a liar, and he, too, would point me in the wrong direction. The problem that had to be solved was how to reduce the liar and the truth teller to the same category. Several friends told me that there were more elegant solutions than mine, but I have long since forgotten what they were.

What I gained from solving the riddle was a notion of unconscious thought processes. The unconscious does much of the heavy lifting. In the literature on scientific discovery, it is easy to find examples of solutions that seemed to emerge quite suddenly—though of course to the prepared mind. This may be, in fact, a primary way scientists arrive at insights. In 1865, a famous solution to a problem in organic chemistry occurred during an afternoon nap. Friedrich August von Kekulé, Professor of Chemistry in Ghent, dreamed of a snake that had swallowed its tail and formed a kind of circle. Upon awakening, he proposed that the molecules of some organic compounds, instead of being linear, were organized into rings. The image of the snake had given him the idea that the structure of benzene could be explained by assuming that a chain of six carbon atoms could form a ring. There are many comparable examples of problem solving among scientists and artists, but this is not to say that creativity springs full-blown from the unconscious mind. Kekulé had obviously been puzzling over the chemical makeup of a particular compound. To put it another way, the process involved in creativity and in problem solving depends to a large degree on some communication between the conscious mind and the unconscious mind.

Of the two way traffic that takes place between the conscious and unconscious, I am much taken with Arthur Koestler's description of the way the mind works:

> One traffic stream continually moves in a downward direction: we concentrate on new experiences, arrange them into patterns, develop new observational skills, muscular dexterities, verbal aptitudes; and when these have been mastered by continued practice, the controls are handed over to a kind of automation, and the whole assembly is dispatched, along the gradients of awareness, out of sight. The upward traffic stream moves in small fluctuating pulses from the unconscious which sustain the dynamic balance of the mind—and in the rare, sudden surges of creativity, may lead to a re-structuring of the whole mental landscape.[4]

The idea of the unconscious long antedates Freud. Koestler quotes Goethe to the effect that: "Man cannot persist long in a conscious state, he must throw himself back into the Unconscious, for his roots live there. . . . Take for example a talented musician, composing an important score: consciousness and unconsciousness will be like warp and weft."

Because creativity is an expression of our deepest nature and is in interplay with the conscious mind, it produces its own kind of pleasure. Sometimes in the lower ranges of creativity, there is a pleasure somewhat akin to stretching a muscle—this lesser kind of pleasure is what I felt when I solved the puzzle. For the artist who creates a masterpiece or the scientist who makes an important discovery, the pleasure of creativity is a veritable exhilaration and a feeling of power. Freud proposed that artists create a world of their own, or, rather, rearrange the constituent parts of the real world in a novel way that provides them (or others) with pleasure. What greater power can there be than to create your own world—or to add significantly to the already existing one?

To express creativity, one needs not only a gift but also courage. One has to take risks—the existing world may have its own say about how welcome a new world or new discovery is. In a way, the risk involved in opening one's creativity to self-scrutiny or the scrutiny of others is a little like the gamble entailed in reaching out to a first love; it can feel overwhelming, and some people are just too timid or beaten down to take it.

Because our creative impulses are facilitated by our ability to surrender to the unconscious, we sometimes feel we have given away the ego, the self. Yet to make use of an emerging vision, insight, or hunch, we must muster the ability, the authority, and the driving force to shape the raw material from the unconscious into a coherent intellectual or artistic product. Passivity, in the form of receptivity to the unconscious, must be coupled with a certain kind of activity. Creativity depends not only on our basic gifts and talents but also on motivation—not just our potential, but the will to exercise it, the willingness to devote a large part of our waking hours to hone our gift, to stretch it to its limits. To do this, process is inevitably involved. By process, I mean the ability to bring together discipline, focus, the ability to be full-out, and perhaps most difficult of all, to discard one's wrong turns, to separate the wheat from the chaff. Then, too, one must nurture one's gift, even though it will appear to wax and wane as the process of creativity moves in fits and starts, and sometimes seems to regress.

For dancers, even those with the ideal body, process entails constant practice and the building of strength and endurance. A dancer and choreographer I know, who has studied, worked and watched dance pieces evolve from their very beginnings with some of the greats of contemporary concert dance, was struck by how the actual creative process varied from choreographer to choreographer and from dancer to dancer.[5] He observes that some choreographers want to make a bold statement about an event in the world while others want to make a subtle statement about the inner life. But to render whatever the original impulse is, one must select music that conveys it and the movements that depict it. When creating a piece himself, he is strict about making sure that his performers have strong technique because he wants them to concentrate on conveying what he is hearing and feeling about a piece of music. He wants them to hear the words he hears, the beats he hears, and to put them together in a signature way. Yet he is unsure how the particular beats or moves first come to mind. Even when he edits what he choreographs, he feels his core impulses remain the same. When he infrequently does something very upbeat—something from the Broadway genre—he still turns to those more subtle beats of music or the sad tone that one seldom finds in upbeat songs. For him, authentic power lies in the ability to experiment, to try new genres and styles—things he has choreographed in a new way that may still be weak, but nonetheless can engage an audience. For the mature artist, the process may be smoothed out, but it depends on bringing together knowledge, expertise, feeling, and the idiosyncratic way each of us sees the world—yet not so idiosyncratic that the artistic product cannot be shared.

FOR CREATIVE PEOPLE, the freedom to pursue a gift, like the gift itself, is usually found early in life. But to persevere, process is inevitably involved. Among other things, this process often entails the ability to sustain the grunt and grind of seeing a project through and polishing it until it is exactly right. Many creative people struggle with inhibitions, which is a way in which feelings of powerlessness come into the equation. The factors that impede potentially creative people include despair that a gift may turn out to be more limited than it initially appeared to be; distractibility; lack of energy; competing goals; and anger at being pushed. Some people who are unsure about the scope of their talent may choose to maintain their belief in their potential by never putting it to the test; therefore grandiosity may be one of the greatest enemies of actualizing one's creative potential.

Even when we find no real support in the external world, there sometimes appears to be a psychic adjustment within our own minds that frees us from vacillation and insecurity. In a passage from her published journal *At Seventy*, May Sarton catches a sense of creativity as personal power. In the course of a talk she gave on old age, she told the audience: "This is the best time of my life. I love being old." Someone in the audience asked, "Why is it good to be old?" Sensing what she described as incredulity, Sarton notes in her journal how she responded: "Because I am more myself than I have ever been, there is less conflict. I am happier, more balanced, and (I heard myself say rather aggressively) 'more powerful.' I felt it was rather an odd word, 'powerful,' but I think it is true. It might have been more accurate to say 'I am better able to use my powers.' I am sure of what my life is about, have less self-doubt to conquer."[6]

Here Sarton is speaking of a kind of power that has little or nothing to do with the domination or control of another person or with subjugation by another person. However, when she talks about the self-doubt she has conquered, I believe she is writing about the silencing of an internal critic. Until such an internal critic is silenced, or at least brought under control, one's creative voice will be stifled. Only when it is unencumbered by fear or timidity can creativity find natural expression as the unified product of our physical, mental, and emotional makeup, stemming from deep sources within our psyches. Thus any creative act is by definition a kind of victory. Our sense of power, or "powers," is the result of that victory.

What I have observed of creativity among psychoanalysts is similar. Several of the most intelligent psychoanalysts I know—certainly gifted enough to have made major contributions to the psychoanalytic literature—have failed to do so because they seem incapable of suspending their critical standards. As a result, they stifle all those little shoots of intuition—as yet illogical, nonlinear, unsubstantiated—that can sometimes flower into new insights and ideas. Intimidated by their own powers of logic, they squelch their creative insights, for fear that inconsistencies in their ideas might embarrass them. They take a pass out of reluctance to face down the internal critic, the naysayer in their minds. Sarton speaks as one who has overcome her internal critic and is thus able to use her powers of creativity to the full.

Of course, one's own self-doubts are often intensified by the comments of external critics—friends and professionals. Here the new critical order, as it exists externally, joins the old order as it exists internally to resist our willingness to gamble on looking foolish. Then, it is no longer simply a question of enduring self-criticism but also of negotiating a path through actual adversaries. For writers, as for other artists, criticism can be devastating. One woman told me about reading a short story aloud in her creative writing class. In the discussion that followed, the teacher, an advocate of a completely different style of writing, attacked her so savagely that she became tongue-tied and was unable to respond. She knew his criticism was motivated by her daring to work in a style completely different from the one he was promoting. Afterward, a number of her fellow students tried to console her, and praised her work, but she never again tried to write. She knows she is overreacting to the criticism, knows that her response has some deeper meaning, but cannot move past the experience. What for some people would simply have been temporarily hurtful—or an occasion for outrage rather than hurt—was for her an annihilation. And it is likely to remain so unless she gains some understanding about why she was so destroyed, what echoes of past experiences were invoked in her by that attack.

One editor at a major publishing house stopped requesting reports on book submissions from a brilliant but critical reader because he never thought anything was fit to publish. And the reader's own creativity was stifled because he never suspended his critical mind long enough to give his creative potential free play. Unfortunately, the brilliant person who sees too quickly the flaws and gaps in someone else's early drafts will miss the kernel of genuine insight or originality that is there and will not be able to provide useful input to his colleagues, no matter how insightful his criticisms are, because only the most self-confident can surmount such unmitigated negativity. This kind of assault on the creative impulse can be deadly, not just on the personal but also on the institutional level. In psychoanalytic circles, for example, there have been periods when the organizational pressure to adhere to one or another theory has stifled many potentially creative people because of their fear that they would be marginalized. This is the external critic writ large.

Internal and external critics are not the only impediments to expressing our creativity. Some of us may be so grandiose that fearing we are not as good as Picasso or Joyce, we retreat from the fray. We maintain our grandiosity by never putting our gifts to the test. Others view creativity as a freely flowing source; if they temporarily run dry, they mistake now for forever and turn a dry period into a perennial drought. Some are so inhibited by the possible envy of others that they obey the internal injunction not to stand out from the crowd. Only when we attain a sufficient degree of self-confidence and independent judgment are we fully free to express our creative powers.

Those who exercise their gifts with what appears to be an automatic feeling of empowerment have most likely already wrestled down the niggling critic who lives inside nearly every one of us. The task of freeing ourselves is often made easier through encouragement by a supportive friend or by a deep intellectual or creative connection to someone else. This person may serve to give us courage, spark an insight, or engage in a full-fledged collaboration. Some creative individuals utilize the evocation of a muse whether literal or figurative. In all these roles, the figure—real or imagined—serves as a transference object, that is, someone on whom we project our hopes for the nurturance that our tentative tender shoots of creativity require. Creativity, which the culture often depicts as a solitary enterprise, is almost always impacted by or even dependent upon a real relationship or one we carry in our heads and in our hearts. And sometimes we can imaginatively invoke a predecessor—someone we may know only through his work—as our inspiration and guide.

FREUD DREW A PARALLEL between the child at play, the adult daydreamer, and the creative artist: "Might we not say that every child at play behaves like a creative writer, in that he creates a world of his own, or rather, re-arranges the things of his world in a new way which pleases him? . . . The creative writer does the same as the child at play. He creates a world of phantasy which he takes very seriously—that is, which he invests with large amounts of emotion—while separating it sharply from reality."[7] Here Freud seems to describes the artist as a solitary figure whose work springs forth full-blown.

Today, however, psychoanalysts and psychologists may be in the midst of a paradigm change in how they think about creativity, attributing more importance to the necessary support an artist requires rather than focusing almost exclusively on the genius of the creator.

For some, play, fantasy, and creativity do seem solitary. More often than not, however, creativity has an interpersonal component. Even in the nursery, children spark each other's creativity in imaginative play. Vivian Gussin Paley says that playacting and storytelling are the primary reality for preschoolers and kindergartners and that their jointly created stories are a way of bonding.[8] Children seek friendships and shared fantasy (as expressed in their joint play) to avoid fear and loneliness, to find a comfortable relationship with people and events, and to address current concerns and future dreads. Friendship and fantasy are the braided paths that lead children into an imaginative world of expanded possibilities.[9] This external connection is as necessary in the development of creativity as in any other developmental process.

During the 1970s and 1980s, a number of analysts observed that certain artists require a supportive and often intense relationship with another person, particularly during a period of creativity.[10] Co-creativity, co-construction, and mutual influence remain important areas of current inquiry into creativity.

The cognitive psychologist Howard Gardner, whose research on the sources of creativity involved biographical studies of some unusually creative people, revealed the important—and to some surprising—fact that social support is critical to many artists' ability to function creatively.[11] Gardner showed that during a time of artistic or intellectual breakthrough, the creator required an emotional support system from someone with whom he feels comfortable and an intellectual relationship with someone who understands the thrust and originality of what he is accomplishing. This may or may not be the same person.[12]

Gardner confesses that he was surprised by the discovery of the social forces surrounding the emergence of creative insights. (Like many of us, he had erroneously thought of creativity as an internal force destined to make itself known.) But he came to compare the relationship between the artist and those who made up his support system to critical relationships earlier in life, whether between caregiver and child, or between a youngster and his peer group. He sees that creative development depends not only on an innate gift, but also on support and encouragement from others. Even if no real person is involved in the support of our creativity, we may draw on the memories of earlier relationships for support and encouragement.

Freud is the first of the creative geniuses Gardner describes. It is an oft-told tale that several emotionally charged alliances were critical in

Freud's creative breakthroughs, but here I will draw largely on Gardner's account.[13] Freud was his mother's firstborn. She showered special attention on him, and she lived until he was over seventy. In addition, his nurse doted on him and is believed to have reinforced the idea that he was special. Freud was, of course, extremely gifted, and this was evident early on. He chose to study medicine but immersed himself in a wide variety of subjects and even taught himself several languages in order to read works in their original language.

Freud always found people in whom to confide his interests and his ideas, including his great friend Eduard Silberstein; later on his fiancée, Martha Bernays; and still later his friend Wilhelm Fliess and his sister-in-law Minna. His biographers have noted that in his early letters he already expressed ambition and extreme confidence that he would achieve greatness. When Freud was seventeen years old, he wrote to his friend Emil Fluss: "You have been exchanging letters with a German stylist. And now I advise you as a friend, not as an interested party, to preserve them—have them bound—take good care of them—one never knows."[14]

Yet while Freud had intense ambition, intellectual gifts, and stunning self-confidence, his talents were not so specialized as to make it clear to him from the start what direction his life's work would take. Choosing medicine as a kind of default career that would at least be practical, Freud worked in the laboratory of Ernst Brücke and wrote articles on neuroanatomy. His correspondence shows that he remained infatuated with the quest for fame as a scientist and with experiments he hoped would win it for him. But his experiment with cocaine, which he dispensed to his friends for medical purposes, nearly ended in disaster when one of his colleagues became addicted to it. Although cocaine did prove to have medicinal powers, it was Carl Koller, not Freud, who was recognized for discovering its usefulness as an anesthetic for eye surgery.

The year after the cocaine debacle, Freud went to Paris to study with Charcot, and it was there, Gardner suggests, that he shifted "his 'ego ideal' from the precise and rigorous neuroanatomical investigator Brücke to the more expansive, charismatic, and psychologically oriented Charcot."[15] Returning to Vienna, Freud attached himself to Josef Breuer, a renowned researcher and internist through whom he began to see patients suffering from hysteria.

Together Breuer and Freud wrote about the "talking cure," a term coined by one of Breuer's patients, and jointly published their *Studies on*

Hysteria.[16] But by the time of the publication, Freud was already boldly soaring ahead to new theories in which sexual factors played a decisive etiological role. Not only was Breuer uneasy with these hypotheses, but Freud's presentation of "The Etiology of Hysteria" to the Vienna Society in 1896 was not well received. The sexologist Krafft-Ebing declared it a scientific fairy tale. As Freud commented later, "The development of psychoanalysis afterwards cost me his [Breuer's] friendship. It was not easy for me to pay such a price but I could not escape it."[17]

Gardner describes Freud's plight quite poignantly "Once an individual who had been virtually canonized by his own family, appreciated and admired by peers and mentors, and able to master vast bodies of information in a veritable library of subjects, Freud had evolved to a most unhappy situation: one where his closest colleagues, like Breuer, were no longer willing to stand with him, while his closest family members, like his wife, could not possibly understand what he was claiming."[18] Of course, it is hard to maintain confidence in one's work without some outside affirmation.

During this time of stress, and in this vacuum, Freud's friendship with Wilhelm Fliess flowered. They corresponded for more than ten years. While Fliess's ideas may seem eccentric and marginal today, they did not appear so at the time, and Fliess was valuable to Freud as someone who was emotionally supportive and intellectually interested in his theories and hunches. Although Freud refers to this period as a time of "splendid isolation," Fliess was for him a major and necessary transference figure, lending him confidence and bolstering his inner convictions and his sense of intellectual strength. Apart from their occasional self-styled "congresses," when the two of them could find a few days to spend together at this or that resort town, their major interaction was by letters, and Fliess, who even Breuer concedes was one of the most brilliant men he had ever met, was willing to read draft after draft of Freud's theories.[19]

Gardner writes that Freud's sharing of "The Project" with Fliess illustrates a theme he encountered repeatedly in his study of creativity: "At times when creators are on the verge of a radical breakthrough, they feel the need to try out their new language on a trusted other individual—perhaps to confirm that they themselves are not totally mad and may even be on to something new and important. . . . I suggest that this desperate effort to communicate may harken back in some ways to the initial communication link between mother and child and to youthful links between peers."[20] After his success, Freud himself became a transference object for idealization and inspiration, and his problems with father figures gave way to problems with rivals and disciples.

How necessary is external support for prodigies and geniuses? In developing his paradigm of how creativity flowers, Gardner includes among his subjects Picasso, the very incarnation of a child prodigy if ever there was one. According to Gardner: "A prodigy always represents a 'co-incidence' of factors. That is, one needs not merely a 'prepared child' and a 'welcoming culture' but also a tremendous amount of social support: good teachers, attentive parents, ample opportunities for performance and display, relief from competing responsibilities, access to avenues of publicity, and a sequence of hurdles that are acknowledged in the domain and over which the child has an opportunity to bound."[21]

Picasso was the son of an artist who encouraged him, and he quickly surpassed not just his father but other local artists. From a very early age, Picasso propelled himself into situations and cities where he traveled in a subculture of artists who stimulated each other, borrowed from each other, and served for each other as the standard for judging themselves. In addition, Picasso chose earlier masters from whom to learn and against whom to measure himself, among them Diego Velázquez. His fascination with Velázquez can be seen in the many variations he painted of Velázquez's *Las Meninas* (1676). These variations are now at the Picasso Museum in Barcelona, the city where Picasso lived after he first left his hometown.

At no time in his life did Picasso lack creative support. He moved from Barcelona to Paris, then the center of the artistic world, where he lived a long life in the company of artists. He was so close to some of them that his paintings of certain periods might be confused with theirs because they experimented together with new modes of expression. Simultaneously, Picasso was involved with a number of lover-muses, whose ascendancy and decline can be traced in his portraits and in his erotic paintings. Still, although Picasso's art did not spring full-blown out of solitude, he did *create* it in solitude.

What of Picasso's innate drive? Unquestionably, he was almost demonically possessed, as can be seen from his massive outpouring of work and in the intensity of his ties to lover-muses. If you were fortunate enough to see his erotic works on display in Paris in 2001, you might concur with Freud that sex is the propelling force in creativity, though for

Picasso sex was decidedly unsublimated, both in his art and in his life. As a matter of fact, the American psychologist Lewis Terman found in his own study of genius that this tended to be the rule: Rather than creativity originating from the sublimation of sex, it sometimes seems that sex and creativity spring from the same innate life force.

GARDNER was writing about creative geniuses, but what he describes is relevant to creativity at all levels. Like other strategies of personal power, creativity often involves another person, in either a fantasized or a real relationship that encourages or catalyzes it. In fact, sometimes a full-fledged partnership is required to help us transcend any sense of creative powerlessness—for example a mentor relationship in which we feel nurtured and supported, or a more egalitarian relationship in which we feel similarly supported, or in an identification with another person who may come to serve as a model for our endeavors.[22]

For most of us, the sense of a strong and independent creative self emerges only slowly, with the accumulation of small successes. It is actually quite rare for a gift to flower spontaneously. As previously suggested, most people must wrestle with internal critics of one kind or another and through these power struggles within themselves hone their gifts in their own way. But negotiating these struggles takes time. Though we may appear autonomous and creative to others, it takes a while before we ourselves can internalize such a sense of self.

In her memoir, A Backward Glance, Edith Wharton writes about her conflicting feelings after the publication of her first two short stories: "Both attracted attention, and gave me the pleasant flutter incidental to first seeing one's self in print; but they brought me no nearer to other workers in the same field. I continued to live my old life, for my husband was as fond of society as ever, and I knew of no other existence except in our annual escapes to Italy. I had as yet no real personality of my own, and was not to acquire one till my first book of short stories was published—and that was not until 1899."[23] She remembers her unbelieving response when that first book, The Greater Inclination, was published: "I had written short stories that were thought worthy of preservation! Was it the same insignificant I that I had always known?"[24] "The insignificant I"—a perfect description of the way many creative people experience themselves before their creative self crystallizes.

In negotiating inner struggle, it can be indispensable to find an external ally. While Freud found a series of allies, Edith Wharton found strength primarily through one friend, the lawyer Walter Berry. She described Berry as "born with an exceptionally sensitive literary instinct, but also with a critical sense so far outweighing his creative gift that he had early renounced the gift of writing."[25] In other words, he was not able to silence his own internal critic. Or perhaps he was not sufficiently creatively gifted. But he proved exceptionally astute at helping Wharton silence her internal critic. Because Berry had found personal fulfillment in another field, he had no competitive feelings toward Wharton and had both the sympathy and the instinct to help her. In her memoir, Wharton recounts how she would begin to write something in a "burst of lyric rapture" and then lose the path. Berry advised her just to write down everything she felt like telling. Once she was finished with a manuscript, "how meticulously he studied it from the point of view of language, marking down faulty syntax and false metaphors, smiling away over-emphasis and unnecessary repetitions, helping [me] patiently through the beginner's perplexities, yet never laying his hand on what he considered sacred: the *soul* of the novel, which is (or should be) the writer's own soul."[26] Clearly, Berry served in many roles, both as a source of emotional support and as an ideal editor. Wharton saw Berry as the instrument for her expansion of herself and says that he followed her "literary steps with the same patient interest" until his death twenty-seven years later.[27]

In some, though certainly not all, mentor/mentee relationships between men and women, the professional may be intricately intertwined with the personal and the sexual. This may be one reason men are sometimes reluctant to take on female protégées—or their wives may be reluctant on their behalf. What Edith Wharton omitted in her memoir is how her professional relationship with Berry evolved into a romantic attachment, something she did not want known while their friends were still alive. Her literary executor placed a stay on the publication of her private papers until 1968, but by 1964 Olivia Coolidge had already written a biography of Wharton that gave a much fuller account of her relationship with Berry. Their relationship appears to have remained platonic until Wharton's troubles with her husband escalated. According to Coolidge, it was after "twenty years of married frustration [that] Edith at last had fallen in love with somebody else."[28] In 1912, Wharton persuaded her husband to enter a private sanatorium after his third mental collapse, and in 1913 she divorced him. He died in 1928 but is described as having been "hardly alive for many years."

It had long been evident that Wharton regarded Berry with great affection. Coolidge identifies Berry as the "soul-mate" in Wharton's short story "The Fullness of Life," and she raises the question why Wharton did not fall in love with him until she was forty-six. Yet when Wharton did turn to Walter Berry "with a passion in strange contrast to her former control," he at first failed to respond and instead went to Egypt with his widowed sister.[29] Berry, a lifelong bachelor, never intended to marry Wharton or anyone else. Yet from 1911 on, after he had retired for reasons of health and settled in Paris, he became Wharton's constant companion. In addition to his friendship with her, Berry "adored flirtations."[30] Wharton apparently made few complaints, and they remained close, even inseparable. Coolidge concludes that Berry's emotional limitations suggest he was a peculiar man: "If he had loved her but renounced Edith, he would have married her on her divorce. If he did not love her, then his behavior was strange indeed. For twenty years he had been willing to play the 'soul-mate' yet he could not be brought to undertake the marriage."[31]

Coolidge was convinced that, whatever his limitations, Wharton loved Berry throughout the latter part of her life. She notes that "some people have felt that there is a trace of Walter Berry in the cultured, selfish dilettantes who appear in her stories now as hero, now as villain. Certainly the type is a persistent one ranging from Selden, too self-absorbed to save Lily Bart [in *The House of Mirth*], as far as to Culwin, the elderly roué of 'The Eyes.' "[32] Berry died in 1926; Wharton lived on until 1937. However complicated her feelings about him may have been, she left instructions that she was to be "laid in the cemetery at Versailles as close to Walter Berry as she could arrange."[33]

Many writers require emotional support just as Wharton did. And many writer-editor collaborations operate in the Wharton-Berry mode, although romance is not always part of the package. Burroughs Mitchell, an editor at Scribner's, wrote that "in the act of writing a book the writer is very much alone. Various people interest themselves in what he is doing—such people as wives and husbands, editors, literary agents, critics, and, now and then, a psychotherapist; but for the most part they remain quite outside the work that holds the writer absorbed." He believes that the legendary Maxwell Perkins (with whom he overlapped at Scribner's for one or two years before Perkins died) was a great editor because he had "the ability to go inside, to enter into the writer's solitary enterprise without intruding."[34] This is exactly what Berry did for Wharton.

Some collaborations become so famous that the public may couple the name of the writer and editor, and some of these collaborations work out very well. Other writer-editor partnerships are not so lucky, and internal tension frequently results in a breakup. There are numerous fault lines that may ultimately destroy many kinds of creative collaborations, whether artistic, commercial, or psychoanalytic. The problem may center on issues of credit and recognition or competition and envy; often the writer finds it difficult to give full credit to the editor, and the editor, in turn, may fail to provide a holding environment for the writer.

Here, then, is another way power enters into creativity—through an old-fashioned power struggle over who contributed what, over whether credit is bestowed or withheld and whether or not appreciation has been expressed. And, of course, over the question of recognition. In good situations, the struggle is somehow resolved and the creative work can sometimes be advanced if the partners weather the contention. But sometimes the struggle is the end of it and the collaboration is over. (Although I am writing here about the struggles between editors and writers, the same potential for conflict is inherent in most creative partnerships, including business and political partnerships.)

Thomas Wolfe and Maxwell Perkins had one of the most noted writer-editor collaborations of the twentieth century. Perkins also worked with other famous writers, including Ernest Hemingway and F. Scott Fitzgerald, but his pairing with Wolfe is legendary. Although Wolfe eventually left Perkins to seek another editor, their breakup was, ironically, a result not of failure but of their colossal success.

Perkins told of the beginning of their collaboration in his Introduction to a reissue of *Look Homeward, Angel* in 1957: "The first time I heard of Thomas Wolfe I had a sense of foreboding. I who loved the man say this. Every good thing that comes is accompanied by trouble. It was in 1928 when Madeline Boyd, the literary agent, came in. She talked of several manuscripts which did not much interest me, but frequently interrupted herself to tell of a wonderful novel about an American boy. I several times said to her, 'Why don't you bring it in here, Madeline?' and she seemed to evade the question. But finally she said, 'I will bring it if you promise to read every word of it.' I did promise but she told me other things that made me realize that Wolfe was a turbulent spirit and that we were in for turbulence. When the manuscript came, I was fascinated by the scene where Eugene's father, Oliver W. Gant, with his brother, two little boys, stood by a roadside in Pennsylvania and saw a division of Lee's army on the march to Gettysburg."[35]

But Wolfe next sent some ninety pages about Gant's life that Perkins considered irrelevant. After consultation with a colleague, Perkins cut out the first wonderful scene and the ninety or so pages that followed, to unify the narrative from a different angle, and he says that for years it was on his conscience that he "had persuaded Tom to cut out the first scene of the two little boys on the roadside with Gettysburg impending." But he need not have fretted, because, as he later discovered, Wolfe incorporated the scene into *Of Time and the River*, and to greater effect. Perkins "began then to realize that nothing Wolfe wrote was ever lost, that omissions from one book were restored in a later one."

Perkins believed that the trouble between them arose when Wolfe dedicated his next novel, *Of Time and the River*, to him in the most extravagant terms: "I never saw the dedication until the book was published and though I was most grateful for it, I had forebodings when I heard of his intention. I think it was the dedication that threw him off his stride and broke his magnificent scheme. It gave shallow people the impression that Wolfe could not function as a writer without collaboration, and one critic even used some such phrase as 'Wolfe and Perkins— Perkins and Wolfe, what way is that to write a novel.'" As Perkins saw it, "No writer could possibly tolerate the assumption, which perhaps Tom almost himself did, that he was dependent as a writer on anyone else." So Wolfe left Perkins and went to another publisher.

According to Perkins's biographer, A. Scott Berg, Wolfe was angry about "the general belief that without Perkins, [he] was unpublishable— a writer manqué," confirming Perkins's own analysis of their rupture.[36] Wolfe had depended on Perkins in many other ways, too, and had revealed too much of himself and his inner life to Perkins, so that the very closeness of their relationship was threatening. Not only had Perkins edited Wolfe and carved out two novels, but he had been Wolfe's mentor, nursed him, wrote and talked him through his crises (including a prolonged rift with his mistress and benefactor, Aline Bernstein), and urged on him (as he did with his other authors) certain of his favorite great books, in particular *War and Peace*. In the end, the break was precipitated when Perkins and Scribner's settled a lawsuit against Wolfe, conceding that he had appropriated someone else's life story for his novel without adequately disguising it. Wolfe felt betrayed, and just as in a marriage when the dependent partner becomes resentful, he turned against his source of strength.

Perkins believed that the switch in publishers did not serve Wolfe well, and many critics concurred. Ultimately, it appears that Wolfe, too, agreed. Before he died (at age thirty-eight), he made Perkins his literary executor.

Some of the essential tension in collaborations between writers and editors include feelings of not "owning" one's own work and fear of dependency on the part of the writer, and envy and desire for glory on the part of the editor. But there are important exceptions—for example, Ezra Pound's famous editing of T. S. Eliot's *The Waste Land*, which has since been replicated in a special edition so that Pound's input is clear. There are also those who once entertained writerly ambitions but ultimately renounced them to become brilliant editors—the late William Shawn of the *New Yorker* being a prime example.[37]

Sometimes it's only the writer who is considered creative by the outside world, and some editors may suffer from a sense of diminishment, unhappy at being a handmaiden, often unacknowledged, and probably not even paid enough. In fact, the best editors are creative in their own right and have no wish to take over the author's role. While no work can be first-rate without the basic ingredients, it may take a brilliant edit to showcase them.

Joel Spingarn, an editor and essayist in the early twentieth century, said that the function of the editor is "to dream the poet's dream." Good editing is transparent, which means that the editor may help to sharpen ideas or, in fiction, help facilitate pace or the emotional flow while seamlessly preserving the underlying integrity of the work. The editor who can discern the meaning and innovativeness embedded in a work functions much as a psychoanalyst or therapist who "reads" a dream. The editor may also combine emotional support with literary expertise, as did Edith Wharton's friend Walter Berry, which in Wharton's case helped her hone her language in such a way as to carry the *soul* of her novel.

The capacity for conflict is much the same, though perhaps to different degrees, in all genres of writing, and the same kind of conflicts can confound the relationship in other kinds of creative partnerships—choreographer and ballerina, director and actor, composer and conductor. Who's the lead horse? Who should get the credit? Who inspires whom? Who is more gifted? Ezra Pound has a different take on the process: "It's immensely important that great poems be written, but it makes not a jot of difference who writes them."

So far, I have emphasized the need most creative people have for some external support to help them overcome whatever internal reservations or sense of inadequacy they may feel. Sometimes, however, inhibition of creativity is a result of a success phobia, which has the same dynamics in creative work as in any other context. The primary problem is not lack of support from the outside world, but rather that the artist is inhibited by the harm he anticipates as a result of success.

There are two forms of success phobia. In the first, people are impeded by a fear that success will draw such envy or disapproval that they will be deserted. Here the problem is not so much a sense of inadequacy as an unconscious fear of emotional, material, or physical harm in retaliation for success. Phobias of this kind prohibit the artist's expression of his gifts, leading others to view them as having let an immense potential for creative fulfillment go to waste.

The second kind of success phobia involves those described as "wrecked by success," in Freud's memorable phrase.[38] One of Freud's cases involved an academic who had long cherished the wish to succeed his mentor when the mentor retired. However, when the older man finally did retire and the teacher was chosen as his successor, he hesitated, depreciated his own merits, began to feel himself unworthy, and fell into a depression that lasted for a number of years. In this kind of situation— which is not at all uncommon—a person is able to dream of success so long as he or she is not in a position to achieve it; but this ambition is interpreted in the inner recesses of the mind as harmful to someone else. Such an inhibition is sometimes related to an early life ambition to succeed a parent by virtue of his death. One of the mysteries in literary circles in Kentucky when I was growing up was why Ross Lockridge, Jr., killed himself after the publication of his novel *Raintree County*, which was a huge success. The suspicion lingered that he was undone by his achievement. Whatever the underlying dynamics in Lockridge's case, there is no doubt that many people are fatally wrecked by success.

THE WAY WE regard creative artists and thinkers has shifted since the nineteenth century and the first half of the early twentieth century. This is easy to discern in the remarks of two original thinkers from the earlier period. Elias Canetti, a prototypical peripatetic European intellectual, and perhaps one of the twentieth century's most original thinkers, wrote a landmark book on social theory, *Crowds and Power*, which he began in the 1920s in Vienna and finished thirty-five years later. Not only was Canetti's subject matter related to Freud's *Group Psychology and the Analysis of the Ego* but he was also psychologically involved with Freud, as he recounts in his memoir, *A Torch in My Ear*: "At the time, I was unaware of how much the manner of my enterprise owed to the fact that there was someone like Freud in Vienna, that people talked about him in such a way as if every individual could, by himself, of his own accord, and of his own result, find explanations for things. Since Freud's ideas did not suffice for me, failing to explain the phenomenon that was most important to me, I was sincerely, if naively, convinced that I was undertaking something totally independent of him. It was clear to me that I needed him as an adversary. But the fact that he served as a kind of model for me—this was something that no one could have made me see at that time."[39]

It was at a farm retreat where he began his study of crowds that Canetti first read Freud's *Massenpsychologie Und Ich-Analyse* (*Group Psychology*): "I was surprised at myself for managing to open up this book out here, even though it repelled me from the very first word, and still repels me no less fifty-five years later. . . ." Manifestly, what Canetti held against Freud was that Freud lacked any personal experience of "falling prey" to the emotional contagion of the crowd. "My rejection of Freud came at the start of my work on [my] book."

Although Canetti acknowledged that he was tangled up with Freud as a necessary adversary, you would never guess it from reading *Crowds and Power*.[40] Quite the contrary. In a book with a voluminous bibliography, no reference to Freud is to be found. There is but a single reference to Freud throughout, and it appears in a footnote describing Schreber's paranoid delusions, which obviously mandated some mention of Freud, since Freud had written extensively about Schriber.

For all Freud's reluctance to abandon instinctual life and Oedipal dynamics as the almost exclusive motivating forces in our lives, in *Group Psychology* he began to emphasize the importance of interpersonal relationships as decisive in shaping inner life. Yet this opening to a broadened view of the essential components of the individual's psyche as essentially linked to life with others which appears in the text is at the same time countermanded by the paradox of Freud's own authorial stance throughout the text. As early as the third chapter of *Group Psychology*, we find Freud inserting a curious statement about his standing alone: "as regarding intellectual work, it remains a fact, indeed, that great decisions in the realm of thought and momentous discoveries and solutions of problems are only possible to an individual working in solitude."[41] Here he expresses the heroic view of creativity typical of his times. Set this comment in juxtaposition to Canetti's own statement, previously quoted, of how much his enterprise owed to the fact "that there was someone like Freud in Vienna" who by himself could "find explanations for things." Nonetheless, both Canetti and Freud shared the wishful fantasy of the independent genius who stood above the crowd.

Contrast their view with the way we now so often view creative life as a joint enterprise—witness for example the great conjunctions of people who come together to make movies. Contrast it, too, with the organization of something like the genome project and the way scientists function as integral parts of a team and how proud they are of the "labs" with which they have been affiliated. While scientists recognize a hierarchy of creativity among themselves, they also acknowledge their involvement in a group endeavor and their dependence on those who have gone before. How paradoxical it is that Canetti and Freud, both dedicated to understanding the essential role of group psychology in the formation of the individual psyche, nonetheless were committed to their belief in the individual striving for genius in isolation. Given that it was the belief system of their time that achievement was individual, this was a position Freud could adhere to despite the fact that he drew on a series of creative collaborators of greater or lesser gifts in the furtherance of his own work— including, of course, Wilhelm Fliess. None of us, not even Freud, is free of the cultural unconscious, the different myths that permeate our thinking in different historical epochs.[42]

It is my contention that creativity, which is sometimes a solitary enterprise, is almost always, at least in part, fueled by our relationships in both the internal world of the psyche and in the external world. And that means, whether we like it or not, that creativity is also caught up, from beginning to end, with issues not only of the freedom of self-expression and other attributes related to personal power, but also from beginning to end with issues of interpersonal power. This is of course easier to see nowadays than it was in Freud's time, since so much of modern creativity, from movie making to scientific research, is transparently a team effort. (Brilliant film directors, recognizing the inspiration of those who have gone before, frequently pay homage to their predecessors in their films.) With these models in mind, we are perhaps more willing to look for the collaborative, cooperative, competitive, conflictual aspects of creative endeavors generally—not only, for example, by taking stock of the editor along with the writer, but also greedily devouring such famous memoirs of scientific rivalries as portrayed in Thomas Watson's *Double Helix*. In the nineteenth century, by contrast, the seemingly solitary artist was iconographic, just as the seemingly solitary scientist like Pasteur or Koch was, in no small part because the ultimate model of power was the single great statesman, be he Napoleon or Bismarck. But the ignored truth of the matter was that Pasteur and Koch had their labs, their assistants, their sources of funding. So, too, did artists. Van Gogh's brother was an art dealer, and Van Gogh, not quite as assiduously but just as effectively as Turner, closely followed the artistic fashion of his time and self-consciously positioned his own work to stay just one brilliant but still assimilatable step in front of it. In fact, the truly solitary artist, like the truly solitary thinker, has always been more personal myth than fact and the poor person who dreamed of shutting himself away on a mountain to complete the great work by his lonesome is probably chasing a will-o-the-wisp. He may temporarily escape this world and all its external power struggles, but he is unlikely to succeed. In fact, despite the artist's quest for solitude, the interpersonal world exists ineluctably in his or her own mind.

None of this is to deny the innate genius of our great painters, writers, and musicians, or of our great scientists and mathematician. It is to argue that power in the sense of a gift is not the whole of creativity, and sometimes may not even be the larger part. There is no successful act of creation which does not entail an ability to assert oneself and one's own vision, along with an ability to draw on others for support and nurturance, patience for the creative process to wind its ways, the courage to face failure, and the inner strength to tolerate the possibility of success.

12

Recognition: Fame and Celebrity, Money and Social Status

"For Hegel, the primary motor of human history is not modern natural science or the ever expanding horizon of desire that powers it, but rather a totally non-economic drive, the struggle for recognition.*"*

Francis Fukuyama, The End of History and the Last Man

Recognition is not something we seek simply to please our vanity. Recognition—confirmation, validation—is something that we require at all stages of our lives. We all need someone who knows us to endorse us as a valuable person. In addition to the connectedness and mutual recognition we find in intimate relationships, some of us try to achieve public or social recognition as an endorsement of our worth.

If our immediate surroundings and situation fail to provide the kind of endorsement we require, we go to great lengths to secure it. An exaggerated need for recognition may be a product of growing up with distant, unexpressive, or even hostile parents. Or it may spring from a fragile narcissism that covers over some basic insecurity. In such cases we crave recognition not for the emotional connection it provides, not as an affirmation of ourselves, our work, or our creations, but as a way of assuaging our self-doubt.

Feeling put down in the family, or believing that a sibling was the parents' favorite in childhood may surface in adulthood as a need to best the other, to top the other's net worth or to garner public acknowledgment from the community. Some people are driven to seek recognition as the result of ambition instilled in them by their parents, or they may be driven by a gift that they feel some internal pressure to express. Some performers are plagued by insecurity, and need applause to feel fully alive; onstage, they may burn bright and feel exalted, but offstage they often feel sad or empty. Many professional comedians are sad if not downright depressed.

The values of the world can also make us feel a need for external endorsement. In a highly competitive milieu, many people seek recognition through political power, celebrity, fame, wealth, or social position. Elias Canetti distinguished among the goals of a rich man, a ruler, and a celebrity: "A rich man collects cattle and hoards of grain, or the money which stands for them. He does not worry about men; it is enough that he can buy them. . . . A ruler collects men. Grain and cattle, or money, mean nothing to him except in as far as he needs them to get hold of men. . . . A celebrity collects a chorus of voices. All he wants is to hear them repeat his name."[1] Being reminded periodically about our accomplishments, money, power, or fame can be just the right medicine to warm our cockles, to compensate for any periodic shortfall in our feelings of self-esteem and self-worth.

Our culture is often said to be overly interested in the signs and symbols of affluence and fame, but the need to be recognized can be found throughout recorded history. Anthropologists have reported that in a tribal society, painting one's face helps provide a sense of individuality and humanity. For example, the anthropologist Claude Lévi-Strauss said of the Kaduevo Indians of Brazil: "The face paintings confer upon the individual his dignity as a human being: they help him to cross the frontier from nature to culture and from the 'mindless' animal to the civilized Man."[2] We may consider self-decoration shallow or narcissistic, but it is a symbolic transformation that marks us as human. The personal adornments so precious to us—our clothes, our braids and curls, our makeup, and the belongings we carry with us—express our individuality and also demonstrate our connection to others. Sometimes we use individual, even idiosyncratic insignia specific to us—for example, a signature ring, a tattoo, a violet streak in the hair, or blue painted toenails—to pin down our individuality. In Freud's parlance this practice might be described as the narcissism of small differences. Our garments, ornaments, and badges let others know who we are or who we want to appear to be. We use these items in almost mystical ways to proclaim our individuality, and, like people in every other culture, to signal our "ability to control energy, to defeat opponents, to command loyalty, to attract attention and envy."[3] In other words, self-decoration announces our power. The insignia, the emblems, the brand names we acquire today are analogous to the uses preliterate people made of body decorations, paints, and tattoos. Many of us take great pleasure in our self-decoration and in an accumulation of possessions that provide status or individuality.

We often choose a car as a statement about who we are. One of the first mistakes I ever made with a psychiatric patient concerned a car. The patient, a former railroad conductor, had been hospitalized for depression at Psychiatric Institute, where I was a resident. He attributed his depression to not having the money to buy the car he wanted. I was still too naive to understand the symbolic significance of that particular car to him. We all have different symbols that confirm our place in the world. And my patient was especially vulnerable because he had just lost his prestigious job on an important run. That made his need for the car even more urgent. He believed adamantly that the first step in his rehabilitation was getting the right car. Fortunately, my naïveté and insensitivity did not destroy the relationship. A year after he was discharged, he wrote to tell me that he had found another job and had bought the car of his dreams. He taught me that we are entitled to our status symbols and to the dreams that give us status and comfort.

Car fever is almost epidemic, or so it seems. I still remember an obituary, decades ago, about a rich girl in Texas who died in her teens. Her last request was to be buried seated in her red convertible—a wish her parents honored. Clearly, what car we prefer—or our preference for no car at all—expresses our values. Some of the old rich still drive station wagons to keep from drawing undue attention to themselves, a kind of reverse snobbery. A Rolls-Royce makes a different statement than a Jaguar. And one of the most brilliant and successful professionals I know doesn't keep a car at all but travels around New York City exclusively by bicycle. (He is not only independently wealthy but also independent-minded.)

Our need for personal markers may have escalated as our sense of a secure place in a defined community has declined. We worry more about brand names in clothing and accessories, and companies devote their advertising to "branding." We use our homes and furnishings to announce who we are and how much power we command. The way we decorate our personal space not only provides pleasure but is often meant to define our place in the world and demonstrate our net worth, whereas traditionally, our homes not only communicated something about us personally but also something about our forebears and our offspring.

Our need to differentiate ourselves through the possessions we accumulate or the groups we associate with may sometimes get out of hand. Some people invest all their energy in being "in," and their behavior is dictated accordingly. Each day's activities are graded in terms of relevance to the ultimate goal—as are the clothes they wear, the places they live in, the church or synagogue they attend, and the people they choose to marry, befriend, work with, and play with. In New York City, such preoccupations can extend to worrying about getting your child into a prestigious nursery school. Common though these pursuits have become, it is risky to make individual achievement, fame, money, or social power our only focus. Since the search for recognition in any of these arenas depends on other people, and they are by their very nature competitive, achieving such a goal is never totally secure. Another risk is that one's ambition, always escalating, may become insatiable; no matter how much we achieve, when we see anyone else doing better, we may still feel envious.

Social Recognition, Fame, and Celebrity

We may possess social recognition by virtue of birth—by being the child of a movie star, a royal family, a CEO, a famous novelist, or the richest family in town. We may have achieved fame through our own accomplishments. Or we may have married someone famous, acquiring fame by association. Fame from any source can build on itself until its origin no longer matters. For example, Sarah Ferguson, the former wife of one of Queen Elizabeth's sons, turns her fame into cash in television commercials, among them ads for Weight Watchers. I am probably not alone in knowing who Sarah Ferguson is but forgetting the name of the prince to whom she was married. I still remember that Gordon Liddy was one of the Watergate burglars, and that James Earl Jones was a remarkable Shakespearean actor and Broadway headliner before he was the voice of Darth Vader, but my sons know Liddy only as the host of a talk show and Jones as the voice of Bell Atlantic.

Every era grants recognition and fame to accomplishments it particularly admires—whether creative, military, financial, or scientific. Toward the end of the nineteenth century, recognition and fame often centered on writers and artists. It was this fashion and the craving it inspired that the writer Max Beerbohm satirized in his story "Enoch Soames." Beerbohm inserted himself into the story as a young man who desperately yearns to attach himself to those who he believes will turn out to be major (or even minor) artists. In the tale, the Beerbohm character meets Enoch Soames in London at the then fashionable Café Royal, where Beerbohm has been taken by a young painter, Will Rothenstein, who cut quite a figure. Rothenstein "knew everyone in Paris. . . . He was Paris in Oxford. It was whispered that 'So soon as he had polished off his selections of dons, those he was going to do portraits of, he was going to include a few undergraduates. It was a proud day for me when I—I—was included."[4] Everyone at the Café Royal is clustered around Rothenstein when in walks a strangely dressed man, Enoch Soames, who circles Rothenstein. When Rothenstein fails to recognize him, Soames patiently reminds him that they have met several times in Paris and that Soames has written a book, *Negations*, and once gave Rothenstein a copy of it.

Despite Soames's odd appearance, Beerbohm is impressed with him: "Soames was quite five or six years older than either of us. Also, he had written a book. . . . If Rothenstein had not been there, I should have revered Soames; even as it was, I respected him. . . . Not to buy a book of which I had met the author face to face would have been for me in those days an impossible act of self denial. When I returned to Oxford for the Christmas Term I had duly secured *Negations*. I used to keep it lying carelessly on the table in my room and whenever a friend took it up and asked what it was about I would say 'Oh, it's rather a remarkable book. It's by a man whom I know.'"[5] But Soames never achieves any real recognition, and by the time he writes his third book, he has to pay to have it published. Beerbohm's acquaintance with him fades away.

Fast forward. A number of years pass and it is now June 3, 1897. Beerbohm enters a small French restaurant and sees Enoch Soames at one table and a Mephistophelian gentleman at another. Soames appears to be in a trance; then he suddenly breaks the silence and murmurs, "A hundred years hence."[6] Soames, come awake, asks Beerbohm if he didn't think that he (Soames) had minded. "'Minded what,' Beerbohm questioned. 'Neglect. Failure,' Soames replies. 'Failure,' Beerbohm replies. 'Neglect—

288 / FEELING STRONG

yes, perhaps; but that's quite another matter. Of course you haven't been—appreciated. But what then?' "[7]

Soames confesses that when he had said some years earlier that it did not matter to him whether or not he was recognized as a writer, it was patently untrue and he implies that Beerbohm was either naive or shallow to have believed him. He goes on to say that while he might have future fame, it would do him precious little good: as a dead man he would not know if people were visiting his grave, commemorating his birthplace, making memorial statues of him. And he moans, "A hundred years hence! Think of it! If I could come back to life *then*—just for a few hours—and go to the reading room and *read*! Or better still: if I could be projected, now, at this moment, into that future, into that reading-room, just for this one afternoon! I'd sell myself body and soul to the Devil for that! Think of the pages and pages in the catalog 'Soames: Enoch.' "[8]

Hearing all this, the gentleman at the other table now reveals himself as the Devil. Beerbohm laughs out loud, but not Soames. And then the failed poet Enoch Soames agrees to sell his soul to the Devil for the privilege of visiting the reading room in the British Museum a hundred years hence to discover whether or not he has made it into the Hall of Fame.

Transported to the British reading room on June 3, 1997—he has been allotted five hours—Soames riffles through the card catalogs, thinking that he must be missing the one in which he is acknowledged; but he eventually comes face to face with the reality that he had not been discovered posthumously as the literary genius he still hopes to have become. His five hours up, he finds himself back in the present, in the very same restaurant where Beerbohm consoles him, suggesting that perhaps he should have waited two or three centuries. Soames confesses this is a thought that has already occurred to him. But worst of all, he reveals that he did find one mention of himself, in a fictional account that Beerbohm has written of a writer's bargain with the Devil. At their parting, Soames, now in thrall to the Devil, implores Beerbohm, "*Try* to make them know that I did exist!" Of course, it is Beerbohm's attempt to do so which is destined to become the fictional piece that Soames had already seen catalogued in the Reading Room. Poor Soames.

Soames is not alone. His longing for fame may be exaggerated, but many of us share it. Gretchen Kraft Rubin, a lawyer who is the author of *Power, Money, Fame, Sex*, divides the contemporary search for fame into four categories: becoming a big fish in a small pond, a household name, a star, or an icon.[9] A significant minority of people aspire to her first category—being a big fish in a small pond. For only in a small pond can our peers really know us and verify for us that our achievements are authentic—and only self-flattery gets better than this. Rubin's last three categories involve achievement in one or another arena that produces varying degrees of celebrity, which involve face and name recognition. They may be achieved through accomplishments but, almost as easily, by being seen with enough important people and in enough important places that one's name and face are impressed on the public's mind. As the writer Dwight MacDonald put it, "A celebrity is a person who is well known for being well known." The fame without the game.

As a consequence, the drive to win recognition for one's achievements (this is what Enoch Soames wants) is often equaled if not surpassed by the urgency to become a celebrity pure and simple, issues of good taste, good manners, or good character be damned. Michael Korda details one of the masters of the game in his hilarious account of how Jacqueline Susann ultimately conquered the publishing world.[10] In 1966, Jacqueline Susann's *Valley of the Dolls* became a huge best-seller. It also "for the first time brought the worlds of Hollywood, T.V., tabloids and Broadway press agentry all together to sell a novel in which they were all the subject."[11]

Susann had always been ambitious; early in her life, she had wanted to be an actress or possibly a model. She married Irving Mansfield—a press agent, promoter, and producer—and he became her entrée to show business and celebrity. According to Korda, Susann hung out so much with celebrities that she herself became a celebrity, relentlessly covered by Mansfield and by Broadway gossip columnists. She hit on the idea of writing a book about her poodle, which she called *Every Night, Josephine!* Published in 1963, it was heavily publicized by her husband, and it made her reputation as a writer. Three years later, at age forty-eight, Jackie wrote *Valley of the Dolls*, which Korda describes as "a brilliant combination of soap opera, show business gossip, and tear jerker, a world wide number-one best-seller in hard cover and mass market paperback and later a successful movie." Korda credits Susann with inventing a new kind of fiction: "shop girl romance, brought up to date with lots of dirty talk, the suggestion of some pretty rough sex, and an unsentimental view of men."[12] Even more important, what she and Mansfield did together was to promote a new way of selling books, shifting wholesale to the Hollywood style of hype.

Susann remained ambitious, and she wanted a prestigious publisher. Simon and Schuster presented Korda, who impressed Susann because his uncle was the movie producer Alexander Korda and his aunt the actress Merle Oberon. So it was with Korda that Susann published her second novel, *The Love Machine*. Korda quotes Susann's basic insight for reaching a wide readership: "I write for women who read me in the goddamn subways on the way home from work. . . . I know who they are because that's who I used to be. Remember *Stella Dallas?* My readers are like Stella. They want to press their noses against the windows of other people's houses and get a look at the parties they'll never get invited to, the dresses they'll never get to wear, the lives they'll never live, the guys they'll never fuck."[13] Her insight cuts to the core nature of celebrity, which is the vicarious thrill it whips up among worshipers of celebrity.

Susann was astute enough to intuit that her readers could be fascinated by the celebrities in her books because all of them ended up badly: "All the people they envy in my books, the ones who are glamorous or beautiful or rich or talented, they have to come to a bad end, see, because *that* way people who read me can get off the subway and go home feeling better about their own crappy lives and *luckier* than the people they've been reading about."[14] Susann was not the dumb broad some people assumed she was—she got it exactly right. Her readers experienced the vicarious thrill of knowing celebrities while also having their envy tamed by the hard luck outcome of the novel's protagonists.

Actually, Susann herself was an authentic heroine. The year she wrote *Every Night, Josephine!* she discovered that she had metastatic breast cancer, and she lived secretly with pain and painkillers until she died. Susann loved *The Love Machine*, and it became an enormous success for Simon and Schuster. As an author, she never underestimated her readers, and while critics found her prose ordinary and her plots contrived, she applied herself to her work with the sincerity and dedication, if not the talent, of a major writer. That was part of her secret. The other was her sense of her audience. Hers was the great insight that celebrity played to widespread fantasies among ordinary people.

Susann's great rule for her heroines—that they had to end badly— helps explain an odd phenomenon of our time: the apparently real grief many people feel at the passing of certain celebrities. Princess Di was one of the latest in a line that includes Marilyn Monroe, Judy Garland, James Dean, Janis Joplin, and Jim Morrison. Some observers say that such figures possess some human quality which comes through and touches each and every one of us. Not so, I think. I do not mean to disparage Princess Di's work or Marilyn's talent or Joplin's incredible delivery; great grief (when not connected to the death of one of our own near and dear) is rather delicious. It is the linchpin of our vicarious enjoyment of celebrity. By dying too soon, these figures successfully forestall our envy—and let us enjoy them all the more in our imaginations. Susann's heroines end badly, but it can be just as effective to end early.

The desire for recognition and celebrity exists in many of us. Just as Sardi's, a restaurant in New York that was once fashionable with the theatrical crowd, has cartoons of theatre people covering the walls, so Della Femina, an "in" restaurant in East Hampton, covers its walls with caricatures, mostly of the minor (and a few major) celebrities who spend the summer there. But the canvas is getting almost too crowded. God forbid someone should be left out. Vincent Sardi had a different way of inculcating loyalty among his patrons: he always had one item on the menu every night that the lowliest actor, working for tips in some Greenwich Village eatery, could afford. You could be as good as broke and still have a bite to eat at Sardi's—and see and be seen. People who made it didn't forget. Of course, the proliferation of caricatures at Della Femina's is matched by that of bronze plaques on hospital walls, and park benches, not to mention the almost ubiquitous "most powerful" lists featured in magazines annually. As The Most Reverend Archbishop Rienard McCarrick, the recently appointed archbishop to Washington, wryly told a reporter, he felt welcome there indeed, as he had been told that he was listed as the thirty-sixth most important man in Washington D.C. Unfortunately, he explained, he failed to recognize the first thirty-five people on the list.

Some celebrities, such as Oprah Winfrey and Rosie O'Donnell, use their fame to support causes they genuinely believe in. But even if celebrities engage in good works primarily for the sake of publicity, they may sometimes provide an impetus for action on an important social issue.

Recognition and respect in one's profession often gives one the power to right a wrong, help a disadvantaged group, or correct an injustice. My friend Alan Trustman—a lawyer, screenwriter, and sometime gold trader—tells about his father, the late Ben Trustman, a respected Boston lawyer who had achieved his distinction the old-fashioned way, by dint of his diligence, acumen, and total scrupulousness. One of the ways he chose to exercise his gifts was to put to bed an old Boston prejudice, an exploit that is recorded in a letter Alan later sent to the President of Harvard University, Neil L. Rudenstine.

October 16, 1996

Dear Neil,

We buried my father on Sunday but there is a story that should not be buried with him: how Jews finally came to be admitted to the Harvard Club of Boston.

The Club remained exclusively Brahmin through World War II and virtually no Jews got past the entrenched Committee on Admissions. By the late 1940s, however, a growing minority of the Club members were finding the situation, in stages, discomfiting, embarrassing, irritating and finally morally repugnant. In 1950, they met with A. M. Sonnabend, one of the few Jewish members and among the most prominent.

A. M. had a simple solution: persuade Club President Lowell and the Admissions Committee that they had to make a concession to the growing discontent by asking Ben Trustman, a "respectable" Jew, one of three Jews out of the 47 lawyers at Nutter, McClennen & Fish, to join the Club and then go on the Committee on Admissions. At the same time, they would tell Ben that they were putting him there to solve the problem.

Ben joined the Harvard Club and was appointed to the Committee on Admissions.

The next meeting of the Committee commenced with a certain degree of tension. The fourth applicant was Jewish. The Committee blackballed him. Ben raised his hand and said his first word, "Why?"

One of the members gave a "character" reason. Ben nodded and said, "That's reasonable," and everyone breathed a sigh of relief; the man was going to "go along" and there would be no confrontation.

Indeed, emboldened by their success at the first meeting, the

Committee members decided to escalate. At the next meeting, the very first name on the list was Jewish. The man was blackballed. Ben again raised his hand and politely said, "Why?"

The Committee Chairman replied at length. "Ben, we have been talking it over since the last meeting and we feel we set a bad precedent. It has always been the policy of this Committee that any member can blackball any applicant without giving a reason."

Ben considered that for a moment. "It seems to me that the policy should be changed and I so move."

There was a silence.

The Chairman said, "A motion has been made. Is it seconded?"

There was silence.

The Chairman cleared his throat, "There has been no second and therefore we cannot vote on the motion. Ben? Do you have any comment?"

Yes," said Ben. "Obviously I disagree, but if that is the policy, I will live with it."

Again, there was a collective sigh of relief. There would be no problem.

They were wrong.

Ben proceeded to blackball every other applicant whose name came up at the meeting.

In fact, he blackballed every applicant whose name came up at the next eleven meetings. The last name presented at the eleventh meeting was that of the son of the Committee Chairman.

"A fine young man," said Ben. "I have heard all sorts of nice things about him." He then blackballed the son.

The news of what had been going on had of course percolated throughout the Club where it was variously greeted with delight and amusement or horror and consternation depending on the member's views on the underlying problem. President Lowell was therefore not surprised when he was visited by the Chairman of the Committee on Admissions.

"This is intolerable," said the Chairman. "We absolutely must get that man off the Committee on Admissions."

"I agree," said the President. "And so does he."

"He does?"

"Yes," said the President. "Ben says the Committee is dysfunctional. But I have no power to remove him. Or any of you for that matter."

The Chairman took the hint. "Are you telling me that he will resign if all the rest of us resign?"

The President said, "I will propose it to him."

And he did.

Ben gave the President without a comment a list of members prepared by A. M. Sonnabend and Sonnie's friends of members who were willing to serve as replacements.

President Lowell got the point and agreed to use the list as the source of Admissions Committee replacements. The entire Committee on Admissions resigned and he accepted their resignations and appointed the replacements.

My uncle, Morton Myerson, '42, was one of those elected at the next meeting.

Best wishes,
Alan Trustman

Money and Social Power

There are those whose entire investment in life is directed toward monetary success. Their fantasy and imaginative lives are as a consequence impoverished, confined to the idea of getting ahead. They believe in the "cash value" of what they do, and their actions are directed accordingly. For some people, accumulating money has become life's sole purpose. The astonishing thing about Michael Milken, finally, was not that he was working sixty, seventy hours a week at this despite the fact that he was already rich beyond anyone's wildest dreams, but that he broke the law trying to amass yet more millions. He was a man more driven than driving.

For other people, it is not money but making connections that drives them, as they strive to climb one or another social ladder. They may be well educated and successful, but they remain concerned with access. The sheer number of useful social contacts is more important to them than the depth of any one relationship. Their day's activities are graded in terms of relevance to the goal of making connections—the appointment book is a battle plan and the telephone appears to have been invented just for them.

Still, I do not want to underestimate the importance of connections. Connections can move us higher on the surgeon's waiting list, get us into the right school, give us an introduction that leads to a job, gain us admittance to a club, or get us scarce tickets for a basketball game. Nor are connections restricted to the upper classes. A maid is able to place her friends in good jobs in private homes through her employer's connections. A girlfriend of a married man persuades him to help her relatives. And so on. Striving for connections only becomes hazardous when we prioritize them over authentic friendship.

Americans' preoccupation with money and riches has from time to time exploded into a veritable lust. Obtaining money through marriage is an old story; in the past, this was one of the few ways in which women could improve their status, because the opportunities to provide for themselves were so limited. In some places marriage was the way people in the social register stayed solvent as new money married into old families—in Boston, for example, Marlborough Street married Beacon Street. The fraternization and mating practices between the old rich and the new rich continues to this very day, with only the external trappings somewhat different. Edith Wharton's novel *The House of Mirth* provides a fascinating example from the late nineteenth century.

In *The House of Mirth*, Lily Bart, the well-bred but insufficiently well-off heroine, has only one way of securing a future—she must find a wealthy husband. One prospective husband is rich enough but she finds him far too pious, serious, and averse to fun. Instead, Lily is drawn to Selden, who is charming and well positioned but he has insufficient means (and perhaps insufficient courage) to take the risk of marrying her. In short Lily is either too refined or too picky, depending on your point of view, and in the end she turns down someone who in today's mind-set may appear to have been her best prospect, Rosendale, a rich Jewish suitor, a man who ultimately cracks into her social world on his own. Lily makes a series of bad decisions that rapidly propel her down the social ladder. She finally loses even her pitiful job decorating hats and dies alone in a single room.

According to Louis Auchincloss, *The House of Mirth* gave Wharton both her medium—the novel of manners—and her subject matter—the assault by new millionaires on the old Knickerbocker society in which she had grown up. Wharton called the new millionaires "invaders." They had come into their fortunes in a boom just after the Civil War, and now they wanted social recognition. Auchincloss identifies one of Wharton's important themes: "[she] saw clearly enough that the invaders and defenders were bound ultimately to bury their hatchets in a noisy, stamping dance, but she also saw the rich possibilities for satire in the contrast afforded by the battle line in its last stages and the pathos of the individuals who were fated to be trampled under the feet of those boisterous truce makers."[15]

Lily, of course, was one of the victims, dead of an infectious illness. That illness was social climbing (and perhaps her inability to close a deal) but Lily's death was real. The ending of *The House of Mirth* may seem contrived—until we remember that health and long life are correlated with nothing so much as money.

In fact, money buys more than access and luxuries. In the *New York Times*, Erica Goode reported that, according to recent research, social class is a better predictor of health than genetic endowment, exposure to carcinogens, or even smoking.[16] The numerous studies documenting this discrepancy were sparked by pioneering research directed by Dr. Michael Marmout, Director of the International Center for Health and Science at University College, London, which tracked 17,530 men in the British civil service over a ten-year period. What makes the study particularly compelling is that the mortality rates varied precisely with the civil service grade the men held—the higher the classification, the lower the rate of death, irrespective of its cause. This finding was counterintuitive insofar as the men were all employed and had equal access under Britain's national health system. Astonishingly enough, the mortality rates in the lowest classification were three times higher than those in the highest grade, results that were substantiated in a twenty-five-year follow-up. Difference in the gradient of mortality by social class lasted past the subjects' retirement, even into the ninth decade of their lives. The class discrepancy was found to be unrelated to habits like smoking. However, prolonged exposure to stress, leading to abnormalities in the immune function and glucose metabolism, might account for it to some degree. Thus Marmout's study suggests a very important conclusion: the lower their social status, the more stress people feel, and it is likely that the stress in their lives contributes to their vulnerability to the diseases that lead to their death.

The link between social status and stress appears to be related to an individual's sense of control. In a second study, initiated in 1985, Marmout and his colleagues looked at civil servants of both sexes. One question they asked employees and managers was how much control they felt they exerted over their job. Not surprisingly they found that control varied directly with how far up in the hierarchy these subjects were. And once again, death rates were greater in the lower pay grades. This seems to be a concrete example of the benefits of possessing at least one kind of power—control over one's work and a certain degree of status.

Similarly, research at Carnegie Mellon found that people who rated themselves low in status at work were more likely to become infected when exposed to a mild respiratory virus than people who ranked themselves higher. Unemployed people were even more susceptible to the virus than those on the lower rungs of the ladder at work.

Other factors involved have to do with the "long arm of childhood."[17] They include not only genetics but nutrition, instances of abuse and neglect, and children's exposure to stressful events. Some, though not all, are also connected to class background, another kind of hierarchy. Lily Bart's death then, for want of marrying up, is not so far-fetched after all.

Nor was Wharton off the mark with her satire of the ways of the wealthy. Indeed, some of the excesses of the 1990s—the worship of celebrity and money—paralleled those of Edith Wharton's Gilded Age. Just as money poured into New York in the 1880s and 1890s, so, too, has it poured in during the 1980s and 1990s, as a result of the stock market boom and the information revolution. That money changed the patterns of wealth and status in the United States, and it resulted in some of the same excesses that Thorstein Veblen wrote about in 1899 in *The Theory of the Leisure Class*.

Ultimately, the possession of wealth has to be confirmed—it must be witnessed by friends and competitors, and so it must be displayed to them through gifts or lavish entertainment. Veblen wrote: "The competitor with whom the entertainer wishes to institute a comparison is, by this method, made to serve as a means to the end. He consumes vicariously for his host at the same time as he is a witness to the consumption of that excess of good things which his host is unable to dispose of 'single-handed,' and he is also made witness to his host's facility in etiquette."[18] This is our version of the potlatch.

From such displays there emerges a "differentiation within the class" that is connected with the inheritance not only of money but also of gentility, which is thought to accompany it. What sometimes happens, though, is that "gentle blood" is transmitted without the money to back it up. Selden—Lily Bart's fainthearted admirer in *The House of Mirth*—plays a gentleman, but without the money needed to fully inhabit the part.

Today, the social register can still be hard to crack. Many people who have become rich through their own efforts lack the connections and the polish to enter "society" on their own. One real estate broker who sells high-end apartments in New York City gives her clients a bonus: when they close a deal with her, they are invited to a dinner at which she entertains a number of socialites. She may be a pale imitation of the social arbiters who paved the way for arrivistes in *The House of Mirth*, but the spirit is there.

The newly rich of today can find their path just as bumpy as Rosendale's. Members of an in-group who feel themselves at a disadvantage and are fearful of being displaced often put newcomers down. The newly rich soon learn that they may need a guide to navigate the treacherous waters of the social hierarchy, so alliances are made between social old-timers who could use some financial perks and rich newcomers who need to be educated and introduced.

Beyond health and social perks, money buys freedom. Sometimes, too, rich people feel an obligation to give something back to the society in which they have flourished; they can be enormously generous in funding a variety of causes, artistic or charitable. Thus an alliance is formed between fund-raisers and socialites, who get "twofers" for their money, buying benefit tickets and thus supporting worthy causes while simultaneously garnering the opportunity to be seen at the event, and perhaps even to be photographed for the styles sections of the *New York Times* or *W*.

Each world has its own special kind of snobbery, slights, and social signals. It may be hard to understand how many different worlds there are until we move from one to another. For many people, the first exposure to another world comes when they leave home to go to college. A working-class boy who arrives at an elite college may discover, for instance, subtle and not-so-subtle differences in table manners and clothes that indicate class background. For some people, a party marks a first visit to a different social world. I remember going with my husband, a lawyer (he was then an associate), to our first Sunday lunch given by a partner in his firm. This was the first time I had ever been invited to a country estate, complete with Black Angus cattle. Where I came from, Kentucky, Sunday lunch was a dress-up affair, so, without thinking to ask someone what might be appropriate, I went so far as to buy a new dress, which I thought was spectacular, a low-cut white dress printed with huge blue roses. I still remember how shocked I was to walk into the house and find the other guests wearing casual country clothes—with boots, so that they could go for a bracing walk after lunch. Of course, looking for some balm to take away the sting of my embarrassment, I salvaged my pride by thinking with some superiority that in Kentucky we would have had better manners and tipped our guests, advising them, "This is very low-key so come dressed down," or alternatively, "I know it's silly but we always get dressed up for Sunday lunch." The blue flowered dress hung in my closet, never to be worn again, until I eventually threw it out.

If there's one recent novel that catches for me, among other things, the degree to which we are steeped in issues of where we and our friends and acquaintances stand in the world, it is Michael Cunningham's novel *The Hours*, an homage to Virginia Woolf and her novel *Mrs. Dalloway*. (*The Hours* was Woolf's working title for what became *Mrs. Dalloway*.)[19] Both works involve self-importance and a discerning stroking of others. Cunningham suggests how we are always adjudicating and calibrating recognition, in our subtle disparagement or acknowledgment of others and in our concern about the way we are being perceived. Like Woolf, Cunningham is sensitive to the signals we choose to send.

Cunningham implies that recognition is worth something only if it comes through an intricate kind of conversational hand-to-hand combat raised to an art form. Social recognition originating in other ways—the kind of recognition that might come easily in a small town—is for that reason all the more worthless. Cunningham's stand-in for Clarissa Dalloway, Clarissa Vaughn, a distinguished book editor with a sixteen-year-old daughter, has lived with a lesbian lover for eighteen years. She is about to give a party and is quite excited about it. Walking down the street, she notices someone who she thinks might be a movie star. Dropping in to see her friend Richard, who is wan and sick, she wonders aloud who the person might be. Richard, however, refuses to discuss it: "Richard, alone among Clarissa's acquaintances, has no essential interest in famous people. . . . It is, Clarissa thinks, some combination of monumental ego and a kind of elitism."[20]

Richard sees specialness not in the famous but in the people he knows: "Richard cannot imagine a life more interesting or worthwhile than those being lived by his acquaintances and himself, and for that reason one often feels exalted, expanded in his presence. He is not one of those egotists who miniaturize others. He is the opposite kind of egotist, driven by grandiosity rather than greed, if he insists on a version of you that is funny, or strange, or more eccentric and profound than you suspect yourself to be—capable of doing more good and more harm in the world than you've ever imagined—it is all but impossible not to believe . . . in that he alone sees through to your essence, weighs your true qualities. . . . It is only after knowing him for some time that you begin to realize you are, to him, an essentially fictional character, one he has invested with nearly limitless capacities for tragedy and comedy not because that is your true nature but because he, Richard, needs to live in a world peopled by extreme and commanding figures." Ah, but what an addictive tonic that is.

Richard, however, is dying, and he will not make it to Clarissa's party. He has always been Clarissa's best friend, her "most rigorous, infuriating companion," and as the party approaches Clarissa muses that if Richard were not dying, "they could be together right now, arguing about Walter Hardy and the quest for eternal youth, about how gay men have taken to imitating the boys who tortured them in high school."[21]

Clarissa herself is aging. She chides herself for caring about not being asked to lunch with Oliver St. Oggs. At the same time she that feels embarrassed that she was not invited, she chides herself for her triviality at a time when Richard may be dying. But she quickly recovers and frets that people don't look at her sexually anymore.[22]

Richard kills himself before Clarissa's party, and she admits two things to herself: her "desire for a relatively ordinary life (neither more nor less than what most people desire)" and how much she had wanted him to come to her party where her guests would be unable to miss his devotion to her. She consoles herself by thinking that she will ask for his "forgiveness for shying away, on what would be the day of his death, from kissing him on the lips and for telling herself she did so only for the sake of his health."[23]

We often try to manage how others see us by invoking symbols of power. Some women professionals might covet Armani or Prada suits as insignia of power. If a woman can afford such a suit, it is a statement that she is part of a powerful group; it is also a talisman—something that will bring more success. Signs and decorations used as insignia of power may reflect reality, or they may reflect no more than an attempt by people who aspire to a position to appear as though they have already reached it. In another world, drug dealers and pimps favor certain cars. People with power have always used symbols—after all, the king has his crown and sceptre.

AFTER ALL of our attempts to be "in," what do we gain once we have acquired money and social power? Some find themselves as disaffected as ever. The novelist James Baldwin said it well: "One of the reasons I had fought so hard, after all, was to wrest from the world fame and money and love. And here I was at thirty-two, finding my notoriety hard to bear, since its principal effect was to make me more lonely; money, it turned out, was exactly like sex, you thought of nothing else if you didn't have it and thought of other things if you did; and love, as far as I could see, was over."[24] Such disdain of fame and money seems to be more prevalent among those who have power than those who don't.

As it turns out, money and status are not something we obtain once and for all. There are many reversals—not only for the middle class but also for the rich. In a competitive, hierarchical society such as ours, a diminution in our status can shake not only our material well-being but also our self-confidence and our belief in our capacity to exert power. In the stock market crash of 1929, some Wall Street traders and bankers who lost their fortunes killed themselves. During the recent bull market, some who failed to participate in the market gains felt threatened and dispossessed. An article in New York Magazine, "To Have and Have More," looked at the psychic plight of people who were doing well but still felt left behind in the boom market of the 1990s: "In another not-too-distant era, we would have been yuppies, scorned for buying up every last exposed-brick two-bedroom in the . . . Village. Now, even though our income has been rising steadily, we may not be able to afford the $650,000 a nice two-bedroom goes for these days—in New York in the late nineties, in other words, you can get ahead and still fall behind."[25] The author, referring to the new breed of instant millionaires, points out that "the

Internet came along and redefined success." In the same issue of the magazine, Ralph Gardner, Jr., in an article entitled "Class Struggle on Park Avenue," argues that "the growing chasm between the really rich and everyone else may be felt most keenly not by the truly poor but by the well-to-do, particularly those who grew up here and who cling to the childish notion that the City should remain theirs. . . . Perhaps most damaging of all to [their] self-esteem . . . is the realization that new money—who in former days relished the opportunity to mingle with impoverished old money—no longer seems to attach much importance to pedigree or refinement."[26]

Downward mobility did not begin in the 1990s, of course. The anthropologist Katherine S. Newman notes that the 1980s witnessed "the first generation since the Great Depression that [could] expect to have a *lower* standard of living than its parents."[27] Writing of a town in northern New Jersey that she calls Pleasanton, Newman says that when those born there in the late 1950s and 1960s came of age, they could not afford to live there, even though they made much more money than their parents. They were exiled from their hometown, just as some natives of New York City are now exiled from *their* hometown.

ANOTHER ASPECT of the drive for social power is a desire to deny status to others. For us to be in, others must be out. This dynamic of exclusion, of nonrecognition, is related to our innate need for recognition in myriad ways. In the displaced theatre of recognition that celebrities play out for us in the tabloids and in *Entertainment Tonight* spin-offs, we thrill equally to discover who is now "out" as well as who is "in" and there is a whole media sub-genre devoted to showing how the stars of another era have sunk into obscurity and mediocrity—or worse, teen idols now grown into middle-aged nobodies. Those whom we no longer recognize are as vital to the celebrity game as those we do. More directly, and painfully, the same dynamic plays out on city streets when we disdain to return the greeting of someone considered beneath us, as though not recognizing an "inferior" is almost as good as being recognized by someone "superior." This dynamic can also be seen in literature, where excluded groups go unrecognized as contributing anything valid to the common cultural experience—a snub so total that for victims to find a voice of their own, they must invert the images and tropes of the dominant group into a kind of anti-prose—as Toni Morrison did with the bitter title of her remarkable novel about the brutally neglected, abused black girl who dreams of being white, *The Bluest Eye*.

Such inversion of literary style, the counterpart of deliberately stylized public greetings among some ethnic groups, has a long tradition of its own. The social theorist Elias Canetti wrote in his autobiography, *The Torch in My Ear*, that he learned from the famous Viennese lecturer Karl Kraus that "one can do anything with other people's words," using an author's own words to catch him out.[28] Such a sophisticated and compelling mode of indictment was brought to bear by the late black writer and critic Joe Wood, who distilled "the autobiography of a race concept," by which he meant the white race, in the ostensibly pluralistic work of the preeminent literary critic Alfred Kazin.[29] Rather than addressing blacks, Wood says Kazin ended up writing "a race concept," which ultimately tells the story of how the children of turn-of-the-century immigrants embraced whiteness. For those immigrants, becoming American and being "white" were the same thing.

Wood dissects Kazin's "race concept" using material from Kazin's *A Walker in the City* and *New York Jew*, "reading" Kazin's no doubt unconscious bias. Wood suggests that because Kazin never came to grips with the literature of nonwhite America, his lifelong project of explaining American literature was left with a gaping hole. In *A Walker in the City*, Kazin writes of Jews that "We were the children of the immigrants who had camped at the city's backdoor, in New York's rawest, remotest, cheapest ghetto, enclosed on one side by the Canarsie Flats and on the other by the hallowed middle-class districts that showed the way to New York. 'New York' was what we put last on our address, but first in thinking of the others around us. They were New York, the capital of gentiles, America; we were Brownsville— . . . the dust of the earth to all Jews with money, and a notorious place that measured all success by our skill in getting away from it. So that when the poor Jews left, *even* Negroes, as we said, found it easy to settle on the margins of Brownsville. . . ." Wood suggests that in *New York Jew* Kazin's attitude had hardened: "My parents still lived in the same Brownsville tenement. News of the big money had not reached this house painter and this 'home and dressmaker.' They were as poor and isolated from America-at-large as the day they had met. . . . But now they were surrounded by poor blacks more than by poor Jews. . . . It was a poisoned spot on the New York map, even to the hundreds and thousands of blacks from the South warily making it into the ghetto vacated by the Jews." Wood contends that in both books Kazin failed to acknowledge blacks as fellow poor people who also longed to share in the American Dream: instead they were used as symbols of "the blackness everybody wanted to discard."

Yet Kazin was no bigot. And that is Joe Wood's point—Kazin, like too many of us, to a greater or lesser degree, had internalized a negative valuation of blacks, even when we consciously hold a deep commitment to end racism. Racism is fed by the desire for power in the form of whiteness. It is this power of racism to infect even liberals that speaks to the way such social and cultural prejudices permeate all of us—and in the past perhaps most tragically, blacks themselves.

To return to my original point: the purpose of bigotry is not exclusively to demean others. Its basic purpose is to elevate the self. We want to raise ourselves even if we need to stand on someone else's back to do it. This is a grim side of our desire for social recognition—this pointedly not seeing people of the excluded social group—thus making the black man into, in the words of Ellison's famous title, *The Invisible Man*.

Recognition from the world is one of the ways power is granted; nonrecognition is one way power is denied. Lacking recognition, some people covet wealth or fame as a substitute. This is how some of us become preoccupied with the rich, the famous, and the powerful. But a fanatic, frantic interest in accumulating more and more recognition, just like the desire for more and more money, ultimately brings doom. The expression "You can't be too rich or too thin" is clever but shallow. It misses the internal devouring hunger—for money, for admiration—that in the end so often destroys those possessed by it. It also misses the fact that the external world may upset our adaptations, when recessions and other calamities shake up what we have come to assume was permanent.

What, then, provides more reliable affirmation? Some kind of recognition is essential to promote authentic power, but it is not always available. Erin, a caseworker in Robert Parker's detective novel *Double Deuce*, has it right when she cites Muslims, Baptists, and the Marine Corps as among the very few sources of personal affirmation—or recognition— available to those who are otherwise deprived of it: the dispossessed, poor kids, ghetto kids, kids with almost no avenues open to them.[30] It may be that some system of belief, religious or ideological, is an important, perhaps necessary, source of personal affirmation, not just for the poor and excluded but for all of us. The next chapter addresses the uses and misuses we make of transcendence, religion, and other belief systems in our search for recognition and authentic power.

13

Transcendence:
The Godfather Fantasy

*"Death is obscene, unmentionable, pornographic; if sex was
nasty, death is a nasty mistake."*

—Rollo May, *Love and Will*

Sooner or later all of us must face
our own mortality. In the same way that a fear of emotional estrangement
stokes the desire for renewing interpersonal ties, our knowledge of our
biological frailty and the brevity of our time on earth leads us to look for
meaning in our lives and, for many of us, to seek some form of transcendence. Establishing meaning in our lives usually depends on feeling that
we have an impact on the future or a stake in eternal life.

We may find meaning through a sense of continuity with our children and their children, providing symbolic survival through succeeding generations. Some of us hope that our intellectual and creative
contributions will stand the test of time, that our work will be remembered. Or we attach ourselves to a shared secular goal, for example, acting to build a good society or overthrowing a bad one. This serves as a
ratification of our worth. But many of us require something more: we
seek transcendence through mysticism or religion that offers the hope
of immortality.

Transcendence seeking generally trumps temporal ambitions because it offers the hope of transformation or life everlasting. Transcendence, however, is not necessarily restricted to the realms of mysticism or religion. Some of us find transcendence through death-defying acts of adventure. In *Into the Wild*, Jon Krakauer describes a young man's journey into the Alaskan wilderness, where he was trying to invent a new life by totally immersing himself in nature. Impulsive and foolish, he took too few precautions and ultimately died. When his story first hit the newspapers, many readers responded angrily to what they saw as his arrogance and carelessness. But Krakauer, who had had similar ambitions as a young man, knew only too well what Chris McCandless was after: the sense that doing something extreme would transform his life, take him out of the humdrum ordinariness of the everyday. Remembering his own youth, he tells us that he "devoted most of my waking hours to fantasizing about, and then undertaking, ascents of remote mountains in Alaska and Canada. . . . Some good actually came of this. By fixing my sights on one summit after another, I managed to keep my bearings through some thick postadolescent fog. Climbing *mattered*. The danger bathed the world in a halogen glow that caused everything—the sweep of the rock, the orange and yellow lichens, the texture of the clouds—to stand out in brilliant relief. Life thrummed at a higher pitch."[1]

Many more of us, however, seek to assuage our existential anxieties through a form of transcendence that invokes the godhead. The role played by obedience and rebellion in our lives—and in the world beyond our personal lives—is pertinent to understanding the psychology of this kind of transcendent experience. While seeking transcendence, we inevitably make use of our innate disposition to both submit to authority and to resist authority.

I see three strategies that we invoke as we try to reconcile our need for transcendence while we are still inextricably tied to the fundamental motives of resistance and submission: we may try to seize for ourselves the power of the gods, that is, we seek the godhead; we try to nestle in the protective embrace of one or another god; or we attempt to cloak a mere mortal in godly power. This third strategy, with a nod to Mario Puzo, I call the godfather fantasy.[2] The secular counterpart to the first two, it encompasses both rebellion and obedience—that is, in invoking this fantasy, we may aspire to become a godfather figure in our own right, or we may want to procure for ourselves the protection of a godfather. Or we may do both.

Seizing the Godhead

Our sense of autonomy begins with our natural resistance to external authority. This innate psychological propensity figures at the beginning of Judeo-Christian religion. It is symbolically depicted in Adam and Eve's disobedience of God. For Erich Fromm, the Adam and Eve story depicts "disobedience [as] the condition for man's self-awareness, for his capacity to choose, and thus . . . this first act of disobedience is man's first step toward freedom."[3] Only because man was expelled from Paradise, Fromm says, was he able to make his own history, "to develop his human powers, and to attain a new harmony with man and nature as a fully developed individual instead of the initial harmony in which he was *not yet* an individual." The Adam and Eve story can be read as a mythic version of the universal plotline by which each one of us emerges from the embeddedness of early life.

But we should remember exactly what the serpent said when he tempted Adam and Eve. The promise was immortality, and "you shall be as gods" was the clincher. This, too, speaks to the human condition. Beyond a natural resistance to authority, and a hunger to achieve power in our own right, there lurks within us an impulse to seek absolute power. Our pursuit of power can become so extreme that we begin to seek the godhead.

The ambivalent project of seeking the godhead runs through classical mythology. In Greek myths, the hero is flawed not just by his failures but by his very aspirations. Many of our basic myths, some as ancient as recorded history, depict our envy-inspired struggle to wrest power from the gods—for example, Prometheus's theft of fire from Zeus.[4] While people throughout history have sought the power of the gods, in classical antiquity they lived more familiarly with their gods than we do with ours. In the myths of antiquity, men danced with the gods, fought with them, and were made love to by them. As a consequence, some among the ancients were believed to be half god, half man—in other words, they were the imaginative link that first gave voice to man's dream of possessing the godhead. Prometheus was a lesser god, the son of a Titan and Titaness. Zeus enlisted Prometheus to provide gifts to all earth's creatures, with the exception of one precious gift—the eternal fire, sacred and reserved for the gods alone. But Prometheus was sympathetic to humans, who, unlike the other animals, were helpless in the natural world. Disobeying Zeus's command, he stole the fire to give to man. In *Prometheus Bound*, Aeschylus tells of Prometheus's other gifts to man—writing, divination, and "dark and riddling" knowledge, gifts which gave men powers far beyond their human limitations. In a rage, Zeus condemned Prometheus to eternal punishment for his act of hubris.

The urge to seize the powers of the godhead, to obtain "dark and riddling knowledge," runs very deep within us. As adults, we learn to be discreet about it, perhaps not even admitting it to ourselves. As children, however, we feed on a steady diet of superheros and fantasy games. Though our culture nervously trivializes our longing for the godhead, Greek civilization did not. The drama critic Walter Kerr pointed out that to be the hero of a classical tragedy, man generally had to have something of a god in him. The entire genre, he wrote, is an exploration of the possibilities of human freedom: "At the heart of classical tragedy, feeding it energy, stands godlike man, passionately desiring a state of affairs more perfect than any that now exists."[5]

For Kerr, the very idea of freedom meant that man must "follow where freedom leads, without foreknowledge, without any sort of certainty, prepared only for discovery and ready for surprise. . . . in Man's mind freedom exists in his godlike capacity for manufacturing the symbols of language and mathematics which Prometheus is so proud to have handed down." Such knowledge and the powers that flow from it, Kerr argued, freed man to move among the stars and to name things that he could not actually see, while his memory extended his powers so as to seem to him he might command the cosmos. Yet such knowledge is two-edged. While it can serve as a bulwark against total obeisance to external authority, it can also ignite our grandiosity such that it seduces us into potentially destructive acts, while equipping us with ever more potent means to carry out our overheated plans.

Knowledge of the stars can sometimes so excite our imaginations that it exacts a heavy price. Cecil Rhodes, the British-born diamond magnate, South African statesman, and financier who changed the map of Africa, once wistfully bemoaned: "These stars that you see overhead at night, these vast worlds which we can never reach. I would annex the planets if I could. I often think of that. It makes me sad to see them so clear and so far away."[6] It would appear that Rhodes understood well the natural limitation to human power, that he understood both the inner temptation to be Icarus or Faust, but also recognized the necessity to resist it. Nonetheless his ambition ultimately undid him. While Prime Minister of the Cape Colony, he organized a conspiracy to overthrow the Transvaal government. As a consequence, he was forced to resign and came to symbolize the overreaching and scheming British capitalist, a victim of his own boundless ambition. Aside from his mixed legacy in Africa, he is probably best known as a man passionately devoted to knowledge, who in his will endowed the Rhodes scholarships. The moral of the story: The man who would be king is the man who would be god.

One of the characters in André Malraux's novel *Man's Fate* meditates on men's lust for power in just these terms: "What fascinates them in this idea, you see, is not real power, it is the illusion of being able to do exactly as they please. The King's power is the power to govern, isn't it? But man has no urge to govern; he has an urge to compel. . . . To be more than a man in a world of men. To escape man's fate. . . . Not powerful: All powerful. The visionary disease, of which the will to power is only the intellectual justification, is the will to the godhead: every man dreams of being god."[7] As Malraux's character so aptly intuits when he speaks of "man's fate," what man is seeking when he seizes the godhead—as messiah, ruler, or tyrant—is to escape from mortality. For absolute rulers, the power to decree death or grant life reinforces the sense of power that they have over mortality. It is the ultimate power. It is also, of course, ultimately illusory. Hans Morgenthau observed it well:

> Those who persist in trying to achieve transcendence through personal absolutism, who seek the God-head through total conquest, are inevitably destroyed one way or another. This is the fate of all world-conquerors from Alexander to Hitler, and is symbolically rendered in the legends of Icarus and Faust.[8]

Submission to God

While aspirants to the godhead are not restricted to classical antiquity (witness the much later emergence of the Faust legend), still and all, a seismic transformation in the way most men regarded themselves appears to have occurred with the birth of the Christian era. While the Greeks believed that they—excluding, of course, slaves and women—partook of the nature of the gods, Christianity said that man was created by God but "not born of him."[9] Many of us, unable or unwilling to claim the godhead in our own right, seek safety and salvation through allying ourselves with and obeying a deity, or with the deity's purported representatives on Earth. With religion, the longing to be one with the cosmos and the desire to put aside individual ambitions offer hope not only for transcendence but also for immortal life.

The submergence of the self into religion and obedience to God creates meaning in our lives. To preserve the ideal of God, the believer must acknowledge his own inadequacy and his sins; thus the saying "It is better to be a sinner in a world with God than to live in a Godless world." The exact opposite of expressing hubris, of aspiring to the godhead, the Christian ideal calls for humility and obedience.

Not just belief, but the transcendent emotional experience that accompanies it is at the heart of what we get from religion. Thomas Merton catches something of the quality of deep religious commitment in this passage from *The Seven Storey Mountain* describing something he felt in a church while he was staying in Havana; this was at a time in his life when he was teetering on the verge of a total immersion in faith:

> It came time for the Consecration. The priest raised the Host, then he raised the chalice. When he put the chalice down on the altar, suddenly a Friar in his brown robe and white cord stood up in front of the children, and all at once the voices of the children burst out:
>
> > "*Creo en Dios* . . ."
> > "I believe in God the Father Almighty."
>
> The Creed. But that cry, "*Creo en Dios!*" It was loud, and bright, and sudden and glad and triumphant; it was a good big shout, that came from all those Cuban children, a joyous affirmation of faith.
>
> Then, as sudden as the shout and as definite, and a thousand times more bright, there formed in my mind an awareness, an understanding, a realization of what had just taken place on the altar, at the Consecration a realization of God made present by the words of Consecration in a way that made Him belong to me . . .
>
> And the first articulate thought that came to my mind was: "Heaven is right here in front of me: Heaven, Heaven!"[10]

While many intellectuals proclaim that religion is dead, the persistence and resurgence of belief in the divine show how wrong they are. Just as for our ancestors, for many of us today religion takes us out of ourselves, gives us access to great and mysterious forces, and provides the hope for control over our destinies through prayers and rituals of worship. For many the only satisfactory refuge from our sense of mortality is God. In fact, we seem to be witnessing a worldwide return to one or another form of fundamentalism.[11]

For centuries, people have sought salvation not through an exploration of human freedom but by means of a personal relationship to God. At the same time, secular rule found its legitimization through the sacred authority vested in it. In certain times and places, secular rule was made more palatable because the church and scripture set explicit limits to earthly power, insofar as God, and no ruler, was accorded absolute dominion. Moreover, each person, weak or strong, had full access to an appeal to God and to divine guidance. The writer Elizabeth Janeway comments: "Though priesthood might claim the power to mediate between God and humankind, it was still assumed that help from on high was available, one way or another, to those who sought it, whatever their station. To believe in the active intervention of the sacred in ordinary life was not abnormal."[12] This belief has comforted many people in times of extreme subjugation and abuse and has acted as a source of inner strength with which to maintain one's own sense of dignity, or, alternatively, to inspire resistance to abuses of power.

While the inner urge to seize the godhead is inherently personal, at least in its most direct manifestation, the longing to submerge oneself in a transcendent union with the deity takes us out of ourselves. Just this, leaving our own sense of self behind, makes it an ecstatic path when—*Creo in Dios*—Heaven seems at hand. But it becomes a most difficult path when fervor subsides and heaven and godhead alike seem like empty abstractions. We are so constructed that we will not cede any sense of personal power, will not genuflect to something that does not seem real to us. In recognition of this difficulty, all the world's great religions interpose a human relationship between man and godhead, be it with a priest, mullah, lama, or guru. Even in Buddhism, where the annihilation of the self is both the path and the goal, the believer is given someone to follow as a mentor and model. It is easier to annihilate the self, it seems, if someone is, however tacitly, cheering you on. (Our need, once more, for recognition is apparent even in this paradoxical situation.) The personal is thus present even when it is being put in abeyance.

Seizing the godhead, on the one hand, and submission to God, on the other—embody the two antithetic tendencies I spoke of earlier: the first to resist and to assert the self, the second to submit. It is as if transcendence can be had by taking one or the other to some ultimate limit while excluding the opposite tendency.

A more complex and darker vision of transcendence, in which both tendencies are present but given a sinister caste, is to be found in "The Legend of the Grand Inquisitor," recounted by Ivan Karamazov to his brother Alyosha in Dostoyevsky's *The Brothers Karamazov*. It is at once a story of corrupted ecclesiastical power, as manifested in the actions of the Grand Inquisitor, who aspired to the godhead, and a portrait of the ordinary Christian's psychology of obedience and servility.[13] Who better to write this tale than Dostoyevsky, a temperamentally religious man, who struggled for most of his life with opposing impulses of submission and rebellion,[14] and who better to appreciate it than Freud, who regarded it as one of the "most magnificent novels ever written"?[15]

According to the tale Ivan recites, Christ reappears in Seville fifteen centuries after the Crucifixion. This is the time of the Inquisition, which Dostoyevsky felt was the epitome of all the evils to be found in the West. That very weekend, the Cardinal, the Grand Inquisitor himself, has had several hundred heretics burned to death. Appearing in human form just as He had looked fifteen centuries earlier, Christ is recognized and welcomed by the people. He raises a girl from the dead at the moment that the Inquisitor appears on the scene. Witnessing the miracle, the Inquisitor orders Christ's arrest and incarcerates Him in a murky vaulted prison of the Holy Inquisition. The submissive crowd, despite the spiritual glow they feel in the presence of Christ, makes no protest.

The night before Christ is to be burned at the stake, He is visited by the Inquisitor, "an old man, of almost ninety, tall and straight, with a withered face and sunken eyes, in which, however, there is still a fiery, spark-like gleam."[16] "Why have you come to get in our way?" he asks Christ, and then launches into a terrible indictment, delivered in the service of a shameless rationalization of the Church's abuse of power.

The Grand Inquisitor accuses Christ of having failed his flock fifteen centuries earlier when, in the desert, he resisted Satan's three temptations (as recounted in Matthew). It was in the name of freedom, the freedom to believe on the basis of one's heart, that Christ refused to succumb to the first temptation in the desert, that of changing stones into bread. This the Grand Inquisitor believes was his first error. The second was His refusal to leap from the pinnacle of the temple, which would have forced God to intervene to keep Him from falling to His death. The third was His rejection of Satan's offer to give Him unimagined worldly power. The Grand Inquisitor's point is that Christ squandered assets—miracles, mystery, authority—that the Church needed.

Men cannot believe when guided only by their hearts, the Grand Inquisitor argues; they need to be convinced of the necessity of worship. Because Christ believed that man should not be moved by miracles, he allowed himself to be crucified like a thief: "You desired that man's love should be free, that he should follow you freely, enticed and captivated by you. Here again you overestimated men."[17] How, he asks, could Christ, who placed such a great moral burden on man's shoulders by offering him freedom, claim to love man?

The Grand Inquisitor understands all too well the psychological longings that give rise to man's obedience to the Church. Had Christ turned stones into loaves, the Inquisitor argues, He would have provided an answer to man's age-old anguished question: "Before whom should one bow down?"[18] He goes further: "Man seeks to bow down before that which is already beyond dispute, so far beyond dispute that all human beings will instantly agree to a universal bowing-down before it. . . . For the sake of a universal bowing-down they have destroyed one another with the sword. . . . You knew, you could not fail to know that peculiar secret of human nature, but you rejected the only absolute banner that was offered to you and that would have compelled man to bow down before you without dispute—the banner of earthly bread, and you rejected it in the name of freedom and the bread of heaven. . . . But only he can take mastery of people's freedom who is able to set their consciences at rest."[19] Here Dostoyevsky presages the totalitarian movements of the twentieth century in which people seem to long for "an indisputable, general, and consensual ant-heap."[20]

The Grand Inquisitor, who acknowledges his allegiance to Satan, accepts the inevitability and legitimacy of the three temptations that Christ rejected. He improves on Christ's model of Christianity by basing it on miracles, mystery, and authority, which the political scientist Dennis

Dalton construes as the metaphorical counterparts of economic power, psychological power, and political power.[21]

The Inquisitor tells Christ that he will be burned at the stake in the morning. Christ, who has not spoken a word throughout the Inquisitor's entire soliloquy, approaches him and kisses his "bloodless, ninety-year-old lips." The old man shivers, opens the door, and says, "Go and do not come back . . . do not come back at all . . . ever . . . ever!" "The kiss burns within his heart," but he does not change his mind.[22] His commitment to temporal power prevails over the power of his belief. He accepts Satan's wisdom.

In the novel, the scene repeats itself between Ivan and his brother Alyosha. Ivan, who tells the story of the Grand Inquisitor, renounces the hierarchical structure of the Church symbolically rendered by the Grand Inquisitor. Like the Grand Inquisitor in the Legend, though in a different key, Ivan renounces God out of love for mankind. So doing, he promptly falls into a delirium and hallucinates himself as the Devil. (Here, according to several critics, is the theme of the Nietzschean superman, one of Dostoyevsky's favorite themes.) Alyosha looks on his brother with horror and sorrow and gently kisses his mouth, just as Christ kissed the Grand Inquisitor.[23] The juxtaposition of this scene with the Legend allows the reader to interiorize the religious drama, to understand it as a psychological struggle taking place within as well as between the characters. The theological backdrop may be noted: it was of the essence of the historical Jesus that he announced that the kingdom of God, not of man, was at hand. The Grand Inquisitor, like the fourth-century Roman emperor Constantine, who made Christianity into an instrument of statecraft, wants to have it both ways. So do we all, Dostoyevsky reveals.

Matters are sometimes different, of course, when it comes to secular religions and secular godheads. The appeal of fanaticism of all sorts lies in part in the fact that the proffer of transcendence, of immortality in whatever form, does not come at the expense of renunciation of this world—or this self. Fanaticism, to put it another way, preys on a frustrated will to power and offers to make its promises of restitution good in this lifetime.

And beyond restitution, there may be the promise of retaliation against our enemies. Nothing makes us want to play god as much as the urge for revenge. We fear death always, but it is especially galling that we should die and those who have damaged us should go on living. The need for revenge must be exacted in this life, not the next. And it needs to be settled omnipotently, that is, as we see fit. Fanatical leaders seem instinctively to know this. And this takes us to what I call the godfather fantasy.

The Godfather Fantasy

The novelist Albert Camus believed that "for anyone who is alone, without God and without a master, the weight of days is dreadful. Hence one must choose a master, God being out of style."[25] It is exactly so with our attraction to one or another godfather. If we do not have a god, let us have the compelling master who has his own share of mystery, miracles, and authority. The fascination so many of us have with Mario Puzo's novel *The Godfather* and its progeny (sequels, films, copycats) is evident in its overwhelming commercial success. (Some extremely ambitious people, including women, acknowledge that they read and reread Mario Puzo's novel *The Godfather*, in an attempt to understand the most intimate workings of the strategies and tactics of power much the way some people still read Machiavelli's *The Prince* [or are advised to do so] for clues to success in business.)

The success of *The Godfather* results from two interlocking fantasies embedded in the plotline. For a few, the Godfather fantasy is about becoming the Godfather, procuring for oneself a secular version of the godhead. But for many more, this fantasy is about seeking vicarious power through a connection to one or another mortal—a godfather or godmother, a titan of industry, a mentor, a totalitarian leader—whom they imbue with the mystique of power and to whom they pledge obeisance. For them the fantasy is primarily about securing riches, knowledge, and vicarious authority in the here and now through attachment to a powerful figure. Sometimes this figure is objectively powerful and possesses such a strong and cogent worldview that an extended group of henchmen and followers are drawn to him.

Such a figure is Don Corleone. Head of a Mafia family, he ruthlessly rules a vast and vicious criminal empire; he uses his power not only for the huge financial rewards, but also for the protection it affords for both his blood family and his crime "family." But of what does the Godfather's power consist? The same stuff as the Grand Inquisitor's, I would argue: miracle, mystery, and authority. Put another way, his power lies in our need for him to be powerful, and not just powerful in an ordinary way, but to be powerful in a transcendent way. The Godfather can command life and death if he wishes; being connected to him—being "connected" is both the path and the goal—allows one to transcend the ordinary rules of right and wrong, to go beyond the ordinary limits of what society allows and does not allow. The Godfather, like the Grand Inquisitor, has a kind of power that makes a mockery of the pieties of those who think they have authority.

In fact, Puzo has said that he was deeply influenced by Dostoyevsky's novel: In his 1997 preface to the reissue of his novel *The Fortunate Pilgrim*, he wrote: "All young writers dream of immortality—that hundreds of years in the future the new generations will read their books and find their lives changed, as my life was after reading *The Brothers Karamazov* at the age of fifteen. I vowed I would never write a word that was not absolutely true to myself and I felt I had achieved that in *The Fortunate Pilgrim*."[26] That book, ten years in the writing, received splendid reviews, but was a commercial failure. Only then did he embark on *The Godfather*, the purpose of which was to acquire money and fame. Yet commercial as its intent may have been, what Puzo renders in *The Godfather* is a secular version of the themes that run through "The Legend of The Grand Inquisitor."

Like the Grand Inquisitor, Don Corleone produces small miracles to secure the adherence of his flock, some of whom he might call upon later for one or another small service in return:

> Don Vito Corleone was a man to whom everybody came for help, and never were they disappointed. He made no empty promises, nor the craven excuse that his hands were tied by more powerful forces in the world than himself. It was not necessary that he be your friend, it was not even important that you had no means with which to repay him. Only one thing was required. That you, you *yourself*, proclaim your friendship. And then, no matter how poor or powerless the supplicant, Don Corleone would take that man's troubles to his heart. And he would let nothing stand in the way to a solution of that man's woe. His reward? Friendship, the respectful title of 'Don' and sometimes the more affectionate salutation of 'Godfather.'[27]

For those who come under his protective wing, the Don's gratification of their humble requests could be considered nothing less than miraculous, veritable stones turned into bread.

Like the Grand Inquisitor, the Godfather is at the center of both knowledge and political power. Between the head of the family, Don Corleone, who dictates policy, and the men who actually carry out his orders, there are three levels of political operatives. At the top is the Consigliere, whose function, in part, is to preserve the mystery. As Puzo tells us:

> The Don gave his orders only to the *Consigliere*. . . . In that way nothing could be traced to the top. Unless the *Consigliere* turned traitor. The *Consigliere* was also what his name implied. He was the counselor to the Don, his right-hand man, his auxiliary brain. He was also his closest companion and his closest friend. . . . He would know everything the Don knew or nearly everything, all the cells of power. He was the one man in the world who could bring the Don crashing down to destruction. . . . But no *Consigliere* had ever betrayed a Don. . . . There was no future in it.[28]

The Consigliere is indeed a possessor of "dark and riddling knowledge."

The internal organization of the family must be cemented by ancillary power. Don Corleone's enforcer, Luca Brasi, is described as "one of the great blocks that supported the Don's power structure."[29] Luca "did not fear the police, he did not fear society, he did not fear God, he did not fear Hell, he did not fear or love his fellow man but he had elected, he had chosen to fear and love Don Corleone."[30] In his portrait of Luca, Puzo provides one of his many astute psychological observations. Even so fearless a man, so cold-blooded a killer as Luca has to find someone to whom he can subordinate himself.[31]

In addition to the internal structure of his organization, the Don has assets outside it. He goes outside to enlist political power through payoffs to police, judges, and even senators. A United States Senator calls the Don to apologize for not personally attending his daughter's wedding, but says he had no alternative because FBI agents were taking down the license numbers of the cars outside. Unknown to the Senator, the Don was well informed by his insiders at the FBI, and he had sent the message warning the Senator not to come.

The Don also wields psychological power, perhaps the most chilling of all. In his secret empire of threat and murder it is indeed better to give than to receive. A prime example of his mastery of this kind of power is demonstrated in the story of his confrontation with a powerful movie producer, Jack Woltz. Woltz has refused the Don's request to give a plum role to singer and movie star Johnny Fontane (a character widely believed to be based on Frank Sinatra). The Godfather sends his Consigliere, Tom Hagen, to negotiate. Woltz greets Hagen courteously, but kisses him off. When Hagen proposes that Don Corleone could help Woltz with some small problems, Woltz responds, "All right, you smooth son of a bitch, let me lay it on the line for you and your boss, whoever he is. Johnny Fontane never gets that movie. I don't care how many guinea mafia goombas come out of the woodwork."[32] As a final display of his power, he adds that J. Edgar Hoover is one of his personal friends.

Unflappable, Hagen responds that Don Corleone knows about Woltz's friendship with Mr. Hoover and respects him for it, after which he takes his leave. Woltz cannot imagine that Don Corleone has the power to threaten him in any serious way. As many will remember from the film if not the novel, Woltz wakes up one morning to find the severed head of his beloved prize horse Khartoum on the pillow next to him: "Woltz was not a stupid man, he was merely an extremely egotistical one. He had mistaken the power he wielded in his world to be more potent than the power of Don Corleone. He had merely needed some proof that this was not true. He understood this message."[33]

Different as they may appear to be, the Catholic Church at the time of the Inquisition and the Mafia as it grew in the United States resemble each other in the techniques they used to keep their subjects in thrall. Through their respective versions of miracles, mystery, and authority, underlined in fear, they both wielded transcendent power.

Let me step back a moment. What I am saying here is that the Godfather fantasy is so compelling not just because we have a wish to dominate and command, but because we have a wish to attach ourselves to power through submissiveness and obedience. Further, I am arguing that these tendencies seek their own apotheosis. The Godfather fantasy allows us to imagine a world in which both tendencies can be lived out to the hilt, directly and personally. Nor is the underlying currency of fear an obstacle to our participation, for the more we fear our godfather the more others in their turn fear us, for we share vicariously in our godfather's power.

THE IMPULSE to cede independence of action to an authority—whether the Grand Inquisitor, the Godfather, the Professor in Milgram's experiments, or the Commander in the cockpit—widespread as it is, requires psychological exploration. Two different frames of reference can be invoked to explain, at least in part, this impulse. The first emphasizes our dependency and sense of powerlessness in early life, the second our sense of powerlessness in the face of death and the need for transcendent meaning as an antidote.

What motivates us to follow those who are drunk on power-lust? Human history gives us the sagas of charismatic leaders and the masses who follow them. While it is traditional to explain the motivation of the followers as the natural response to the aura and charisma projected by leaders, psychology provides a different explanation. The leader's charisma is only effective in conjunction with the propensity in many people for subordination.

We may sometimes experience a desperate temptation to surrender to authority.[34] Psychoanalysts understand the individual's propensity for selfsubordination and surrender as a manifestation of his or her charismatic overvaluation of the parents of early childhood. Freud's genius allowed him to see the infant's helplessness but also to see beyond it and grasp that there is an active love of the power of the Other. This concept can be used to understand the links between religion and mysticism, heroworship, and our immersion in hierarchical organizations, all of which share in our human need to vest some part of ourselves in a higher authority. These different modalities constitute the variety of ways by which we seek to overcome our human frailties.[35] Yet simultaneously we all harbor an opposing impulse in our natural resistance to authority.

Our conflicting predilections to submission and resistance to authority nearly always coexist in us side by side. In a group, dominance and submissiveness are no longer merely antagonists in an internal psychological conflict. Taken together, not only do they propel us into group life, but they are fundamental to the power gradient that stabilizes our position in hierarchical structures. A predilection for both domination and submission allows us to integrate into a hierarchical structure, whether familial, corporate, or even psychoanalytical.

Freud turned toward an exploration of man's "thirst for obedience" and the nature of the group-mind in *Group Psychology and the Analysis of the Ego*.[36] He had previously explored the psychological meaning of hypnosis in terms of erotic submission and used this insight to explain the patient's transference to the psychoanalyst. He saw both phenomena as evidence that people have a craving for direction and authority originating in earliest life—one that ultimately derives from our evolutionary past in Freud's view. This craving is assuaged by what he believed was an "erotic" tie to, and identification with, first a father and, later, a chief of one or another sort. He believed the longing for a father, behind whom lurked a primal father, explained the "uncanny and coercive characteristics of group formations."[37] The chief is a "dangerous personality, toward whom only a passive-masochistic attitude is possible, to whom one's will has to be surrendered."[38] This is because man has "an extreme passion for authority"[39] and "wishes to be governed by unrestricted force."[40] For Freud, these wishes arise out of unconscious erotic longings: ". . . a group is held together by a power of some kind: and to what power would this feat be better ascribed than to Eros, which holds together everything in the world."[41]

Many psychoanalysts have concurred with Freud that the individual's propensity for self-subordination and surrender to a leader is yet another manifestation of that charismatic overvaluation of parental power so necessary when one is young and truly powerless. The leader-follower relationship, whether expressed in hero-worship in the mentor-protégé relationship, in transference, or in any of its other forms, is indeed partly—but I would argue never wholly—inspired by the longing for something to counter the weakness and helplessness of childhood.[42]

While Freud brilliantly elaborated the group mind in *Group Psychology*, what he omitted was not just the urgent need so many of us have to unite with others but to do so in an "ant-heap" of shared belief. Such a need for ideology takes us beyond Eros. The function of the group mind—as distinct from transference—is to provide transcendent meaning. The model of transference is based on early childhood and leaves out any acknowledgment of the new anxiety later in life that is related to our fear of death and oblivion. To counter our death fears, we attempt to find transcendent meaning. Some of us become highly ambitious and counter such anxiety by striving for immortality through our achievements or through attempting to seize the godhead in our own right. More often, however, we counter anxiety by allying ourselves with a transcendent group. The transcendent function of the group mind is achieved through vicarious participation in the godhead: one is part of a chosen people or a master race, a descendant of Allah or the sun god, a follower of Jesus, Muhammad, or Buddha, or a warrior in a conquering army. Submission to a group leader or a group ideal is often facilitated by the invocation of an outside enemy—Christ for the church hierarchy in Dostoyevsky's rendition of the Inquisition, rival Mafioso for Corleone. What is at stake is affiliation with an elite group that confers real or symbolic survival. A transcendent group encompasses a shared credo, a belief system, and a corollary code of behavior. Participation in the group mind assuages the fear of meaninglessness, not the terrors of childhood.[43]

In the contemporary world, science offers the hope of a new approach for participating in the godhead. As a result of our newfound technological wizardry and the dream of vastly extending the duration of life, we fall prey to the illusion that our control of the physical world will be without limits. If a meteor hits Earth, we will climb into our spaceships and flee to a faraway galaxy. If our body parts wear out, we look forward to replacement parts à la the Bionic Man.

What shatters transcendent groups? Sometimes they fall prey to outside enemies. But sometimes they are victims to internal dissent, to the natural resistance invoked in response to power and particularly to its abuses. Such resistance to authority can set a limit to the indefinite perpetuation of any one ideology and, in the process, can sometimes give rise to the creation of a new ideology or faith. We find this kind of resistance in the back-to-Jesus movements and in fundamentalist movements of all kinds, whether Christian, Jewish, or Islamic. Here the faithful find a reason to resist the hierarchical structure of official churches, which interpose a layer between God and individual.[44]

Resentment of and resistance to authority were also pivotal in the birth of the Mafia. In Puzo's novel *The Godfather*, Michael Corleone, Don Corleone's idealistic youngest son, tries to separate from his father's world, only to have a rival Mafioso's attempted murder of his father abruptly bring him back. It is then that he becomes cognizant of "the roots from which his father grew." Through the voice of Michael Corleone, Puzo shares with us the actual story of how the Mafia was born, romanticized only a little bit:

> The word "Mafia" had originally meant place of refuge. Then it became the name for the secret organization that sprang up to fight against the rulers who crushed the country and its people for centuries. Sicily was a land that had been more cruelly raped than any other in history. The Inquisition had tortured rich and poor alike. The landowning barons and the princes of the Catholic Church exercised absolute power over the shepherds and farmers.

The police were the instruments of their power and so identified with them that to be called a policeman is the foulest insult one Sicilian can hurl at another.

Faced with the savagery of this absolute power, the suffering people learned never to betray their anger and their hatred for fear of being crushed. . . . They learned that society was their enemy and so when they sought redress for their wrongs they went to the rebel underground, the Mafia. And the Mafia cemented its power by originating the law of silence. . . . *Omerta* became the religion of the people.[45]

We cannot grasp the full power of our psychological need either to seize the godhead, to annex the stars, or to participate in transcendence-oriented groups simply by looking backwards to the fears and terrors of childhood. The history of the world is the history of groups that compete not only for natural resources, trade advantages, and monopolies but also for a transcendent meaning that confers significance on life. Authority that attaches to nationalistic fervor or religious belief gains compliance because its precepts are accepted as legitimate or true and this because they are cloaked in a shared belief system taking the form of ideology.[46] Because ideology rationalizes and legitimates power, thus transforming it into authority, it reduces the amount of power that must be applied to attain compliance. This is the meaning of the Grand Inquisitor's insistence that people long for "an indisputable unanimous ant-heap" that ratifies a belief system and in doing so gives meaning to life. Thus is produced an apparently endless cycle of devout causes, each protected by an honor guard ready to die in its defense or to kill in the service of its propagation. Stability is threatened either internally, through resistance to authority, or externally, through the clash of two incompatible ideologies.

Taken together, resistance to (or co-option of) authority and obedience to ideology provide a major engine for the historical changes and upheavals that punctuate the human journey.[47] Ironically, we kill more people in the name of an ideological cause run amok than we destroy by virtue of thwarted passion, personal vendettas, criminality, or greed. While many of the world's greatest glories derive from one or another of our belief systems, so, too, do some of the most horrific chapters in human history.

14

Standing on Your Own
Two Feet

"Insist on yourself; never imitate."
RALPH WALDO EMERSON, "Self-Reliance"

W hen we think about our individ-
ual power, we often think, reasonably enough, in terms of the ability to go
forward whether it is simply with our plans, in our career, or in our lives.
This kind of success through forward motion is an important aspect of
both interpersonal power and personal power. Indeed, our dreams about
power—and when put in these terms, they are typically more hopes than
reality—often have to do with getting ahead, or with overtaking someone,
as in a race, or getting to the finish line with someone we love. Even more
fantastically, we see power in terms of taking off, or soaring or streaking
like a comet. As the business writer Harriet Rubin tells us: "The word destiny is a sailor's term meaning to align your ship with nothing earth-
bound, to point yourself in the direction of the stars."[1]

But though real power may be perceived as "taking steps," or even
"taking a first step," or "getting going again," it involves something more
than movement. It involves, first, having the ability to stand up for oneself, and one's own point of view. (As the song goes, straighten up and fly
right.) Standing on our own two feet entails not only forming an intention, but also resolving to stick with it to the best of our ability. The nec-

essary ability to keep chugging along to our destination was celebrated in *The Little Engine that Could,* a story about huffing and puffing up a hill, symbolically the story about the perseverance of the little guy, the one who is seen as weak but turns out to be a winner.

Metaphors of power and powerlessness that indicate position infuse our language and are readily entwined with other assessments of value. Just as heaven is above, so hell is below. Just as right connotes good and left evil, so does "up" designate power, while "down" denotes powerlessness; up is good whereas down is bad. In addition to their power and moral connotations, "up" and "down" also carry class connotations— upper and lower class, highborn and low.

Metaphors and phrases that denote personal power are regularly cast in terms of the upright position, of locomotion, of forward momentum, and sometimes of the ability to soar. Standing on your own two feet. Sitting tall in the saddle. At work one wants to be at the top of the ladder or at the top of the heap, not at the bottom of the barrel.

Similarly, interpersonal power is sometimes depicted as being top dog (not underdog or low man on the totem pole). We are enjoined to stand up to someone; Stand up and fight like a man. Stand up for what you believe. Stand up and be counted. And nobody needs a partner, in friendship, marriage, or business, who will not stand up for themselves. What one wants in a friend is for him to be a stand-up guy.

In contrast, metaphors and phrases that denote powerlessness are often cast in terms of down, cast out, or below the salt: "Nobody wants you when you're down and out." Flat broke. Flat on your back. Flatter than a pancake. The whole point of boxing is to stand on your feet and knock someone off his feet so that he goes down for the count. A business that can't pay its bills goes belly-up.

Kneeling and genuflecting are gestures that concede power, though they may confer derivative power if we are willingly submitting to a higher authority. Our appreciation of someone else's power or charisma is expressed in phrases such as: Bowled over, Swept off my feet. A beautiful woman can be a knockout.

All these metaphors that connote power and powerlessness appear to be rooted in our early life experiences and in the design of our bodies. When as toddlers we express our will in the battle of the spoon or in the battle of the pot, our power is largely restricted to naysaying. We cannot yet escape from the offending personage who makes unwelcome and outrageous demands on us, and who has the power to swoop down on us from above. Greater freedom comes only with locomotion, which is itself dependent on our ability to reach a vertical position. When it comes to power, standing and walking are clearly superior to crouching and crawling.

Becoming vertical is connected with forward movement in infancy and with the inherent design of our cognition. Once we become vertical, we are able to form an intention, which we express through either forward or backward movement. People speak of get-up-and-go, a single phrase. Sometimes the going, though purposeful and deliberate, is movement away from something. Turning one's back on someone and walking away is a declaration of freedom, of the power to be one's own person and be dismissive of the person who has offended us. But in order to do this, we first have to get up, whether we get up from our chair, or rouse ourselves from somnolence, or simply get off our derriere. First up, then forward or backward as the situation warrants.

Moreover, "up" and "down" refer to different body halves, with different connotations. The upper half of our bodies, including head and heart, is emotive, expressive, and sometimes cerebral, whereas the bottom half involves excretion and reproduction. Thus, the upper half is more celestial, the bottom half more bestial. "Down and dirty" denotes power, but a "no holds barred" kind of power.

While our spacial metaphors clearly derive and survive from infancy and childhood, they may also represent basic biological organizing principles. Research suggests that people vary not only in the way they use the space around them, but more specifically in how they integrate their gestures and postures in terms of up-down, forward-backward, and side-to-side. A person who reaches out his hand to shake yours and leans or steps forward in the same motion is often a go-getter, someone who puts himself forward, who is friendly or outgoing, or pushy or aggressive, depending on your taste in people and whether or not he likes you. But a person who stands up straighter as he reaches for your hand, whose handshake is more up and down than not, whose gesture of acknowledgment is a nod of the head up and down—this is a true decision maker, an executive type, perhaps a strong silent type, who is very much his own man. Then again, a person whose "posture-gesture mergers," to use the technical term for these things, is in the horizontal plane, whose gestures and movements are organized from side to side or reaching left and right across the midline is typically more of an explorer, ponderer, and negotiator.[2]

Standing on your own two feet is an apt metaphor for self-reliance and authentic power, provided the expression is understood to mean that you must find the courage to stand on your own two feet even if you don't have two good feet. The importance of amending the metaphor was made clear to me early in my professional life by a patient who showed me how my liberal prejudices sometimes blindsided me. Hugh, a black man about the same age as I was, had made it out of the ghetto into reform school because of his violent tendencies. But a psychologist at the reform school saw his human potential and helped him to find a rewarding career in graphic design that took advantage of his abundant artistic gifts. After achieving initial success in design, Hugh encountered a dry patch. At the urging of his mentor, Hugh came into treatment with me to take a look at his creative block and especially at his flash-point temper.

From our first meeting, I knew that I would get as much out of Hugh's therapy as he would—and, as it turned out, he taught me a great deal about authentic power. At the time, my office mate, the psychoanalyst Dr. Robert Liebert, was treating several members of the revolutionary group Students for a Democratic Society (this was in the 1970s). Hugh, contemptuous of all kinds of cant, figured out that some of Dr. Liebert's patients were radicals, and ran his own experiment to test their mettle. Every so often, he would come to his session early, sit in our waiting room, and begin screaming that someone was trying to kill him—all this just to see if he could smoke out any of the young radicals (or our neighbors) to come to his aid. In effect he set out to prove that what had happened to Kitty Genovese was no fluke, that even the self-proclaimed good guys would not go too far out of their way to help someone else. No one ever answered his screams for help—not the neighbor, not the SDS'ers, not even Dr. Liebert, who interestingly never even asked me about the periodic screams emanating from our waiting room. I could hear Hugh through my office door, as could Dr. Liebert and whoever was in his office. But, then, Dr. Liebert was extremely respectful of patients' privacy and probably intuited what was going on. As far as Hugh was concerned, he had made his point. He was also testing me to see if he could get me to tell him his behavior was unacceptable—that is, to smoke out how uptight I might be. Since no one else seemed to notice, I decided to let him run his intermittent experiment. He may well have needed this latitude in order to settle into treatment. Hugh was very much a stand-up guy, or rather he was trying very much to become one without letting his rage become his undoing. It seemed important to satisfy himself that whatever else the other people in and around my office had going for them, they were not stand-up people.

That Hugh responded to the SDS'ers in this way speaks to his dynamics. But we must remember that those scraggly adolescent "revolutionaries" were a lightning rod for people's conflict about power and authority generally. Hugh was not the only one interested in them. Bob Liebert and I found a policeman in our waiting room one morning when we came to open up the office. He claimed he had been called because of a suspected robbery. In fact he had entered through a locked door. It was the time of Daniel Ellsberg's revelation of the Pentagon Papers, and the FBI had broken into Ellsberg's office. Bob and I believed the policeman was there to get a look at our files, particularly Bob's. Apparently, we had arrived just in time to thwart his plans, and, as a consequence, I have coded and scrambled the names of my patients ever since.

All people, including patients, test others to gauge their mettle—to smoke out their strengths and weaknesses. Hugh tested me in a lot of different ways. One morning, he staggered into my office a little late wearing a bloodied shirt and then pulled out a bloody knife. He said he had just come from a late-night bar, basically an after-hours joint, where a man sitting on the stool next to him had relentlessly taunted him. Hugh finally shut him up by stabbing him, and he was unsure whether the man was dead or alive. This alarmed me, but not as much as it might have had I not grown up in Louisville, where there were plenty of knife fights in bars, a couple of which my father happened to own. I was inclined to stay cool, but was frightened enough not to want to be alone with Hugh. I told Hugh that I was uncomfortable because I was frightened, but that, if he liked, we could continue our session in a coffee shop down the street. He laughed at me and said I was silly: "Don't you know that I would never stab a woman?" While appreciative of his assurances, I insisted that I would feel more comfortable in the coffee shop. He agreed to go with me. Once we got there and talked over the events, he was able to accept my suggestion that he go back to the after-hours club—this was a place where the police did not go and accordingly where people managed their own affairs and their own violence—and find out how badly hurt the man he had stabbed was, indeed whether he was dead or alive. He was willing to do this and we rescheduled an appointment later in the day. He came back, considerably sobered up, to tell me that luckily he had not killed the man. I took him at his word, and I think he was as relieved as I was. The event appeared to be a turning point for Hugh. To the best of my knowledge, for as many years as I knew him afterwards, he never again became so rattled in a public or private confrontation that he had an outburst of rage such as he had experienced in that after-hours bar. That last blowout, the realization of its potential consequences, his willingness to suffer the consequences had the man died, and his genuine feelings of guilt greased the path toward his consolidation of feelings of genuine strength. Henceforth, he managed to express his explosive feelings through the use of shocking bursts of color in his graphic art.

I learned a lot from Hugh. For example, he taught me how to walk the streets safely (keeping a distance from both doorways and parked cars, so it sometimes means walking in the middle of the street provided there is no traffic). He also taught me about standing up. One day, Hugh was telling me about his encounter with a young friend, who was convalescing at home and feeling very sorry for himself after losing a leg in a near lethal knife fight with a neighborhood rival. Hugh, disgusted with his friend's whining, bluntly told him to get up on his one good leg and take a walk around life. At first, I was horrified by his seeming callousness. Hugh, who liked to point out to me how lily-white my judgments often were, argued that confrontation was the only way to get an angry enough response from his friend to jump-start his assertive juices into flowing. My spontaneous response would have been to comfort the young man, not confront him. But when Hugh made his case he convinced me. I was, in fact, guilty of a white liberal turn of mind that might well have been construed by the amputee as condescension or pity—surely the wrong medicine.

This all comes back to me now because of a recent accident. While trying to track down a particular reference, I was too impatient to get the library step stool in the next room and climbed up on a chair to reach almost to the top of a floor-to-ceiling bookcase. I had done this a couple of hundred times before, but this time I lost my balance and went crashing to the floor, ending up with a serious fracture of my left leg and a complication called a compartment syndrome, all of which ended up requiring three surgeries. The last surgery was on September 9th, two days before the September 11th terrorist attack on the World Trade Center. I am still recuperating from my fracture, even as I write this chapter some months later. Though I am far enough along to know that I will eventually walk normally and have complete function of my leg, I now know what it is to lose the sense of being vertical in the world, unable to stand or walk.

The minute I landed on the floor, I knew I had experienced one of those moments when one's life is turned topsy-turvy by an event from out of the blue. For me, one of the occupational hazards of being a psychoanalyst is that the first lens I use to explore mishaps is generally psychological. So I mentally twisted and turned and strained to find some reason that I had done myself in—some lurking depression or discontent, some disturbance I had not cottoned to, maybe a success phobia, and so on. This train of thought proved futile, so I scoured my memory for some previously unnoted indication of an incipient, hopefully slight neurological deficiency that might explain why I tipped off a chair. But I was unable to find a physical cause either—no prior areas of numbness, no muscle weakness, no balance problems. One of my exceptionally witty patients later asked me if I had needed a break, picking up on the fact that both of us can get carried away with whatever we are doing and find ourselves verging on exhaustion. I ended up attributing my fall, in part, to restlessness and, in part, to laziness in not walking into the next room to get a proper library ladder. I'm left with a less cause-oriented, more philosophical view—that we are all subject to the fickle finger of fate.

The vicissitudes of fate that we are all potentially subject to every day was surely brought home to me on September 11, when the Twin Towers were destroyed. After experiencing horror and sorrow at the lives lost and shock that our government could have been so caught off guard, the next things that grabbed my attention were the accidents of chance, the random roll of the dice—the fact that some people who would have normally been in the towers were saved because they had been late coming to work. One man had taken his son to school, someone else had overslept, a woman had gone on vacation—and so on. But many people died because they were in the buildings by fluke; they were there this one time only because of a breakfast meeting or a job interview. Of course, fate can touch us for bad or for good—but even if for bad, not always in such deadly form as occurred in the World Trade Center tragedy.

What does it mean, then, to exert power when we have so little control over our ultimate destiny? We pride ourselves on being able to stand up tall, and yet there are times when the building, indeed the whole world it seems, is falling down around us. One aspect of authentic power is being able to cope with adversity that comes in the form of accidents and other vicissitudes of fate, as well as the ability to cope with its blessings.

WITH MY RECENT EXPERIENCE of being unable to walk, of losing the vertical dimension even if temporarily, and with the knowledge that we are now engaged in a war of such possible magnitude that it may rival World War II, not surprisingly my thoughts turned to Franklin Delano Roosevelt. For me, it became important to understand how he faced the task of standing on his own two feet both physically and metaphorically after polio had rendered him paralyzed in both legs—permanently paraplegic in fact—and how he came back to lead our nation through a treacherous war.

Roosevelt was one of the heroes of my earliest childhood. I was just old enough to be overcome with grief when I heard of his death, though perhaps this was in response to my parents' reaction. I have been a great admirer of Roosevelt ever since, without, as it turns out, knowing very much about him. During my enforced immobility, I found myself reading about him and asking what it meant to him to find himself paralyzed, how he managed to live with his handicap, return to political life, and be elected Governor of New York and then President of the United States.

The political columnist Joseph Alsop observed that when you went back to the opinions of those who knew Roosevelt in his youth, "there is always the same note of astonishment about what Franklin Roosevelt became."[3] Corinne Robinson Alsop, who was Theodore Roosevelt's niece, recalled that she and her friends had privately called Franklin the "feather duster" because he was altogether too good-looking, too chatty, too eager to please. Alice Roosevelt (Theodore's daughter) was even more brutal: "He was the kind of boy whom you invited to the dance but not the dinner," she said, "a good little mother's boy whose friends were dull, who belonged to the minor clubs." Once when Roosevelt was asked what he wanted to do, he said he thought he might one day be president. Someone then asked, "*Who else* thinks so?" Later, Alice Roosevelt would say that they used to call him "poor Franklin," although in the end "the joke was on us."[4] But at the time, his contemporaries viewed him as a "high-spirited, pleasant companion, full of energy and ambition, a good fellow in all respects, but fairly superficial and wholly without the strength and largeness of character, the depth of judgment and the other qualities that are needed to make a great man, or at least a man both great and good."[5]

To understand Roosevelt's character at this stage of his life, it is important to appreciate that despite his wealth and privileges, he did not come from the very highest tier of the Roosevelt clan or society generally. His branch of the family had residences in Hyde Park, but most people of his background had not just country houses but houses in New York City as well. Another branch of the Roosevelt clan had residences in Oyster Bay and counted among its members Theodore Roosevelt.

Teddy, the former President and Eleanor's uncle, attended Franklin and Eleanor Roosevelt's wedding, a guest of a stature not every young couple can command. But it was Teddy who held court at the reception and everyone gathered around him, until finally Franklin and Eleanor figured out that if they wanted anybody to congratulate them, they would have to make their way over to that side of the hall.[6] At Harvard, Roosevelt had not been invited to join the exclusive, elite Porcellian Club, though Teddy had been its president. And whereas Teddy wrote and published a book while still an undergraduate, the best Roosevelt could claim was to have been the editor of the *Crimson* during his senior year. This could have won him a job at any newspaper in the country upon graduation, but it was a trifling achievement considering his aspirations.

How Roosevelt dealt with his situation is reasonably clear. As was famously remarked of him, he had a second-rate intellect, but a first-rate temperament, and he became even more social, outstandingly so. The person who is not first, not even tenth, on the guest list, had better learn how to act as though he still belongs at the party; this calls for affability and discernment, as well as continual attention to connections, but not necessarily resolve. We might think of Roosevelt at this stage of his life as so many of his contemporaries did—as a lightweight—and can only ponder how he metamorphosed into an unambivalently powerful personage.

There are different routes to achieving authentic power. Ralph Waldo Emerson, our nineteenth-century essayist, who embodied something of the ethos of the independent, even iconoclastic spirit that Americans traditionally treasure, proposed nonconformity and self-reliance. In his essay "Self-Reliance," he writes about the pressures of conformity brought to bear by socialization:

[Resolve and self-reliance] are the voices which we hear in soli-tude, but they grow faint and inaudible as we enter into the world. Society everywhere is in conspiracy against the manhood of every one of its members. Society is a joint-stock company in which the members agree, for the better of securing his bread to each share-holder, to surrender the liberty and culture of the eater. The virtue most request is conformity. Self-reliance is its aversion. It loves not realities and creators, but names and customs.

Whoso would be a man, must be a nonconformist. He who would gather immortal palms must not be hindered by the name of goodness, but must explore if it be goodness. Nothing is at last sacred but the integrity of our own mind.[7]

For Emerson, independence from the pressures to conform was prerequi-site to being a man, to what I call authentic power.[8]

Yet Emerson's is but one way to achieve authentic power. Roosevelt followed a different course. Very definitely a conformist in his own way, he developed great gifts in the art of getting along with people, of arranging to be included in other people's plans and of keeping himself informed of what was going on around him. His affability was studied, no doubt, but it was also real. It is said that when he was running against Wendell Willkie, whom he sincerely liked, that he would take time out to listen to Willkie's speeches. And when Willkie would say something politically inadvisable, Roosevelt would be pained. "Oh no, we shouldn't have said that . . ." he would murmur or "No, don't say it that way." He was in short rooting for the fellow to make a better show of it.

Affability, social judgment, sheer nosiness—these are a politician's virtues, not a philosopher's. But they fall well short of what is required of a leader. While Roosevelt advanced steadily upward on the strength of these virtues, he appeared to most politicians to lack weight. Clearly something changed, to give us the man who became one of our towering wartime presidents. Alsop suggested that two unhappy—even tragic—events contributed to the metamorphosis: a doomed love affair and a crippling case of polio.

Alsop's first thesis refers to Roosevelt's unhappy love affair with Lucy Mercer, who met him in her position as part-time social secretary to Eleanor Roosevelt and who later married Winthrop Rutherford. Although

Roosevelt and Lucy Mercer saw a great deal of each other, with and without Eleanor present, Alsop is quite certain that it remained a chaste relationship, if for no other reason than the fact that Lucy Mercer was a devout Catholic (and also because the sexual mores of the first quarter of the twentieth century were far more restrictive than our own). Alsop believes it was Roosevelt's mother who advised him that a divorce from Eleanor and a subsequent marriage to Mercer would be politically unwise; in any case, Mercer would never have given up her Catholicism in order to marry a divorced man. Alsop's point is that for the first time Roosevelt encountered an obstacle that would not yield to his charm, his persuasiveness, his connections. The world was not his oyster. He had been passionately in love; now he must accept a loss. Limitation, a new kind of reality, had to be faced.

Whether or not this affair had the impact Alsop believes it did, most of Roosevelt's biographers concur that his character underwent a profound change during the decade-long hiatus in his political career brought about by his illness.

Although viewed as lightweight, Roosevelt had always been ambitious. In 1907, while clerking in a Wall street law firm, he told a mightily surprised fellow employee that he wanted to become president of the United States. His game plan was to get into the New York State Legislature, this to be followed by an appointment as Assistant Secretary of the Navy, and finally he would run for the Governor of New York in a Democratic year. At that time, to be a Democratic Governor of New York was considered a good route to aim for the presidency. For Alsop, Roosevelt was distinguished by his "longsightedness," a kind of life trajectory that he had carved out early in his life. (Surely it was no coincidence that the sequence he had in mind paralleled the actual political career of his cousin Theodore Roosevelt.)

As it turned out, Roosevelt's career closely followed his game plan. Beginning in 1910, he spent four years in the New York State Senate, triumphant as the Democrat who had been elected in a Republican district. It was in Albany that he connected with Louis McHenry Howe, a politically astute newspaperman who made it his self-appointed role to shepherd Roosevelt to the Presidency. In 1914, President Woodrow Wilson appointed Roosevelt to be Assistant Secretary of the Navy and in that post Roosevelt prepared the navy such that it had achieved military readiness in time for World War. I. In 1920, still following the path of Teddy Roosevelt, Roosevelt was nominated as the Vice-Presidential candidate to run on the ticket with James M. Cox of Ohio. But Cox lost the election, and Roosevelt failed to become vice-president as Teddy had. But he had done himself no permanent harm. He was recognizable and respected nationwide and had every reason to look forward to an important political career. Roosevelt returned to his work as a businessman and lawyer but kept up a heavy speaking schedule to stay in the public eye.

It was at this juncture in his life, in August 1921, that he and his family left for their traditional summer holiday at Campobello, an island in the Bay of Fundy. He was already tired at the outset of the holiday, and the first three days were exhausting: the first day he brought a yacht into the bay in difficult seas; the second day he superintended a major fishing expedition and fell into the icy bay; and the third day he swam in the freezing water with his sons and then jogged two miles in a wet bathing suit to get home. In retrospect, he believed that the polio had developed before he first left the yacht.[9] When he became sick and feverish, a local doctor diagnosed a heavy cold, although paralysis had already begun. Between Thursday, when the doctor saw him, and Saturday, Roosevelt became completely paralyzed from the chest down, his upper extremities were weakening, and his skin and muscles were extremely painful to the touch. A specialist from Bar Harbor was called in; he diagnosed "a clot of blood from a sudden congestion . . . settled in the lower spinal cord, temporarily removing the power to move, though not to feel" and prescribed massage.[10] Ten days later the family brought in Dr. Lovett, a specialist from Boston who diagnosed polio. He stopped the massages, which were probably harmful, suggested hot baths, and prescribed bromides. The slightest pressure on Roosevelt's body caused intense pain, and his upper trunk as well as his lower body remained weak.

Though their marriage had been an affair of the heart only for a short time, if at all, and had been damaged by Roosevelt's love for Lucy Mercer, Franklin and Eleanor appear to have formed a new bond during his illness, becoming working partners. Roosevelt was also nursed by Louis Howe, the political guru who had already decided that Roosevelt would be president.

Roosevelt insisted—and perhaps believed—that he would recover fully. Eleanor said later that he never discussed death or permanent disability. Whatever he might be fearing or feeling, he kept up a show of good spirits. After four weeks at Campobello, Howe arranged transport to Hyde Park, shielding Roosevelt from the scrutiny of reporters. Roosevelt was transferred, painfully, on a stretcher, but by the time the reporters saw him on the train, "he was arranged in his berth, resting on pillows, his famous cigarette holder cocked at a jaunty angle in his mouth"[11] The newspapers reassured the public that he would definitely recover. Roosevelt went to a hospital for six weeks, then returned to Hyde Park in November, still in agony. But he had already begun to strengthen his upper body by using a trapeze suspended over the bed to move himself. He learned how to sit in a wheelchair wearing a corset for back support, and he was able to move himself from bed to a chair and vice versa. As his pain receded, his energy and endurance grew.

This was the beginning of what became a long and unsuccessful project of recovery.[12] While his hoped-for recuperation became his career for almost a decade, Louis Howe and Eleanor Roosevelt would keep up Roosevelt's political contacts and made sure his name remained before the public.

Eventually, Roosevelt regained control of his bowels and his bladder; and gradually he regained sensation in his entire body and muscular strength in his upper body. But the only way he could stand erect was with crutches, braces, and a pelvic band for support and stability. Walking became both his full-time preoccupation and occupation. He "tried massage, salt water baths, ultraviolet light, electric currents, walking on braces with parallel bars at waist height, walking while hanging from parallel bars mounted above his head, also horseback riding and riding an electric tricycle, not to mention exercises in warm water and exercises in cold water."[13] (Whether or not he retained sexual function is not a question I found addressed; I have been told by several neurologists that it generally is preserved in conditions such as his, but not in all cases.) He had a regular routine of morning exercise and afternoon walking, which he kept up for seven years, even though he must have sensed that his total recovery was becoming less and less likely.

Roosevelt discovered Warm Springs, Georgia, in 1924, through a friend, George Peabody, who was a part owner of what was then a rundown spa, though famous for its natural hot springs. Roosevelt's exercise in the warm pool helped him, and he discovered that with the support of the warm water, he could walk in the pool. This encouraged him to hope that he would someday be able to walk normally. He spent mornings in the pool and motored or worked out in the afternoon. He had a car with hand controls that he could drive: this in part restored his sense of independence. He was so enthusiastic about Warm Springs that he put two-thirds of his net worth, $200,000—then an enormous sum—into upgrading it. Other polio patients flocked there and, in essence, Warm Springs became a rehabilitation center, though it was never profitable. Roosevelt learned to stand erect for a period of time, even though it caused him pain and he needed a heavy steel brace to keep his legs from buckling. Ever conscious of appearances, he learned to give the impression that he could walk by leaning on his son, a difficult trick that took months to master. And he presented to the world the smiling face that we see in nearly all his photographs. Reporters—out of respect, and according to the ethos of a bygone day— kept his secret.

Despite all his efforts, Roosevelt required constant assistance for the rest of his life. He was "forced to train himself to remain for hours on end wherever he had settled himself for work or for amusement. . . . until the time came for another move, when he would need help again—unless it was just a matter of hoisting himself back into his wheelchair and propelling himself to the luncheon or dinner table."[14]

Roosevelt's courage was undoubtedly a form of authentic power. Where had it come from? The reporter and author Bonnie Angelo quotes Roosevelt's daughter, Anna, to the effect that while Sara Roosevelt was overcontrolling of her only son, Franklin had the "self-assurance of a pass . . . he spoke from security." Anna believed that "the man who would rally America" had that confidence in him "from the cradle."[15]

Alsop proposes another explanation. A complete admirer of the kind of tough obstinacy that refuses to accept defeat, Alsop believed that the paralysis did not create these qualities in Roosevelt, but brought them to the surface. In his view, polio gave Roosevelt the opportunity to make himself into the man he became, in large part psychologically, but also because polio also kept him out of political life at a time when he would likely have been totally defeated.

Accidents again: serendipity, in the form of polio, kept Roosevelt from making the wrong moves in his political life. Without polio, according to Alsop, Roosevelt would have challenged Alfred Smith for the governorship of New York in 1922 and lost. Instead, he was invited to put Smith's name into nomination at the Democratic National Convention in 1924.

By then he had mastered crutches and could stand erect at the podium to give his "happy warrior" speech—a speech that made him an important player in the Democratic Party. In 1928, it seemed doubtful that the Democrats could carry New York state, since Smith would have to give up the governorship. Smith asked Roosevelt to run for governor. Ironically, while Al Smith was defeated by Herbert Hoover, Roosevelt was elected governor and was back on the trajectory he had originally laid out for himself. In 1932, he defeated Al Smith to win the Democratic nomination for president, and then the presidency.

A noteworthy feature of Roosevelt's leadership was his flexibility. The writer Garry Wills notes that what a "leader most needs is followers" and that a leader is "one who mobilizes a goal shared by leader and followers."[16] Roosevelt realized that he could not dictate policy but must acknowledge interdependence and nudge his constituency when he could. In confronting the Great Depression, Roosevelt felt free to try one thing and then another. This was the same course he took in World War II. He had resolve, but he expressed it not from a fixed vision but through a constant scrambling for new ad hoc plans. Emerson, who wrote, "A foolish consistency is the hobgoblin of little minds, adored little by statesmen and philosophers and divines," would have approved.[17] Roosevelt, like Emerson, did not feel bound to consistency and preferred to trust his emotional reactions.

Emerson was no worshiper of famous men. He argued that only when men express themselves genuinely do they take on luster. Original actions must be grounded in what he calls Spontaneity or Instinct, such primary wisdom constituting Intuition, which he contrasts with all later teachings—tuitions. Emerson's entreaty is to do what you can do best: "Where is the master who could have taught Shakespeare? Where is the master who could have instructed Franklin, or Washington, or Bacon, or Newton? Every great man is unique. The Scipionism of Scipio is precisely the part he could not borrow. . . . Do that which is assigned thee and thou canst not hope too much or dare too much." Roosevelt seems to have understood this though he could use conformity when necessary.

Alsop, for his part, believed that with hindsight Roosevelt's polio must be seen to have been an advantage: "It is a rule of life in this weary world that few experiences an individual can encounter are ever wholly wasted—unless the individual is destroyed thereby; and for an intelligent and resilient man, even the harshest survived experiences are somehow liberating." Alsop proposed that Roosevelt's polio finished the job of making him the man he became, which had been begun by his strong but disappointed love. My contention is similar: meeting some challenge, overcoming some obstacle, struggling with the latest vicissitude of fate is surely one route by which we achieve authentic power. Standing up for oneself entails facing down the random blows of fate.

Roosevelt gave us a phrase that is particularly relevant to our individual search for authentic power: "The only thing we have to fear is fear itself." Strength follows from facing down our fears—fear of success; fear of failure; fear of our parents, spouses, children, or bosses; fear of death, illness, or impoverishment. In fact, the poet Rainer Maria Rilke instructed us to follow our fear:

> We have no reason to mistrust our world, for it is not against us. Has it terrors, they are *our* terrors; has it abysses, those abysses belong to us; our dangers at hand, we must try to love them. And if only we arrange life according to that principle which counsels us that we must always hold to the difficult, then that which now still seems to us the most alien will become what we most trust and find most faithful. How should we be able to forget those ancient myths that are at the beginning of all peoples, the myths about dragons that at the last moment turn into princesses; perhaps all the dragons of our lives are princesses who are only waiting to see us once beautiful and brave. Perhaps everything terrible is in its deepest being something helpless that wants help from us.[18]

Only when we seek to overcome our fears do we position ourselves to achieve authentic power. No longer merely counterpunchers, we can initiate.

To do so, we must trust in ourselves as a credible, self-contained center of authority. Even after we have committed ourselves to this resolve, there are still moments when a decision seems overwhelming. In her diary, Sojourner Truth describes how once freed from slavery she became exhausted, experiencing freedom as so difficult that she decided to sell herself back into slavery, to be taken care of. But on her way back to her former master, a second voice stopped her: "I have two hearts inside me."[19] The inner conflict between the wish for autonomy and the wish for dependency is something we must resolve in order to feel strong. This sometimes entails giving up our illusion of security. We must sometimes gamble, not always put safety first. We must be responsive to inner guidelines. We must act—not just react but initiate—and sometimes we must be able to stand alone. (Here I echo Emerson's warning about conformity.) And, as Goethe believed, we must "Live for the moment, live in eternity."[20] Only when our emotions are in synchrony with our actions do we feel fully alive.

AS FOR ME, my surgeries went well and I am recovering from my injury. I am still working with a brilliant physical therapist who has the unlikely but wonderfully appropriate name of Job. He told me that what he likes about his work is seeing people at a critical moment just after something sudden and unexpected has interrupted the flow of their lives. He also says that the road back from a serious injury elicits as many different responses as a Rorschach test. Whatever the behavioral response, the psychological response is just as complicated. I know exactly what he means—some people rise to the occasion; some are too frightened to push themselves; some are in such denial that they push too hard and sometimes aggravate their injuries. What most caught my attention, though, was Job's story of one patient, an artist, who was distraught over his injury but somehow reached deep down into his creative self and produced his most widely acclaimed work. What effect my injury and recuperation will have on me I do not yet know. It has been traumatic, but I hope some indirect benefit will come from it—that is, I hope I will be among those who can use adversity to stoke inner growth.

As I ponder things from my immobility, I am struck by how much sheer movement there is in all of us all the time. Whether sitting in a chair or lying in bed, we are always moving—shifting, turning, straightening, curling up, rebalancing—just to stay what we think of as still. I am aware of this, because right now I cannot do it, not really, not as I would like. Indeed, to stay comfortable at all, I need people to help me shift about.

Where is my sense of authentic power now? The reader is entitled to ask this; certainly, I am asking it myself. As luck, bad luck, would have it, a close friend has just this very week broken his leg. We consult on the phone, and I am worried about him; his attitude is that he will do nothing for six weeks, two months—doctor's orders—and then everything will be fine. I am positive that it will not work that way, but I have to be careful how I put this to him. When I ask myself how I know this, ask why I envision a grimmer, or at least more trying course in front of both of us, I find the counsel of the nanny who raised me. Her highest praise was that so-and-so was "Nobody's fool." So I rehearse all the negatives in my mind, go down every path that leads to worst-case scenarios, in order to prepare myself. Be nobody's fool, I say to myself, get ready. Of course, I did not prepare for breaking my leg in the first place. But I can prepare for what might happen next.

However, I also hear Hugh's advice to his friend, the amputee: Get up on that one good leg and take a walk around life. This brings me to the assortment of people—attendants, aides, and technicians—who have lent their time and muscles to help me do this to the extent I have so far. I am impressed by how little impressed they are by signs of outward success in my life—my profession, my friends who come to visit. They take me as I am. Equally, they take themselves as they are. They have abilities that matter in this situation, including sheer simple physical strength, and also the feel of how to handle a body not their own, and they are surprisingly dignified in their use of those abilities. Some of them I believe—a couple of them I know—are fundamentally religious, and their work fits in the scheme of charity toward others. But there are those who are only making a dollar, just doing it well and with a sense of pride that is, as I see at very close quarters, justified. Their sense of personal power, Hugh's altruistic rage, my nanny's canniness, my family's unconditional support—I lean on all of these. Standing on your own two feet sometimes involves leaning on others, metaphorically and literally.

Meanwhile in the larger world, events continue to unfold. The nation, it seems, has found a new set of heroes—New York City firemen. It somehow has struck people that New York City is not, finally, composed only of financiers and celebrities. The people who died in the World Trade Center were equally financial and business people, working men and women: security guards, secretaries, messengers, restaurant workers, policemen—and firemen. It is the firemen who somehow speak most directly to us. I think it is because, like the aides and physical therapists who tend to the disabled, they use their abilities in the service of others. As we know, it takes courage to go into a building that is burning and may collapse. That there are people who make it their job to do this speaks to how interdependent we all are. This touches us. And that people take pride in doing this, and do it for only a little more than a workman's wages, strikes us as admirable.

What, then, of power? Realism, however grim, counts. So does an understanding of our inevitable dependence. And then there is determination, whether it be a patient, quiet one, or a bold courageous one, or something in between. These are all necessary ingredients in authentic power. When people think about power, they tend to think in terms of limitless ability and limitless resources and control over others. When they fantasize about having power, they fantasize about what they will be able to do that they cannot do now, and how it will be so easy. Life does not work that way, however. But there is such a thing as authentic power. It comes from standing up, on your one good leg if need be, and taking a walk around life. The striving for inner strength, for authentic power becomes real when it is anchored in a sense of facing what needs to be faced and doing so in the context of an interdependent world. As I watch New York City come back to life, I see it literally all over the place.

Epilogue: The Failure to Theorize Power in Psychoanalytic Theory

"There is and can only be one Führer, Freud, the founder of *psychoanalysis."*

FRANÇOIS ROUSTANG

Despite its clinical importance, power (and its perversions) is not a major concept in psychoanalysis. Following Freud's lead, most analysts have regarded the power motive as a relatively minor component of aggression or narcissism or as a derivative of infantile fantasies of omnipotence.[1] The exception is Rollo May, who emphasized its importance in interpersonal life.[2] The reality, however, is that power extends beyond interpersonal concerns to encompass self-control and self-mastery, autonomy and agency, mastery of the physical world, and the search for transcendence.

Neither psychoanalytic therapy nor other psychotherapies are immune to issues of power. In the therapy situation, power interactions are an intrinsic part of transference and countertransference. If, as Alfred North Whitehead says, "intercourse between individuals and between social groups takes one of two forms: force or persuasion," then power is as much an issue for the therapist and patient as it is in any other relationship.[3] Therapists, as the designated authority, command the power position in the treatment situation. The therapy takes place in the therapist's office, and the therapist sets the fee and establishes the ground rules and the guidelines. It remains the therapist's responsibility to help the patient, and no matter how resolutely he or she assigns responsibility for change to the patient, both parties are aware that if the patient fails to improve, that failure becomes part of their joint discussion. Of course, like all relationships, the therapeutic relationship evolves over time, sometimes in the direction of mutual empowerment when the collaboration is going well, sometimes in the direction of stalemate or struggle.

Therapists recognize that the power interaction in any therapeutic dyad, no matter what the therapist's theoretical orientation, is specific to that pair. Most therapists are simply trying to be helpful, scanning their own reactions to pick up any distortions on their part. But some therapists dominate or infantilize their patients. Some are paternalistic (though with adolescent patients, a bit of parental solicitude may not be misplaced). A few may be disparaging or condescending in their interpretations, and a few may be competitive or envious. Some are oversolicitous. Others are too passive.

Patients, too, bring their own predilections with regard to power into the relationship. As Richard Almond writes: "Our patients are continually trying to *do* things to us and get us to *do* things to them—to get us to *answer* and *ask* them questions or *make* us feel things toward them. Analytic exploration of the meaning of such motives often reveals that the patient's thinking and behavior derive their compelling quality from a wish to actualize a fantasy in which a sense of power is central."[4]

Since issues of power pervade not only the therapeutic dialogue but also professional organizations of psychoanalysts and of psychiatrists, one would think that no psychoanalytic theory could ignore power (as expressed or wished for) or powerlessness (as experienced or dreaded) as a major plotline in the theater of the mind. Yet the pervasive role of power in motivation is generally unexplored in the psychotherapeutic literature, with the exception of couples' therapy, where it is emphasized. Even when issues of power are addressed in therapy, they are generally discussed not in terms of power per se, but in terms of authority, persuasion, dominance, and submission.

Why has power been so little theorized in psychology, and particularly in psychoanalysis, even as it was and is being discussed extensively in political science and philosophy? The answer lies in part in the personality of the founder of psychoanalysis, Sigmund Freud. It lies in part in the early history of the psychoanalytic movement. And it lies, too, in a fear that the concept of power—especially willpower—detracts from the primacy of the unconscious. However, this marginalization of power as a motive and a concern has negatively impacted on both psychoanalytic theory and psychoanalytic organizations.

AS THE PSYCHIATRIST and psychoanalyst John Mack pointed out, Freud failed to examine the subject of power head-on—he simply never brought to it the same dispassionate intelligence that he used to explore so many other areas of psychic life.[5] Mack sees further evidence of Freud's avoidance of the recognition of power as a force in individual psychology in his "flawed" response to Nietzsche, the great philosopher of the "will to power" and a thinker whose works were studied thoroughly in the student groups Freud belonged to during his university years. Although Freud later credited Nietzsche with anticipating some of his own discoveries, he strongly resisted Nietzsche's writings—claiming to be blocked by a "surfeit of interest"—and was unable to study and assimilate them effectively. This was in marked contrast to his easy mastery of the intellectual contributions of many other writers.

Mack speculates that Freud's personality and "the circumstances of his life" played a large part in his failure to bring his critical acumen to bear on power issues. He focuses particularly on Freud's pain in response to his father's powerlessness and in his response to his own experiences of powerlessness. Mack bolsters his interpretations with biographical material from a variety of sources, but primarily from Freud's own writings. In a vignette in The Interpretation of Dreams, Freud recounted a painful conversation when he was about ten or twelve in which his father told him of an incident from his own youth. Their interchange is now famous as part of Freudian lore. Wearing a new fur cap, Freud's father went out for a walk. A gentile approached him, knocked his cap into the mud, and shouted: "Jew! Get off the pavement!" Freud wanted to know how his father had responded. "I went into the roadway and picked up my cap," his father replied. Freud judged his father's behavior as unheroic. He contrasted it with another incident "which fitted [his] feelings better: the scene in which Hannibal's father, Hamilcar Barca, made his boy swear before the household altar to take vengeance on the Romans." Freud goes on to say that "Ever since that time Hannibal had had a place in my phantasies."[6]

Mack believes that Freud was traumatized by his father's failure to fight back against this episode of anti-Semitism. He speculates that Freud's painful recognition of his father's personal and political impotence might well have lingered in his preconscious, especially because a pubescent boy is vulnerable when he becomes aware of his father's humiliation in the outside world—even if that world was a hostile one, as was the anti-Semitic Vienna of Freud's time. In fact, Freud recalled his father's humiliation in the course of writing associations to four dreams about Rome, at a time when he had yet to visit Rome. In fact, Freud introduces his father's story by saying that he had been "brought up against the event [in his] youth whose power was still being shown in all these emotions and dreams."

Freud, like his boyhood idol Hannibal, "the favorite hero of (his) later school days," seemed "fated not to see Rome." "Like so many boys . . . I had sympathized in the Punic Wars not with the Romans but with the Carthaginians. And when in the higher classes, I began to understand for the first time what it meant to belong to an alien race, and anti-Semitic feelings among the other boys warned me that I must take up a definite position, the figure of the Semitic general rose still higher in my esteem. To my youthful mind, Hannibal and Rome symbolized the conflict between the tenacity of the Jewry and the organization of the Catholic church." According to Freud, his dream wish to "go to Rome," in identification with Hannibal, had "become in [his] dream-life a cloak and symbol for a number of other passionate wishes." And yet Freud had a phobia about going to Rome.

Mack understands Freud's "passionate wishes" to be Freud's ambitions (the identification with Hannibal) as the antidote to the frustration and humiliation he felt in response to the limitations placed on him in his own young manhood by the anti-Semitic Viennese medical establishment.[7] He suggests that Freud's own experience of professional powerlessness due to anti-Semitic prejudice is linked to his father's powerlessness in similar circumstances. The lack of a revered father figure may well have stoked Freud's manifestly ambivalent need for a powerful father-figure, leading him to promote a series of mentors and, later, collaborators—Charcot, Breuer, Fliess, Jung—to positions of reverence, only to break with them subsequently.

Mack's hypothesis is plausible. Children and adolescents often hate any sign of weakness in their parents because they see their parents as their protectors, the guarantors of their safety and their very survival. Not only is their safety at stake, but also their pride.

The psychoanalyst Gail Berry suggests additional sources of Freud's devaluation of his father. His father was not very successful as a business-man during Freud's early life, and the family lived in relatively straitened circumstances. Berry suggests that Freud's father's relative lack of success could easily have bred intrafamilial devaluation, which came to serve as a stimulus for Freud's family romance fantasies, among which was his iden-tification with Hannibal. She furthermore believes that the senior Freud's response to young Freud after he had urinated on his parents' bedroom carpet ("That boy will never amount to anything!") was "a terrible affront to [Freud's] ambition." She speculates that Freud silently decided that it was his father—not him—who amounted to nothing.[8]

The intellectual historian Carl E. Schorske, an authority on fin-de-siècle Vienna, also concluded that Freud was beset by feelings of power-lessness due to being Jewish in an increasingly anti-Semitic Vienna.[9] Schorske, too, uses Freud's self-reported dreams and his associations to them (in *The Interpretation of Dreams*) to demonstrate how Freud anguished over having been denied some of the signs and substance of power that might rightfully have been his had he not been Jewish. In Schorske's view, Freud retreated from a preoccupation with worldly ambi-tion because of organizational and social barriers that were preventing him from scaling the ladder of professional and academic achievements in Vienna. Freud turned instead to a searching self-analysis, which is woven into his masterwork—*The Interpretation of Dreams*. Whereas Mack and Berry focus on the personal element of Freud's associations, Schorske cites the numerous references to contemporary political figures and other prominent figures in *The Interpretation of Dreams*, demonstrat-ing that while Freud may have been cut off from full participation in the power hierarchy of his time and place, he kept well abreast of events and indeed, as his own self-analysis attests, was deeply involved with them on an emotional level.

Schorske proposes that "by reducing his own political past and present to an epiphenomenal status in relation to the primal conflict between father and son," Freud avoided having to acknowledge his own conflicts about power—while simultaneously fashioning his own end-run by creat-ing psychoanalysis: "Sigmund Freud by family background, conviction, and ethnic affiliation, belonged to the group most threatened by the new [social and political] forces: Viennese liberal Jewry. . . . Freud needed no specific political commitment to make him feel the lash of resurgent anti-Semitism; it affected him where he was already hurting—in his professional life. . . . In response to his professional and political frustrations, Freud retreated into social and intellectual withdrawal. He actually stepped down the social ladder. . . . The more Freud's outer life was mired the more winged his ideas became. . . ." Schorske goes on to suggest that "Freud gave his fellow liberals an ahistorical theory of man in society that could make bearable a political world spun out of orbit and beyond control." And fittingly, as another historian, Dennis Klein, has pointed out, the first versions of his new theory were presented not before professional audiences but at lectures to the local B'nai B'rith by "brother Freud."[10]

Schorske asks, however, if there was nothing left of Freud's ambitions, of his identification with Hannibal as clearly portrayed in his dreams, or of his identification with other powerful people. He believes that "the Latin legend on the title page of *The Interpretation of Dreams* suggests an answer: Flectere si nequeo superos Acheronta movebo (If I cannot bend the higher powers, I shall stir up hell [the river Acheron]).[11] Thus, in Schorske's view, Freud's masterwork becomes his protest and his justification. His thwarted desire for power in the academic establishment was subsequently transferred to his ironclad control of organizational psychoanalysis, with ramifications that have continued right up until the present. So it is that we identify with the power of the aggressor.

HOWEVER personally and intellectually uncomfortable Freud may have been with the subject of power, he was adept enough in exercising it that he was able to ban the intellectual contributions of the one analyst of his time who did important work on power—Alfred Adler.

The story of Sigmund Freud (1856–1939) and Alfred Adler (1870–1937)—their friendship, their collaboration, and their falling-out—involves not just a theoretical disagreement about the nature and importance of power in the psyche but is itself the tale of a major power struggle, in which Freud ultimately purged Adler from the psychoanalytic movement.[12] It is in part as a consequence of Freud's disaffection with Adler's attempt to place his concept of the "will to power" at the center of the psyche that the concept of power has remained marginalized.

Following the publication of *The Interpretation of Dreams* in 1900,

Freud enjoyed a period of fulfillment. His creativity flourished, and he began to gather adherents, what the psychoanalytic historian Paul Roazen describes as a "small band of loyal followers." Even though Freud proposed a policy of "intellectual communism" to his local compatriots and subsequently to his Swiss supporters when they appeared on the scene, Freud remained jealous of his priority, as is apparent in his published references to his colleagues' work. For example, in a passage added to the 1909 edition of *The Interpretation of Dreams*, he notes that "a large number of dreams have been published and analyzed in accordance with my directions in papers by physicians who have decided to adopt this psychoanalytic therapeutic procedure, as well as by other authors." Among those mentioned are Carl Jung and Wilhelm Stekel. But Freud pointedly remarks that "these publications have merely confirmed my views and not added anything to them."[13]

Freud's break with Alfred Adler was the first of the many infamous quarrels within the psychoanalytic movement. Subsequent to their rift, Adler was dismissed not only as a defector, but as someone who failed to credit infantile sexuality as the core discovery of psychoanalysis. But Freud and Adler had at one time been close colleagues. Adler, who was fourteen years younger than Freud, became a member of Freud's circle in 1902 when Freud invited him, along with Wilhelm Stekel, Max Kahane, and Rudolf Reitler to meet weekly at his house to discuss issues of mutual interest. First known as the Psychological Wednesday Society, the enlarged group reconstituted itself as the Vienna Psychoanalytic Society in 1908.

Freud wanted psychoanalysis to grow and to expand to more and more countries. As is common in any emergent movement, everyone in Freud's circle was "enlisted in proselytizing and preaching."[14] Freud worried that psychoanalysis might be identified as almost exclusively Jewish, and therefore he made a point of enlisting and promoting gentiles. In accordance with his desire to expand the movement and yet keep it under his control, Freud prompted the Hungarian psychoanalyst Sandor Ferenczi to give a speech in Nuremburg in 1910, on the occasion of the second international meeting of Freud's followers, proposing that they create a formal organization. Ferenczi proposed that an international association of analysts, designated as the International Psychoanalytical Association (IPA), should be created with different societies in different countries. On Freud's instructions, Ferenczi proposed Carl Gustav Jung, a non-Jewish Swiss, as its President and also proposed that as President, Jung, who was

Freud's closest associate and editor of the only existing psychoanalytic journal, have complete power over all psychoanalytic publications, clearly a form of censorship.

With the new president based in Zurich, the center of psychoanalytic power would inevitably shift there. Organizational transparency and intellectual diversity be damned; it was going to be Jung's show, with Freud holding power behind the scenes. Freud's original Viennese supporters, including Adler, naturally feeling excluded, held "a protest meeting in Wilhelm Stekel's hotel room" in Nuremburg.[15] Freud, who needed to make peace with the Viennese, went to the hotel room and pleaded for their continuing loyalty. According to Ernest Jones: "He laid stress on the virulent hostility that surrounded them and the need for outside support to counter it. Then dramatically throwing back his coat, he declared: 'My enemies would be willing to see me starve; they would tear my very coat off my back.'"[16]

Freud once had been impressed with Adler—having repeatedly praised his work at the Wednesday night meetings and even referring his sister-in-law to Adler for analysis—but now he was suspicious about his friend's loyalty. Even so, he still wanted to keep his Viennese supporters. To promote that accord, he backed down on the censorship issue and also on making Jung President for life. He even relinquished his own Presidency of the local Vienna Society whereupon Adler and Stekel were elected president and vice-president. Adler's election as President of the Vienna Society, according to Freud, was justified on the grounds that "after all he is the only personality there." Adler became coeditor, along with Stekel, of the Central Journal for Psychoanalysis (Zentralblatt Für Psychoanalyse), founded on their initiative. Freud continued to feel nervous about Adler and expressed the hope that in these positions of power, "Adler might possibly feel an obligation to defend our common ground."

However, Adler in his new positions, did not become any more compliant to Freud, any more dedicated to their "common ground," but appeared even more intent on further exploring his own insights. No doubt Adler was ambitious, but he was also gifted and had genuine intellectual differences with Freud. He felt that the time had come to make those differences clearer than they had been.

Up to that time, Adler's major original work had been focused on what has since been called, somewhat inaccurately, the "inferiority complex." Adler theorized that if nature burdened a person with an organic defect or weakness, that person might well develop a neurosis as a kind of camouflage. Alternatively, the person might learn to compensate for it, and here Adler began to consider the role of assertion and, ultimately, the will to power. The idea was that in certain favorable conditions an individual's defect or shortcoming might stimulate him or her to achieve greatness. This might be said to be the story of Adler's own life. Having endured a sickly childhood, and gone on to enjoy great success, it is no surprise that he had insight into the role of compensation for early defects, or what he called a sense of "organ inferiority." Freud himself could be understood in this way, according to Alder, who believed that a sense of inferiority on Freud's part led him to greatly overestimate the dangers faced by the psychoanalytic movement.

Adler's formulation challenged the traditional Freudian belief that libidinal conflict was the whole of neurosis, and Adler pointed out that sexual behavior itself could have symbolic meaning. He observed further that both males and females tried to avoid feminine characteristics and characterological passivity through struggles toward masculinity. This he called "masculine protest." He recognized that much of private and public life rests "upon the prejudice of the superiority of the male."[17] (This is, of course, an important insight, foreshadowing the intellectual rationale of the women's movement. It is unclear, though, whether Adler thought this was solely a cultural bias or whether he believed masculinity to be innately superior.) In essence, Alder stressed the importance of self-assertion and the will to power, in the form of the masculine protest, as an antidote to the fear of passivity and femininity. In this scheme, the development of a neurosis could be seen as a kind of psychic trick whereby individuals assert themselves through illness, thus getting their way while secretly gratifying their disavowed passive, feminine longings (an insight into what I have described as one of the powers of the weak).

Adler's presentation of his latest ideas about the will to power in two lectures he gave in early 1911 ignited the smoldering power struggle between him and Freud. In trying to be rid of Adler, Freud attacked his friend's key insight: "We must not be misled by the term 'masculine protest' into supposing that what the man is repudiating is his passive attitude [as such]. . . . Such men often display a masochistic attitude—a state that amounts to bondage—toward women. What they reject is not passivity in general, but passivity toward the male. In other words, the 'masculine protest' is in fact nothing else than castration anxiety."[18] Freud viewed the will to power as no more than a superficial derivative of the aggressive instinct, which was a drive covalent with libido.[19] For Freud, Adler's focus on the power machinations of neurotics was made irrelevant by Freud's own discoveries about libidinal urges and their repression.

Freud objected that Adler, in focusing on the masculine protest and the will to power, spent too much time on surface psychology and the ego. Although Freud acknowledged that power had been neglected by psychoanalysis, he believed that dissecting the workings of power had more to do with common sense than with psychoanalytic excavation.

But Freud did not do justice to the deep rootedness of power dynamics in all areas of our lives. Adler had intuited something important about motivation—that conflicts of personal and interpersonal power, self-assertion, and mastery might have as great a role in neurosis and character pathology as conflicts about sex. Moreover, Freud failed to see that conflicts involving power could be every bit as unconscious as conflicts about sexuality were.

The disagreements between Adler and Freud came to a head in early 1911. Freud was extremely critical of the two papers Adler presented. His criticism was not just scientific but also personal. Shortly thereafter, Adler and Stekel resigned as president and vice president of the Vienna Psychoanalytic Society, though at first they remained members of the Society. In May, Freud asked for Adler's resignation as coeditor of the Journal. Only then did Adler resign from the Society as well. He founded his own society, taking three members with him, and called it the Society for Free Psychoanalysis. Freud commented bitterly on Adler's "tasteful" choice of a name. Later Adler renamed the group the Society for Individual Psychology.

The following fall, Freud called for a vote on how to handle the split. The Vienna Psychoanalytic Society passed a resolution, by eleven votes to five, with five abstentions, that psychoanalysts belonging to the Vienna Society could not attend Adler's group if they wished to remain in Freud's group. This vote resulted in the resignation of six more members from Freud's group. Hanns Sachs, who was loyal to Freud, reported that those who withdrew did so not out of any commitment to Adler's theories, but on grounds of scientific freedom.[20] The irony of this outcome should not be lost on us. The ambitions, competitiveness, and power struggles of the first generation of analysts played a significant role in the theoretical marginalization of power in psychoanalytic theory.

Max Graf, a freethinking musicolgist (he was the father of Little Hans, the subject of one of Freud's famous case studies), was present at the meeting. He saw the expulsion of Adler as an excommunication in reprisal for Adler's refusal to give complete priority to the libido theory. He made a stunning analogy: "Freud . . . insisted . . . that if one followed Adler and dropped the sexual basis of psychic life, one was no more a Freudian. In short, Freud—as the head of the church—banished Adler; he ejected him from the official church. Within a space of a few years, I have looked through the whole development of church history."[21] Jung's recollections also confirm how militantly Freud was attached to the libido theory. "I can still recall how Freud said to me, 'My Dear Jung, promise me never to abandon the sexual theory. That is the most essential thing of all. You see, we must make a dogma of it, an unshakable bulwark.' He said that to me with great emotion and the tone of a father saying, 'And promise me one thing, my dear son: that you will go to church every Sunday.'"[22]

From the testimony of his followers, Freud, in engineering Adler's resignation, finally accomplished something he had wished to do for some time. As early as November 1910, he had written to Jung expressing his desire to be done with Adler. To his intimate correspondents, Freud spoke frankly of his relief after the resignations were received and the Society was "purged." In 1914, in his essay "On the History of the Psycho-Analytic Movement," written while he was "fuming with rage,"[23] Freud described not only his troubles with Adler but his fight with Jung, which followed shortly thereafter.[24]

Contemporaries describe Freud as knowing how to hate. When Adler died in 1937, some twenty-five years after their split, Freud remained unforgiving. Adler died while on a speaking trip to Scotland, and, in a letter to Freud, Arnold Zweig mentioned that he was moved by the news. Freud replied, "I don't understand your sympathy for Adler. For a Jew boy out of a Viennese suburb a death in Aberdeen is an unheard-of career in itself and a proof of how far he had got on. The world really rewarded him richly for his service in having contradicted psychoanalysis."[25]

If Freud had been reluctant to admit the concept of power into psychoanalysis in 1911, he understood how to exert it. If he failed to make the will to power a part of his canon, he certainly possessed an iron will himself. His later works show that at some point he did think deeply about power and he made a major contribution to understanding it. For example, in *Group Psychology and the Analysis of the Ego*, written in 1921, Freud described the power of a group leader:

> A group is an obedient herd, which could never live without a master. It has such a thirst for obedience that it submits instinctively to anyone who appoints himself its master. Although in this way the needs of a group carry it halfway to meet the leader, yet he too must fit in with it in his personal qualities. He must himself be held in fascination by a strong faith (in an idea) in order to awaken the group's faith; he must possess a strong and imposing will, which the group, which has no will of its own, can accept from him.[26]

Freud might be describing himself here—a leader possessed of indefatigable purpose, gripped by his faith in an idea, and so powerfully persuasive that he could impose his ideas on an "obedient herd"—at least once the heretics had been "purged." As he demonstrated, he knew full well the benefits that sometimes accrue from getting rid of one's enemies. Thomas Szasz came to characterize the organization of psychoanalysis under Freud's leadership as a kind of tyranny: "Freud's essential concept of leadership seemed to be to bestow tokens of power on his competitors, only to discredit them if they dared to use it."[27]

Even posthumously, Freud generated enough power to dictate for many years to come the contours of the official history of the psychoanalytic movement. The very psychoanalytic historians who first documented his need for absolute dominance were hesitant to judge him negatively. As late as 1971, Paul Roazen softly characterizes Freud's behavior to Adler as "understandable," arguing that it was rooted in a genuine intellectual concern for the integrity of his work:

> Despite the disagreeableness of the fighting, especially following such a successful decade, it was understandable of Freud to worry lest the core of his original findings get lost in the tendencies Adler represented. . . . From Freud's point of view, Adler's concern with ego processes was endangering everything Freud had worked on.[28]

Roazen endorses Erik Erikson's view that Freud "had to establish one thing at a time, and his great contribution was psychosexuality. It is a mark of a great man that he watches jealously over the expansion of his field. He makes sure that certain principles do not get lost before they can be superseded."

True, Freud was trying to preserve key psychoanalytic insights, but probably not only the theory of sexuality. Rollo May suggests that Freud's foremost contribution was his demolition of the concept of willpower that had pervaded the Victorian era. Freud described the motor force in our lives as our instincts, not our will.[29] Like Groddeck, who first said explicitly that each person is "lived by the unconscious" and who resurrected Nietzche's term—the id—to embody this insight, Freud's major point was that unconscious factors govern our lives. As Alan Wheelis put it: "Among the sophisticated the use of the term 'will-power' has become perhaps the most ambiguous badge of naiveté. . . . The unconscious is heir to the [former] prestige of will. As one's fate was formerly determined by will, now it is determined by the repressed mental life. . . ." Wheelis goes on to say that "The image that emerged was of man as determined— not *driving*, but *driven*."[30]

When Adler emphasized will and the will to power, he did more than threaten to downgrade sexuality. To Freud's way of thinking, Adler had also downgraded the primacy of the unconscious.

THE OUTCOME of the Freud/Adler contretemps still finds echoes in the ongoing power struggles within psychoanalysis and in the continued theoretical marginalization of the power motive. Freud did not rid himself of organizational controversies by abandoning his Viennese colleagues in favor of Jung. Quite the contrary. The falling-out between Freud and Jung that followed so quickly on the heels of Adler's excommunication was perhaps Freud's most devastating confrontation with a defector and precipitated a reorganization that had profound consequences for the psychoanalytic movement. Richard Webster, a critic of Freud, describes the orthodoxy imposed in the reorganization: "It was in response to the anxieties . . . aroused [by the imminent break with Jung] that Ernest Jones wrote to Freud in July 1912 to put forward a proposal . . . that the future of the movement should be safeguarded in a different way. . . . He proposed that a secret committee should be formed in order to protect Freud and his doctrines. One of the implicit aims of this committee would be to monitor Jung as well as any future dissidents."[31] Freud responded to Jones, "What took hold of my imagination immediately was your idea of a secret council composed of the best and most trustworthy among our men to take care of the further developments of and defend the cause against personalities and accidents when I am no more. . . . I dare say it would make living and dying easier for me if I knew of such an association existing to watch over my creation."[32] Jones replied that the committee would be secret and unofficial but would keep "in the closest possible touch with you for the purposes both of criticism and instruction." The signature bond was Freud's gift to each committee member of an antique Greek intaglio which was to be set into a ring. The committee was charged with ensuring that psychoanalysis would continue after Freud's death. This "band of brothers," consisting of Jones, Karl Abraham, Sandor Ferenczi, Otto Rank, and Hanns Sachs, was meant to supersede the need for a single heir. As Webster points out, however, the effect was to confer importance on the group itself. Inevitably, competition and the need of each member to make an important statement in his own right led to dissension within the group. Otto Rank, for instance, was eventually purged because of his emphasis on the birth trauma. And this same pattern was repeated over and over again within psychoanalysis long after the gradual dissolution of the committee.

François Roustang, in "Dire Mastery: Discipleship from Freud to Lacan," demonstrates how theoretical conformity became embedded in the very structure of organizational psychoanalysis through insistence on complete discipleship. As Roustang suggests:

> Obedience to Freud and to the cause, the search for refuge in the founder, the paternal understanding, the demands for loyalty, the solicitude regarding money (once someone has entered the circle, he must be helped, be sent patients, be lent money, etc.), and the acceptance into Freud's family that changed the disciples into clients in the Roman sense of the term (i.e., dependents of a patrician family)—the conglomeration of all these features presents to us the figure of a very intricately organized society. . . . Such features did not arise by chance in the relationships between the first psychoanalysts, but were codified when the International Psycho-

analytic Association was founded in 1910. Freud proposed that the Association be given a chief (*ein Oberhaupt*) who, on the death of the founder (*der Führer*), would be his successor, his *Ersatz*, prepared to instruct and admonish.

Roustang, like Graf, invokes the church analogy:

There is nothing to prevent us from admitting that all this amounts to laying the foundations of a new church. There is and can only be one *Führer*, Freud, the founder of psychoanalysis. After his death, the *Führer* will be replaced by an *Ersatz*, who must obediently submit, for if Jung was a failure in this respect it was because Freud [here Roustang quotes Freud] "had lighted upon a person who was incapable of tolerating the authority of another, but who was still less capable of wielding it himself, and whose energies were relentlessly devoted to the furtherance of his own interests." . . . Such clichés can also be heard in religious societies: the right to command is in proportion to the perfection of the obedience.[33]

Part of Roustang's contribution is to show how the same perverted power relationships that plagued Freudians have surfaced among Lacanians: "In group discussions, for example, a quotation from Lacan acts a concluding point or verdict, as the last word, which no one dares to criticize, analyze, or assess from a subjective viewpoint."

Does this history affect the current structure of institutes and organizational psychoanalysis? For the prominent contemporary psychoanalyst Otto Kernberg, as for Roustang, continuity from the early dictatorial structure to the present is inevitable. The institutional legacy became embedded, during the last years of the committee, in the guidelines for training: "psychoanalytic education attempts to maintain the transference that psychoanalysis tries to resolve."[34] Many commentators concur with Kernberg that the perpetuation of discipleship (with its religious connotations) derives from unresolved transference to the training analyst, who is generally a member of the same society (or institute) in which the future analyst will spend his or her entire professional life. Such shared transferences to a few powerful people in an institute are at the heart of some theoretical wars in psychoanalysis today. Given the tripartite model of training that has been almost universally adopted in training institutions worldwide, analysis, supervision, and class work are all conducted within the boundaries of an institute where there is often only one overriding point of view. Consequently, a young analyst's prospects, as with Freud's disciples, often depend upon adhering to whatever "doctrine" is specific to that institute.

The power struggles and purges that still plague organizational psychoanalysis persist in part because of our failure to treat psychoanalysis as a scientific discipline. In order to minimize the "religious" elements in psychoanalysis, psycholanalysts must assert the principles of verification that are intrinsic to scientific endeavors.[35] Psychoanalysis illuminates the schemata of meaning and their association with emotions (affects) in a given segment of time.[36] From the correspondence between meaning sets and affects, we generate psychoanalytic hypotheses, that is, hypotheses about unconscious wishes and defenses, conflicts and aspirations. The psychiatric researcher Gerard Klerman observed that psychoanalysis has been rich in generating hypotheses but has not been sufficiently committed to verifying them.[37] To be sure, validation in the broadest sense cannot come in the consulting room. One must design controlled longitudinal studies—and this analysts have only recently been willing to undertake.

To hold to theories without such validation is to invite contamination by value biases and to guarantee that the political or religious takes the place of the scientific. One need only consider the psychoanalytic studies of sex and gender to uncover such biases. To take but one example, the idea of penis envy as the primary organizer of female development is now discredited, thanks to contemporary research into child development, complemented by feminist critiques within and outside institutional psychoanalysis. Yet this idea, as well as other outmoded ideas about gender development, persisted for at least three decades longer than it should have—especially since it had already been effectively demolished by the arguments of neo-Freudian and interpersonal theorists. Far too many psychoanalysts discredited their critiques as merely culturalist. They objected to the theories of the interpersonal school because this school implied that subjectivity mirrored the external world and seemed to endorse a perspective that undermined the hard-won recognition of the importance of intrapsychic and unconscious factors.

Only recently have the theoretical assumptions of psychoanalysis been enlarged to a point where earlier critiques of female psychology could be assimilated. Before this could happen, the question of whether "the unconscious has a history," in Stephen Marcus's phrase, had to be addressed.[38] What was required was a theory that could account for how external reality is internalized and becomes organized and reorganized in the individual psyche. What was required, then, was a shift away from a theory which posited that development was exclusively the preordained outcome of libidinal development—that is, a shift away from reducing mental processes to biology—and a shift toward a theory that acknowledged object relations and internalization as major psychic organizers. As the psychoanalyst Joseph Sandler observed, we are now more amenable to considering multiple motivational systems, rather than reducing motivation to two drives. This shift has had relevance for the way we now theorize about sex, gender, and fantasy. It is also relevant to how we might better theorize about power.

It is both sad and ironic, but perhaps inevitable, that Freud, who had to struggle with professional and personal powerlessness by virtue of being born Jewish, should mistake the pervasive personal and professional marginalization suffered by the women of his era by virtue of being born female, the concept of "penis envy," as the core of female psychology. This misunderstanding doomed his theories of female and male sexuality, of femininity and masculinity and of homosexuality. It also impaired other theories, as well, including theories of object relations, intersubjectivity, interpersonal relationships, and, what is relevant here, theories of power.

ONE STILL SEES few references to power in the psychoanalytic literature. Given the extent to which the first psychoanalysts were driven by their own ambitions and their lust for power, and the degree to which the movement was saturated with ongoing power struggles, some of which persist into the present, it is as though psychoanalysis itself is in denial.

However, the importance of power as a motive is implicit if not explicit in classical psychoanalytic theory. In the male Oedipus complex, we observe not only the boy's sexual wish for his mother but his wish to replace the father in the family hierarchy of power. It may even be the latter wish that is the impetus for the former.

Will and the will to power—the issues with which Adler was concerned—eventually made their way into psychoanalysis through the invocation of the aggressive instinct as of equal importance with libido. In his paper of 1924 on masochism, Freud for the first time speaks of "the destructive instinct, the instinct for mastery, or the 'will to power'" in terms more or less coequal with libido.[39] It has been argued that Freud transformed Adler's preoccupation with power into a larger theory of aggression. Unfortunately, power is still considered a derivative of the aggressive drive—a formulation that misses the broad scope of power as a motive. Whereas aggression implies destruction, the power motive encompasses mastery and agency, which are fundamentally not destructive but constructive.

Why is it necessary to theorize that power is a desire or drive rather than a secondary ego phenomenon? The most basic form of power is agency; in fact, agency is prerequisite to our ability to express our other drives. It is in this exact sense that Winnicott speaks of the inherent "ruthlessness" of drives and of "aggression."[40] Unfortunately the word *aggression* is too steeped in an outmoded instinct theory to express the full sweep of the power motive. Throughout this book, I have described power as an innate force that moves us toward self-control, self-mastery, and mastery of the external world, on the one hand, and, interpersonal power on the other (whether through the powers of the strong or the powers of the weak).[41] I have also suggested that power as a motivational force is analogous to sex, bonding, and aggression in its central importance in our lives.

From early childhood on, we process our dual concerns about personal independence and our relationships with others both in conscious awareness and in the preconscious ranges of our mind. Indeed, dealing with issues of power is an inescapable part of finding our sense of self. Our involvement with people extends beyond our external relationships into our innermost sense of self. As Freud astutely noted in *Group Psychology and the Analysis of the Ego*, in the recesses of our minds, "Someone else is invariably involved as a model, as an object, as a helper, as an opponent; and so from the very first individual psychology, in its extended but entirely justifiable sense of the words, is at the same time social psychology as well."

The impulse toward power is both innate and shaped by teaching and experience. The basic drive (in the form of agency and rudimentary interpersonal strategies of power) is augmented or compromised, depending on our experience. I have previously emphasized that our need for power is intensified by the weakness that is our common lot. Here is an important link not just to Adler but to the insights of our philosophers. Man is driven not by instinct alone but also by the need to create meaning in the face of his mortality. The fear of death is an impetus for many attempts to exert power and sometimes even for an attempt to seize the godhead.

In thinking about the way power becomes an intrinsic part of who we are, an analogy to gender suggests itself. We now know that while the ability to differentiate male and female begins almost at birth and may well be innate, the ability to categorize the self as one gender and not the other is comparatively slow to develop and begins to be consolidated only around the age of eighteen months. It is also relatively clear that this development, which becomes an essential part of a child's identity, is based on biology—at least in part—but comes to be cognition driven. It is not solely the result of any innate drive to become masculine or feminine. But no one would contend that gender identity is any less important for this reason. We know gender, as acquired, gives rise to the rich and deeply meaningful motives and conflicts which may well be unconscious as well as conscious. The same is true of power. While there is an intrinsic drive toward power, a great deal of social learning is involved in the way issues of power are assimilated in development. Issues of power do not become any less central to our sense of self and to the unconscious agendas we bring to our experience of the world and interpersonal relationships because they partake of developmental issues and social learning.

WE CANNOT UNDERSTAND the integration of individuals into families, groups, and political structures without reference to dominance and submission, and to hierarchies We cannot usefully build on Freud's insights into group psychology without recourse to the concept of power. Transference to the leader of a group—or to a religious leader, or to a god—protects us not only against powerlessness in our daily lives but also against our powerlessness in the face of death and decay. The illusions we adhere to in groups give us a sense of both safety and importance. This same phenomenology of power can be observed in psychoanalytical organizations. It is the need for absoluteness and for meaning that sometimes conflicts with the critical mind-set necessary to keep the psychoanalytic profession within the boundaries of "historical" science and to allow it to utilize the findings of scientific disciplines adjacent to its own.

Acknowledgments

Like most of us, I first learned about power from my parents. They were a successful couple, but in some ways an odd one. At a time when most women went to normal school if they went past high school, my mother earned a master's degree in mathematics from Columbia University. While my grandfather supported his three sons through college and postgraduate degrees, he thought higher education superfluous for girls. My mother did not agree. She paid for her college tuition by working as a telephone operator on the nighttime shift. Even so, she had just enough money left to take the bus to the University of Louisville or to buy lunch—never enjoying both luxuries on the same day. She was a gifted woman, a linguist who spoke three or four languages fluently, a good amateur pianist, and a poet who was published in the *Louisville Courier Journal* and other local publications beginning in her teens. For all her gifts, she was not at ease in the world; she felt too different from her peers and not as pretty as her sister.

My father had a different kind of courage and drive. In his mid-teens, he traveled alone from Eastern Europe to Buenos Aires, then up the West Coast of the United States, and on to New York City. Like my mother, he could do mathematical calculations in his head and spoke several languages, but he never learned to read or write English. My parents met in New York City while my mother was studying at Columbia University and my father boarding in the family home of my mother's best friend. They married and moved to Louisville. I don't know how my father got together a stake, but he was flush enough to buy a bar, and then several more. Despite my maternal family's emphasis on education, they loved my father more than my mother. Perhaps it was because my mother was contained, my father one of the great charmers of his day. My parents shared few interests except in one another, in me, in the business, and in world events. They even liked different movies. But their marriage worked extremely well and gave lie to the reigning gender stereotypes of the day.

My mother gave me the freedom to pursue my dreams. In fact, she shaped them. To protect me from identifying with the traditional female role, she refused to let me do any housework, which was fine with me. She also discouraged me from learning how to type, which was a big mistake, one that I rectified only as an adult. My father's influence was decisive for my life, even though he died when I was twelve. He felt more comfortable in the world than my mother, and could find enough common ground to engage anyone in animated conversation. My social skills, such as they are, come from him. He was the one who possessed an authentic sense of power, and it was through his example that I acquired a sense of ease in the world.

My interest in power is undoubtedly connected to the somewhat atypical power valences in my immediate family—the fact that my parents' roles and strengths were far from the norm. Whatever the reasons, the subject of power has played a supporting role, if not the leading one, in my books on love, fantasy, and sex and gender. It is, of course, impossible to study sex and gender without stumbling onto issues of power.

Thanks go to a number of friends, colleagues, and relatives for their input and support. Beth Rashbaum critiqued and helped shape my book proposal. Gladys Topkis and Judith Rossner read and helped refine the focus of the first few chapters. John Atwood, Dr. Jack Barchas, Dr. Gail Berry, Jessica Diamond, Nancy Diamond, Lori Dickstein, Morris Dickstein, Betty Gaylin, Dr. Willard Gaylin, Vicki Goldberg, Molly Haskell, Dr. Alex Holder, Denise Lefrak, Dr. Moisés Lemlij, Dr. David Levine, Dr. Paul Lippman, Dr. Barbara Rocah, Lucy Simon, Catherine Stimpson, Anna Stoessinger, Caroline Stoessinger, Daniel Stern, Toby Talbott, Dan Talbott, Alan Trustman, Larry Young, and Dr. Claudia Zanardi pointed me to important source material, discussed ideas, or helped me iron out some apparent contradictions. Anne Roiphe read and critiqued the intimacy chapter in its earlier incarnation as a lecture. Hilma Wolitzer read several chapters with a kind but critical eye; and in playing with book titles, we arrived at the book's subtitle, "The Achievement of Authentic Power."

The person with whom I spent the most time discussing power is the psychologist and editor John Kerr. We met by chance when I was chair of the publications committee for the International Psychoanalytical Association and he was the publisher's editor for a volume in an IPA monograph series I was editing. Because he lives in New England and I live in New York, we communicated almost exclusively by phone. We shared many interests, so we kept on talking, becoming friends in the process. Our conversations were decisive in my thinking through some basic distinctions about the nature of power, among them, how ethology both is and is not a useful frame of reference.

Because power has social dimensions as well as interpersonal and intrapsychic ones, I have benefitted from work in adjacent fields—philosophy, political science, ethology, psychology, and sociology. In particular, the late Hans Morgenthau educated me about how to think about power from the vantage point of political theory.

To decipher how power was viewed in different fields, I needed to do a considerable amount of research. This was facilitated by the staff of two libraries, the Amagansett Free Library on Long Island, and the Society Library in New York City. Special thanks go to Judy Mars, librarian at the Columbia University Psychoanalytic Center, who supplied me with an endless flow of books and research material from the various Columbia University libraries, and who helped check the bibliography.

Thanks also go to my very competent assistant, Joshua Widick, who typed and retyped the manuscript, kept track of my bibliographical references, and in one cogent conversation helped me better understand the creative process (he is a dancer and choreographer).

My agent Kris Dahl not only found this book its proper home, but also assuaged my anxiety at a few critical moments. Thanks go to Arnold Dolin for an excellent copy edit. For this book, I wanted a male editor in his thirties or forties. And I was lucky enough to find him. Not only did Henry Ferris force me to think through some elusive issues and pull out all the stops in the last half of the ninth inning, but he supplied what it was that I was looking for—he proved a corrective to my sometimes generational and female bias.

I am grateful to my patients, past and present, for what they have taught me, and I am especially grateful to those who have generously agreed to let me recount their stories. For the sake of confidentiality, as I have done in previous books, I disguised the actual life situations or used composites, with every effort to preserve psychological authenticity.

In a different vein, I want to thank the orthopedic surgeon Dr. Mathias Bostrum, who put back together my badly shattered leg in what must have been a major high-wire virtuoso performance. And Job Becerra, not only a gifted physical therapist but also a natural born healer, enabled me to go the distance in a sometimes arduous process.

Most of all, I owe a debt of gratitude to my husband, Stanley Diamond, who is my most critical reader and my most ardent supporter. He has a more disciplined mind than I do, and he uses his legal logic to nudge me to argue my case rather than to state it. And he, too, nursed me through a stressful year. I am grateful, too, to my sons, Louis Sherman and Lloyd Sherman, who know better than any one else in my life how to persuade or manipulate me, and who sometimes know what I'm up to, even when I don't. Without their expertise in raising me, I would have lacked the experience to write this book.

Several of the chapters in this book first saw the light of day as lectures. Chapter 4, "The Powers of the Weak and the Powers of the Strong," was originally given in April 1998 as a lecture in Lima, Peru, at the conference "At the Threshold of the Millennium," sponsored by Comisión de Prompción de Peru, Interdisciplinary Commission of Andean Studies, and the International Psychoanalytical Association. An earlier version of Chapter 5, "Intimacy and Power," was given as a lecture "Distortions of Power in Love and Sexuality" April 17, 2000 as part of the summer program, Lindauer Psychotherapywochen, in Lindau, Germany. Chapter 6, "Sex, Gender, and Power," was presented as the Virginia Clower Memorial Lecture, February 26, 2000, at Emory University. Chapter 13, "Transcendence," draws on ideas I first presented in my plenary address, "Knowledge and Authority: The Godfather Fantasy," at the winter meetings of the American Psychoanalytic Association in New York City, December 2000. The Epilogue, "The Failure to Theorize Power in Psychoanalytic Theory," was first presented in Hamburg, Germany, at the DGPT Conference, September 1999.

Notes

Introduction

1. Rollo May, 1998, [c. 1972], *Power and Innocence: A Search for the Sources of Violence*. New York: Norton (paperback), p. 122.
2. Adolph Berle, 1969, [1967], *Power*. New York: Harcourt, Brace, and World, p. 37.
3. Walter Benjamin, 1979, *Reflections: Essays, Aphorisms, Autobiographical Writings*, ed. and intro. Peter Demetz. New York: First Harvest/ HBJ Edition, p. 65.
4. Sigmund Freud, "Group Psychology and the Analysis of the Ego," *The Standard Edition of the Complete Psychological Works (S.E.)*, ed. and trans. by James Strachey. London: Hogarth Press; New York: W. W. Norton, vol. XVIII, p. 129.
5. Hans Morgenthau, 1962, "The Demands of Prudence," in *Politics in the Twentieth Century: Volume III, The Restoration of American Politics*. Chicago: University of Chicago Press, p. 15.
6. Bertrand Russell, 1938, *Power: A New Social Analysis*. New York: W. W. Norton, p. 12.

Chapter I

1. Webster, *New International Dictionary*.
2. John O. Whitney and Tina Packer, 2000, *Power Plays: Shakespeare's Lessons in Leadership and Management*. New York: Simon and Schuster, p. 25.
3. Michael Korda, 1975, *Power: How to Get It, How to Use It*. New York: Random House, p. 48.
4. Depression is sometimes a result of a biological predisposition, but it is just as likely to be psychological in origin, the consequence either of turmoil or deprivation in early life or of a current life situation that makes our well-being seem precarious.
5. Quoted in "Life of the Party: Journalist/Hostess/Washington Insider Sally Quinn Issues a Manners Manual," in W, November 1997, pp. 62–64.
6. Gore Vidal, 1995, *Palimpsest: A Memoir*. New York: Penguin, p. 62.

7. Our current fascination with the Mafia (*The Sopranos, Falcone, Analyze This*) may have replaced our earlier preoccupation with the Old West.

8. Camille Paglia, May, 1997, "At Home with Mario Puzo: It All Comes Back to Family," *New York Times*, p. 8.

9. Mario Puzo, 1997, *The Fortunate Pilgrim*. New York: Random House, p. xii. In the interview with Paglia, he elaborated: "My mother was a fairly ruthless person."

10. Quoted in Felicia R. Lee, 2000, "A Feminist Survivor with the Eyes of a Child," *New York Times*, 4 July, p. E-1.

11. Erik Erikson and Joan Erikson, 1953, "The Power of the Newborn," *Mademoiselle*. Quoted in John Mack, 1994, "Power, Powerlessness, and Empowerment in Psychotherapy," *Psychiatry*, 57:179–199.

12. Althea Horner, 1995 [1989], *The Wish for Power and the Fear of Having It*. Northfield, N.J.: Jason Aronson, pp. 84–85.

13. René A. Spitz, 1957, *No and Yes: On the Genesis of Human Communication*. Madison, Conn.: International Universities Press.

14. Judith Viorst, 1998, *Imperfect Control: Our Lifelong Struggle with Power and Surrender*. New York: Simon and Schuster, p. 63.

15. Ibid., pp. 33, 34.

16. Horner, op. cit., p. 14.

17. Thomas Moore, 2000 [1998], afterword to *Stalking the Soul: Emotional Abuse and the Erosion of Identity* by Marie-France Hirigoyen. Canada: Helen Marks Books. Paris: Éditions La Découverte et Syros, p. 202.

18. D. W. Winnicott, 1950–1955, "Aggression in Relationship to Emotional Development" in *Collected Papers*, ch. 16.

19. Michael Schulman, 1987, "On the Problem of the Id in Psychoanalytic Theory," *International Journal of Psychoanalysis*, 68:161–174.

20. Viorst, op. cit., p. 64.

21. Robert W. White, 1959, "Motivation Reconsidered: The Concept of Competence," *Psychological Review*, 66 (5):320, 322.

22. Viorst, op. cit., p. 29. The psychoanalytic paradigm reigned supreme for some decades, but more recently the evolutionary psychologists (evo-psychos, as the science writer Natalie Angier calls them) are currently in vogue.

23. Bertrand Russell, 1938, *Power: A New Social Analysis*. New York: Norton, p. 18.

24. Alexander Thomas and Stella Chess, 1977, *Temperament and Development*. New York: Brunner/Mazel.

25. Jerome Kagan, 1984, *The Nature of the Child*. New York: Basic Books, p. 65.

26. Ibid., p. 68.

27. I'm grateful to my colleague Bennett Simon, who in a discussion of my paper "Male Sexuality and Power" (1983) elaborated on the diversity of fantasies involved. (See Bennett Simon, 1986, "The Power of the Wish and the Wish for Power: A Discussion of Power and Psychoanalysis," *Psychoanalytic Inquiry*, ed. Joseph Lichtenberg, Analytic Press, vol. 6, no. 1, p. 127.) The Jungian analyst James Hillman similarly advocates viewing power in terms of fantasy: "Rather than a *theory* of power, ours is a *phenomenology* of power, even a phenomenology of the fantasies of power" (James Hillman, 1995, *Kinds of Power: A Guide to Its Intelligent Uses*, New York: Currency/Doubleday, pp. 105–106).

28. Henry James, 1909, "The Beast in the Jungle" in *The Altar of the Dead, The Beast in the Jungle, The Birthplace, and Other Tales*. New York: Scribner.

29. Hugh Walpole, 1984 [1940], "James's Friendships," in *Henry James: Interviews and Recollections*, ed. Norman Page. New York: St. Martin's, pp. 22–26. Originally published February 1940 as "Henry James: A Reminiscence" *Horizon*, 1: 41, 76–80.

30. Edmund Gosse, 1984 [1920], "The Mayor-Elect of Rye," in *Henry James: Interviews and Recollections*, pp. 83–85. Originally published 1920 as *Henry James*, London: *Mercury* 11, pp. 32–34.

31. In Gosse's account, James was "standing on the pavement of a city, in the dusk, and gazing upwards across the misty street, watching, watching for the lighting of a lamp in a window on the third storey. James stood there . . . and through bursting tears he strained to see what was behind it. . . . The mysterious and poignant revelation closed, and one could make no comment, ask no question, being throttled oneself by an overpowering emotion" (ibid., p. 85).

32. Charles H. Thomas. "Zimmerman's Bookstore" in "First History/The Old Thompson Block: A Touch of Bohemia," *Filson Club History Quarterly*, October 1997, pp. 415–421.

33. Hans Morgenthau, 1962, "Love and Power," in *Politics in the Twentieth Century: The Restoration of American Politics*. Chicago: University of Chicago Press, p. 8.

34. Ibid., p. 8.

35. A feeling of transcendence may be achieved through the replication of some of our DNA in our offspring; sometimes through a sense of merging with nature, religion, or the cosmos; and sometimes, too, through romantic love. In love, as in religion, there is an object of worship, a means of communion, a route to union with something larger than the self. Not surprisingly, there is a striking overlap between the language of love and that of religion. See Ethel S. Person, *Dreams of Love and Fateful Encounters: The Power of Romantic Passion*. New York: W. W. Norton, 1988.

36. *The Letters of Gustave Flaubert, 1830–1857*, selected, ed., and trans. Francis Steegmuller, 1980 [1977]. Cambridge, Mass.: Belknap Press of Harvard University Press, p. 158.

37. Ibid., p. 215.

Chapter 2

1. Rollo May, 1998 [1972], *Power and Innocence: A Search for the Sources of Violence*. New York: Norton, p. 21.

2. Walter Kerr, 1967, *Tragedy and Comedy*. New York: Simon and Schuster, pp. 148–149.

3. Ibid., pp. 172, 173.

4. Ibid., p. 174.

5. Marie Brenner, 2000, *Great Dames*. New York: Random House, pp. 239–240.

6. Philip Rahv, 1966, *The Myth and the Powerhouse*. New York: Farrar Straus and Giroux, Noonday Ed., p. 141.

7. Alex Kuczynski, 2000, "Oprah, Coast to Coast: A Phenomenon Struts Herself on the Newsstand," *New York Times*, October 2, p. C1.

8. Gene Stratton-Porter, 1910, *A Girl of the Limberlost*. New York: Doubleday.

9. Althea Horner, 1995 [1989], *The Wish for Power and the Fear of Having It*. Northfield, N.J.: Jason Aronson, p. 84.

10. Ernest Becker, 1973, *The Denial of Death*. New York: Free Press, pp. 13–15.

11. Ibid., pp. 19–20.

12. Among others, the writer Elizabeth Janeway also observes the near universality of nightmares and night terrors. Janeway, 1980, *Powers of the Weak*. New York: Knopf, pp. 81–82.

13. Of course, we also worry about more realistic threats. We worry about health and financial security. We may also be troubled by an array of much smaller worries—burning the dinner, missing the bus, not being invited to a special party, threats to an important friendship, an unmanageable weight gain. Here what is often at risk is our sense of importance, our narcissistic wholeness, a fear of ineptness or rejection clouding our horizons.

14. Willard Gaylin argues that feelings can be the very instruments of rationality: "Emotions . . . are not just directives to ourselves, but directives from others to us, indicating that we have

been seen; that we have been understood; that we have been appreciated; that we have made contact." Gaylin, 1979, *Feelings: Our Vital Signs*. New York: Harper and Row, p. 9.

15. Feelings are the experiential aspect of emotions. Emotion encompasses not only a subjective feeling but also a biophysiological state and the underlying chemical changes accompanying the feeling.

16. Eugene O'Neill, 1963, [1946, 1952] "The Iceman Cometh," reprinted in *Best American Plays: Third Series, 1945–1951*, ed. John Gassner. New York: Crown, pp. 164–165.

17. For example: "I did it because of a gut feeling." "I did it because I loved him." "I was angry at her betrayal, so I struck out." "My guilt immobilized me." "I was so anxious [or depressed] that I couldn't go to the party." "I was so disgusted at the way I look in a bathing suit that I won't go to the beach until I lose weight."

18. Alfie Kohn, 1999, "In Pursuit of Affluence at a High Price," *New York Times*, 2 February, p. 7.

19. John Lahr, 1999, "Making Willie Loman," *New Yorker*, 25 January, pp. 47ff.

20. Sigmund Freud, 1927, "The Future of an Illusion," Chapters 3 and 4. S.E. See also Freud, 1926, "The Problem of Anxiety." S.E.

21. Maslow's argument is that we fear both the external world and the internal world: "We tend to be afraid of any knowledge that could cause us to despise ourselves or to make us feel inferior, weak, worthless, evil, shameful. We protect ourselves and our ideal image of ourselves by repression and similar defenses, which are essentially techniques by which we avoid becoming conscious of unpleasant or dangerous truths." Abraham Maslow, 1963, "The Need to Know and the Fear of Knowing," in *Journal of General Psychology* 68:111–125.

22. Hannah Arendt, 1958, *The Human Condition*. Chicago: University of Chicago Press.

23. William James, 1958, [1902] *The Varieties of Religious Experience: A Study in Human Nature*. New York: Mentor, p. 121.

24. John Lahr, 2000, "The Whirlwind: How Kenneth Tynan Reinvented Theatre Criticism—and Himself," in *New Yorker*, August 7, p. 42.

Chapter 3

1. Jonathan Lear, 1999, *Open Minded: Working Out the Logic of the Soul*. Cambridge, Mass.: Harvard University Press.

2. Anne Roiphe, 1987, *Lovingkindness*. New York: Summit, p. 120.

3. Mario Puzo, 1997 [1964], *The Fortunate Pilgrim*. New York: Fawcett Columbine/Ballantine, p. 115.

4. John Kenneth Galbraith, 1983, *The Anatomy of Power*. Boston: Houghton Mifflin, pp. 72-73.

5. Paul Kennedy, 1987, *The Rise and Fall of the Great Powers*. New York: Vintage. Katherine Newman notes, "Few empires have mastered the fine art of decline; few nations have developed the cultural means of letting themselves down gently when the tide of history turns against them." Newman, 1993, *Declining Fortunes: The Withering of the American Dream*. New York: Basic Books, p. 25.

6. Philip Rieff, 1961, *Freud: The Mind of the Moralist*. New York: Doubleday/Anchor, p. 168.

7. Stanley Milgram, 1974, *Obedience to Authority*. New York: Harper and Row, p. 166.

8. Beforehand, Milgram had asked a group of psychiatrists what they thought the outcome would be; they predicted, essentially, that all the subjects would refuse to obey the experimenter. When this experiment was repeated in Italy, South Africa, and Australia, the proportion of obedient subjects was even higher, and in Munich it reached 85 percent.

9. Milgram, op. cit., p. 167.

10. Ibid., p. 131.

11. Toni Morrison, 1970, *The Bluest Eye*. New York: Penguin, pp. 107–109.

12. John Loughery, 1999, *The Other Side of Silence: Men's Lives and Gay Identities—A Twentieth-Century History*. New York: Holt/John Macrae, pp. 447–448.
13. Ruth Goetz and Augustus Goetz, 1975 [1946], *The Heiress*, Dramatist's Play Service.
14. Ibid., p. 19.
15. Ibid., p, 10.
16. Ibid., p. 11.
17. Ibid., p. 56.
18. Ibid.
19. Ibid., p. 57.
20. Katherine Graham, 1997, *Personal History*. New York: Knopf.
21. Ibid., p. 15.
22. Ibid., p. 31.
23. Ibid., p. 32.
24. Ibid., pp. 110–111.
25. Ibid., p. 131.
26. Ibid., p. 214.
27. Ibid., p. 140.
28. Ibid., p. 324.
29. Ibid., p. 420.
30. Ibid., p. 421.
31. Ibid., p. 422.
32. J. B. Priestly, 1960, *Literature and Western Man*. New York: Harper, p. 4.
33. Henrik Ibsen, 1961 [1879], *A Doll's House*, trans. and ed. James Walter McFarlane. New York: Appleton, pp. 197–286.
34. See Ethel S. Person, 2000, "Change Moments in Therapy," in *Changing Ideas in a Changing World: The Revolution in Psychoanalysis—Essays in Honor of Arnold Cooper*, ed. Peter Fonagy and Robert Michels. London and New York: Karnac.
35. Malcom X with Alex Haley, 1965, *The Autobiography of Malcolm X*. New York: Grove Press. Quotes from pp. 187, 189.
36. Hans Morgenthau, 1970, *Truth and Power: Essays of a Decade, 1960–1970*. New York: Praeger, p. 15.
37. Ben-Avi was a supervising analyst at William Alanson White Institute in New York City. Quoted by the psychologist, analyst, and editor John Kerr.

Chapter 4

1. F. Scott Fitzgerald, 1934, *Tender Is the Night*, New York: Scribner, p. 277.
2. Domination consists of enactments of what the psychoanalyst Carl Gustav Jung called the power complex: "the total complex of all those ideas and strivings whose tendency is to range the ego above other influences, thus subordinating all such influences to the ego." Quoted in Hillman, 1995, p. 95.
3. Susan Isaacs, 2001, *Longtime No See*. New York: HarperCollins, p. 222.
4. John Kenneth Galbraith, 1983, *The Anatomy of Power*. Boston: Houghton Mifflin, p. 25.
5. Ethel S. Person, 1995, *By Force of Fantasy*. New York: Basic Books.
6. Charles Lindholm, 1990, *Charisma*. Cambridge, Mass.: Basil Blackwell, p. 5.
7. The pull of charisma can lead us to make choices that shape the rest of our lives, long after the object of our enthusiasm is dead or we have become disenchanted. In Washington today, you will still find brilliant and now-aging private-practice lawyers, who as idealistic young professionals came in on the Kennedy tide only to find themselves stranded like beached whales when the tide moved out.

8. Bobby Baker, quoted in G. Wills, 1978, "A Guy Like I," *New York Review of Books*, xxv (20 July), p. 12.
9. Elizabeth Janeway, 1980, *Powers of the Weak*. New York: Knopf.
10. However, in humans this basic mechanism sometimes fails because culture overrides it. In China, for example, girl babies are so devalued that their parents often abandon them to die.
11. Janeway, 1980, ibid. Still, such power is tricky to wield and often comes at the cost of self-esteem.
12. Sometimes, ingratiation and flattery are necessary modes of survival and may even be raised to an art. The proverbial Uncle Tom was no fool. He was securing his safety by being as non-confrontational and abject as possible—while occasionally indulging in the pleasure of sabotaging his master's plans through his "incompetence." The same could be said of the title character in *The Good Soldier Schweik*.
13. Irvin Yalom, 1999, "Mama and the Meaning of Life," in *Tales of Psychotherapy*. New York: Basic Books. The quotations are from pp. 1–13.
14. Sharon Olds, "The Takers."
15. Frank Sulloway, 1996, *Born to Rebel*. New York: Pantheon.
16. Michael Korda, 1975, *Power: How to Get It, How to Use It*. New York: Random House, p. 6.
17. Daniel Stern, personal communication.
18. This kind of research raises the possibility of being able to link observational microanalysis of mother-child interactions in infancy between mothers and infants to patterns of behavior in childhood and even adulthood.
19. Robert Timberg, 1966 [1995], *The Nightingale's Song*. New York: Touchstone, pp. 6–64.
20. The way we internalize submissiveness or dominance is shaped in part by the cultural unconscious—shared fantasies and narratives specific to particular cultures in particular epochs that become part of the individual's inner world. Person, 1995, *By Force of Fantasy*, pp. 197–217.
21. On the basis of an animal model, one might say that we are hardwired to respond in both a dominant and a submissive mode. An evolutionary force must be at work to provide hierarchical stability for the group.
22. John Cheever, 1991, "Journals," *New Yorker*, 21 January, pp. 34–35.
23. *Time Out New York*, 1999, 4–11 February, p. 14.
24. H. Clayton Foushee and Robert L. Helmreich, 1988, "Group Interaction and Flight Crew Performance," in *Human Factors in Aviation*, ed. Earl L. Wiener and David C. Nagel. New York: Academic Press. Quotations are from pp. 189–227, 193, 195–196.
25. Quotation from a report submitted to the AAFA/FAA aviation safety reporting system. Eugene Tarnow, 2000, "Self-Destructive Obedience in the Airplane Cockpit and the Concept of Obedience-Optimization," in *Obedience to Authority: Current Perspectives on the Milgram Paradigm*, ed. Thomas Blass. Hillsdale, N.J.: Lawrence Erlbaum, p. 112.
26. R. L. Helmreich, J. A. Wilhelm, S. E. Gregorich, and T. R. Chivster, 1990, "Preliminary Results from Evaluation of Cockpit Resource Management Training: Performance Ratings of Flight Crews," *Aviation, Space, and Environmental Medicine* 61:576–579.
27. J. B. Sexton, E. J. Thomas, and R. L. Helmreich, 2000, "Error, Stress, and Teamwork in Medicine and Aviation: Cross-Sectional Surveys," *British Medical Journal* 320 (7237): 745–749.
28. A. M. Rosenthal, 1999, *Thirty-Eight Witnesses: The Kitty Genovese Case*. Los Angeles: University of California Press.

Chapter 5

1. Marilyn French, 1985, *Beyond Power: On Women, Men, and Morals*, New York: Ballantine, p. 541.

2. Deidre Bair, 1990, *Simone de Beauvoir: A Biography*. New York: Summit.
3. John Bowlby, *Attachment and Loss. Volume 1: Attachment* (1969). *Volume 2: Separation, Anxiety, and Anger* (1974). *Volume 3: Loss, Sadness, and Depression,* (1980). New York: Basic Books.
4. Daniel Stern, 1984, *The Interpersonal World of the Infant: A View from Psychoanalysis and Developmental Psychology.* New York: Basic Books.
5. Stern's theory of intersubjectivity refers to a field between the self and the other; consequently it is different from, though not incompatible with, earlier theories of psychic development. Essentially, the infant's growing awareness of separateness develops in tandem with an increasing appreciation of the other. Stern's observations suggest that the capacity for consolidating a cohesive self with healthy self-esteem rests on recognition and validation from an other.
6. Blaise Pascal, 1958, *Pensées* (paperback ed.), with an introduction by T. S. Eliot. New York: Dutton.
7. As Bowlby puts it, "Intimate attachments to other beings are the hub around which a person's life revolves, not only when he is an infant or a toddler or schoolchild, but throughout his adolescence and his years of maturity as well, and on into old age. From these intimate attachments, a person draws his strength and his enjoyment of life and through what he contributes, he gives strength and enjoyment to others. These are matters about which current science and traditional wisdom are as one." Bowlby, *Attachment and Loss. Volume 3: Loss, Sadness, and Depression,* p. 442.
8. This material draws on A. Scott Berg, 1988, *Lindbergh.* New York: Putnam. See also Eric Pace, 2001, "Anne Morrow Lindbergh Is Dead at 94," in *New York Times,* February 8, p. A 29 (obituary). Quotations are from these sources: see esp. Berg, p. 379.
9. The Atchley Pavilion there is named for him.
10. Deborah Tannen, 1989, *You Just Don't Understand: Women and Men in Conversation.* New York: Ballantine.
11. Sigmund Freud, 1921, "Group Psychology and the Analysis of the Ego." *S.E.,* vol. 18, p. 101, footnote. Freud suggests one possible exception—the relationship of a mother to her son, which he believes is based on narcissism, "is not disturbed by subsequent rivalry, and is reinforced by a rudimentary attempt at sexual object-choice." This view was based on his view (now discredited) that a boy is a mother's surrogate penis.
12. Peter Lawner, 1988, "Trust and Testing in Love Relations," in *Love: Psychoanalytic Perspectives,* ed. Judith Lasky and Helen Silverman. New York: New York University Press, pp. 133–146.
13. Jessica Benjamin, 1988, *The Bonds of Love: Psychoanalysis, Feminism, and the Problem of Domination.* New York: Pantheon, p. 28.
14. *East Is East,* directed by Damian O'Donnell. Written by Ayub Khan-Din, based on his play. Released by Miramax Films, 2000.
15. D. W. Winnicott, 1958, "The Capacity to Be Alone," in *The Maturational Process and the Facilitating Environment.* New York: International Universities Press, 1965.
16. This section draws on my earlier work on passionate relationships. (Ethel S. Person, 1988, *Dreams of Love and Fateful Encounters.* New York: Norton, Chapter 7.)
17. Francisco Alberoni, 1983, *Falling in Love,* trans. Lawrence Venuti. New York: Random House, pp. 12–13.
18. Hans Morgenthau, 1962, "Love and Power," in *Politics in the Twentieth Century: Volume III, The Restoration of American Politics.* Chicago: University of Chicago Press, p. 10.
19. Ibid.
20. The desire for possession and dominance, effected through the power of the strong, has its roots both in early psychological life and in the lineaments of the culture. But sadism, like

masochism, is invariably a product of distorted relationships in early life and is often connected to a history of physical abuse. Clinical scrutiny usually reveals that neither sadism or masochism is pure; each is generally mixed with the other.

Chapter 6

1. In the Western world, the three big sex and gender stories of the twentieth century were sexual liberation, gay liberation, and the women's movement. Describing the twentieth-century reaction against Victorianism as "sexual modernism," the intellectual historian Paul Robinson discussed how modernist sex reformers, researchers, and theorists affected a sea-change in contemporary attitudes. Unlike Victorian sexologists who were proponents of sexual repression, the current practitioners are "sexual enthusiasts," advocating tolerance for pluralism in sexual practices, legitimization of some common behaviors previously considered deviant (particularly homosexual sex and masturbation), and recognition of the sexual desires and capacities of women. They have also, of course, challenged the idea that the aim of sex is primarily procreation. To Robinson, removing sexuality from the institutional context of marriage and reproduction is the core of modernism. (Robinson, 1976, *The Modernization of Sex*. New York: Harper and Row, p. 3.)

2. Lionel Tiger, 1999, *The Decline of the Male*. New York: Golden Books. John MacInnes, 1998, *The End of Masculinity: The Confusion of Sexual Genesis and Sexual Difference in Modern Society*. Buckingham and Philadelphia: Open University Press.

3. See Ethel S. Person, 1991, *The Sexual Century*, New Haven, Conn.: Yale University Press.

4. See, for example, Jeffrey Weeks, 1979, "Movements of Affirmation: Sexual Meaning and Homosexual Identity," *Radical History Review* 20:164–179. See also Weeks, 1986, *Sexuality*, New York: Routledge.

5. The benefits of orgasm extend beyond pleasure. Orgasm provides relief of mental as well as genital tension, and strengthens the ego, regression in the service of the ego, and so on. (Nathan Ross, 1970, "The Primacy of Genitality in the Light of Ego Psychology," *Journal of the American Psychoanalytic Association*, 18:267–280.)

6. Kurt Eissler, 1958, "Notes on Problems of Technique in the Psychoanalytic Treatment of Adolescents: With Some Remarks on Perversion," *The Psychoanalytic Study of the Child*, 13:223–254. Eissler, 1958, Problems of Identity," *Journal of the American Psychoanalytic Association (JAPA)* 9:131–142.; Heinz Lichtenstein, 1977, "Identity and Sexuality," *JAPA* 9:179–260.

7. Eissler, "Notes on Problems," ibid., p. 237.

8. Whereas psychoanalytic theory customarily derives the emergence of identity from early object relations (the separation-individuation phase) and from the infant's development of a body image, Lichtenstein proposes that both identity and the sexual theme are transformations of the infant's perception of its instrumental use by the mother. He considers this process a version of "imprinting."

9. One analyst has gone so far as to suggest that the sex drive is primarily object seeking rather than pleasure seeking. Sexuality may also symbolize union with the love object; it may be the primary expression of intimacy in a culture in which so many other expressions of physicality are proscribed. See W. R. D. Fairbairn, 1952, *An Object-Relations Theory of Personality*. New York: Basic Books.

10. Vivian Gornick, 1999, "*The Second Sex* at Fifty," *Dissent*, Fall, pp. 69–72. Quotation is from p. 69.

11. Susan Bordo, 2001, *The Male Body: A New Look at Men in Public and in Private*. New York: Farrar, Straus and Giroux, p. 143.

12. Ibid., p. 143.

13. Ibid. This and the previous two quotes are from p. 147.
14. Pedro Almodovar (Director), *All About My Mother*. Culver City, Ca.: Columbia TriStar Home Video, 1999.
15. This photo accompanied a column: Geraldine Bedell, 1999, "Nothing's Weak about Women," *London Sunday Express*, 14 March, p. 34.
16. Natalie Angier, 1999, *Woman: An Intimate Geography*. New York: Houghton Mifflin/Peter Davidson, pp. 334–345.
17. Bernard Zilbergeld, 1978, *Male Sexuality*. New York: Bantam, p. 23.
18. Kate Millet, 1970, *Sexual Politics*. Garden City, N.Y.: Doubleday.
19. Susan Brownmiller, 1976, *Against Our Will: Men, Women, and Rape*. New York: Bantam, p. 320.
20. That men frequently ask their partners "Did you come?" is evidence of this. Sexual anxiety is also manifest in the obsessions some men have with their partners' past lovers: "Was he better? Did you have more orgasms? Better orgasms?"
21. See an early report of this problem. George Ginsberg, William Frosch, and Theodore Shapiro, 1972, "The New Impotence," *Archives of General Psychiatry*, vol. 26, pp. 218–220.
22. Sigmund Freud, 1920, "Beyond the Pleasure Principle," *S.E.* 18. Karen Horney, 1932, "The Dread of Women: Observations on a Specific Difference in the Dread Felt by Men and Women Respectively for the Opposite Sex, *International Journal of Psycho-Analysis* 13:348–360. Joyce McDougall, 1980, *Plea for a Measure of Abnormality*. New York: International Universities Press. Janine Chasseguet-Smirgel, 1984, *Creativity and Perversion*. New York: Norton.
23. Freud, 1925, "Some Psychical Consequences of the Anatomical Distinction between the Sexes," *S.E.* 19:248–258.
24. Ethel S. Person, 1986, "The Omni-Available Woman and Lesbian Sex: Two Fantasy Themes and Their Relationships to the Male Development Experience," in *The Psychology of Men*, eds. G. Fogel, F. M. Lane, and R. S. Liebert. New York: Basic Books.
25. Richard Farmer, as told to Rebecca Gooch, 1999, "Atlas Drugged," in *Maxim for Men*, June, pp. 95–98.
26. Letter to the editor, *Maxim for Men*, June 1999.
27. Quoted in Bordo, op. cit., p. 73.
28. Ben Brantley, 1999, "Grim Waltz of Desire," *New York Times*, 26 March, p. E1.
29. See J. Money, F. Schwartz, and V.C. Davis, 1984, "Adult Erotosexual Status and Fetal Hormonal Masculinization and De-Masculinization: 46, XX Congenital Virilizing Adrenal Hyperplasia and 46, XY Androgen-Insensitivity Syndrome Compared," *Psychoneuroendocrinology* 9:405–415. R. Friedman and J. Downey, 1995, "Biology and the Oedipus Complex, *Psychoanalytic Quarterly*, 64:234–264. M. Diamond and H. K. Sigmundson, 1997, "Sex Reassignment at Birth: Long-Term Review and Clinical Implications," *Archives of Pediatrics & Adolescent Medicine*, 151:298–304.
30. Nancy Chodorow, 1994, *Femininities, Masculinities, Sexualities: Freud and Beyond*. Lexington: University of Kentucky Press.
31. Ethel S. Person, 1995, *By Force of Fantasy: How We Make Our Lives*. New York: Basic Books, chap. 9.
32. Vivian Gornick, 1999, "*The Second Sex* at Fifty," in *Dissent*, Fall, pp. 69–72.
33. Ibid., p. 70. Each was able to use her insight to understand the role of hierarchy in social arrangements.
34. For this reason, Beauvoir criticized women more harshly than blacks. This is an important distinction that Gornick highlights in her essay.
35. Like the standard-bearers of women's liberation who had preceded her, Friedan was schooled in other liberation movements—in her case, the civil rights movement and the student

revolts of the 1960s. Before that, she had been a labor writer for ten years and a left-wing advocate of the working class.

36. Cynthia Epstein, 1999, "The Major Myth of the Women's Movement." *Dissent*, Fall, p. 85.

37. Molly Haskell, 1977, *Holding My Own in No Man's Land: Women and Men and Film and Feminists*. New York: Oxford University Press, p. 44.

38. Toby Talbot, *Gone* (unpublished novel), p. 9.

39. Haskell, op. cit., p. 9.

40. As in "Come on over here, girl."

41. "'Girl' Just Wants to Have Fun," *New York Times*, 28 December 1997. "Zena, the Warrior Princess" and "Hard Candy" nail polish are both of recent vintage.

42. Simon Doonan, Executive Vice-President for Creative Services, Barney's quoted in "'Girl' Just Wants to Have Fun," *New York Times*, 28 December 1997.

43. Felicia R. Lee, 2000, *New York Times*, 6 March, City section 14, p. 1.

44. Neal Gabler, 2000, "Male Bonding: Why Is James Bond So Popular? He's a Baby Boomer Writ Large," *Modern Maturity*, January–February, pp. 52ff. Quotations are from pp. 54 and 55.

45. Quoted in Judith Shulevitz, 1999, "The Fall of Man" (review of *Stiffed*), *New York Times Book Review*, 3 October.

46. This is not to suggest that Freud is irrelevant to contemporary thinking about sex and gender. Perhaps Freud's most important contribution to understanding sex and gender is his fundamental insight that what people do is not identical with what they fantasize about doing, nor are their underlying self-identifications or preconscious motives or behaviors necessarily congruent with their conscious beliefs (consider, for example, the occasional sexual lapses of men of the cloth or of psychoanalysts). In studying fantasy, Freud discovered both the complexity and the diversity of desires that fuel our sexual lives and mold our sense of self. The behavioral observations on which the studies of liberationists, sexologists, and academics are based are not always sufficient to explain the layering of motives that impels specific sexual acts or gender role behavior or to account for the feelings that accompany them.

Chapter 7

1. Frank Browning, 1994, *The Culture of Desire: Paradox and Perversity in Gay Lives Today*. New York: Modern Library, p. 82.

2. Ibid., p. 84.

3. Lillian Faderman, 1991, *Odd Girls and Twilight Lovers: A History of Lesbian Life in Twentieth-Century America*. New York: Columbia University Press.

4. Susan Sontag, 1980 [1974], "Fascinating Fascism," in *Under the Sign of Saturn*. New York: Anchor/Doubleday, p. 105.

5. Ethel S. Person, 1995, *By Force of Fantasy*. New York: Basic Books/HarperCollins.

6. John Leo, 1995, "The Modern Primitives," *U.S. News and World Report*, vol. 119, 31 July.

7. Dominique Aury (pen name Pauline Réage) quoted in John De St. Jorre, 1994, "The Unmasking of O," *New Yorker*, vol. 70, 1 August. Quotations are from pp. 43 and 45.

8. Ibid., p. 45.

9. Daphne Merkin, 1997, "Dreaming of Hitler," in *Dreaming of Hitler*, San Diego: Harvest/Harcourt Brace, pp. 346–363. Quotations are from pp. 346, 351, and 363.

10. Daphne Merkin, "Spanking: A Romance," in *Dreaming of Hitler*, pp. 49–65. Quotations are from pp. 54, 59–60, and 61.

11. Daphne Merkin, 2001, "The Black Season: Reflections of Life in an Institution," *New Yorker*, 8 January, pp. 32–39.

12. Gloria G. Brame, William D. Brame, and Jon Jacobs, 1996, *Different Loving: The World of Sexual Dominance and Submission*. New York: Villard/Random House, p. 5. These authors

agree with George Bastaille's statement: "The kind of sexuality [de Sade] has in mind runs counter to the desires of other people. . . . They are to be victims, not partners . . . The partners are denied any rights at all: this is the key to his system." See George S. Bataille, 1986, *Eroticism: Death and Sexuality*, trans. Mary Dalwood. San Francisco: City Lights, p. 167.

13. Brame et al., op. cit., p. 5.
14. Ibid., p. 71.
15. Ibid., p. 72.
16. Ibid.
17. Ibid., p. 74.
18. Ibid.
19. Ibid., p. 75.
20. Ibid., p. 77.
21. Ibid., p. 78.
22. Ibid., pp. 81–82.
23. Robin, Liza, Linda, and Tiffany, (as told to Jenny L. Frankel, Terrie Maxine Frankel, and Joanne Parrent), 1995, *You'll Never Make Love in This Town Again*. Beverly Hills, Calif.: Dove (distributed by Penguin U.S.A.).
24. James Elroy, 1997 [1996], *My Dark Places: An L.A. Crime Memoir*. New York: Vintage /Random House.
25. Ibid., p. 101.
26. Ibid., p. 112.
27. Ibid., p. 120.
28. Ibid., p. 122.
29. Ibid., p. 124.
30. Ibid., p. 127.
31. Ibid., pp. 251–252.
32. Ibid., p. 260.
33. Ibid., p. 354, p. 358.
34. Ibid., p. 382.
35. Ibid., pp. 386–387.
36. Ibid., p. 388.
37. Marie-France Hirigoyen, 2000 [1998], *Stalking the Soul: Emotional Abuse and the Erosion of Identity*. Canada: Helen Marks. Originally published by Éditions La Découverte et. Dyros, Paris
38. An abuser is often a perverse narcissist, a type first elaborated by Racamier. "Perverse narcissistic individuals are those who come under the influence of their grandiose self [and] try to create a bond with a second individual, specifically attacking the narcissistic integrity of the other with the goal of disarming him/her." Quoted in Hirigoyen.
39. Hirigoyen says that there are three steps in this process: (1) an active appropriation, by dispossessing another person of her will; (2) an act of domination whereby the other person is kept in a state of submission and dependency; (3) an element of branding, whereby one leaves one's mark on another.
40. The psychoanalyst Janine Chasseguet-Smirgel believes that perversion is a buffer against rage: with the disappearance of genital sexuality, which is characteristic of perversion, aggression becomes transformed into sadism, masochism, or both. Robert Stoller also conceptualized perversion as the erotic form of hatred—previously, it had generally been considered a product of sexual conflict only. One is reminded, too, of Anna Freud's description of a masochistic beating fantasy ultimately transformed into altruistic surrender. Anna Freud, 1974, "Beating Fantasies and Daydreams" in *The Writings of Anna Freud*, Vol. 1 (1922–1935). Madison, Conn.: International Universities Press.

41. From this perspective, Veronique experienced herself as what self psychologists call a vulnerable or fragmentation-prone person. See Anna Ornstein, 1991, "The Dread to Repeat: Comments on the Working-Through Process in Psychoanalysis," *Journal of the American Psychoanalytic Association* 39(2):381.

42. Susan Faludi, 1999, *Stiffed: The Betrayal of the American Man*, New York: Morrow, pp. 8–9, Faludi understands the powerlessness that motivates the batterer: "Men cannot be men, only eunuchs, if they are not in control." A description of the reciprocal psychology involved between the battering husband and the battered wife is found in an Anna Quindlen's novel *Black and Blue*. New York: Random House, 1999.

43. See, for example, Leslie Fiedler, 1986 [c. 1960], *Love and Death in the American Novel*, rev. ed. New York: Stein and Day.

44. How does anger fit in with sadomasochism? Though anger, or an angry exchange, is what people ordinarily think of when they hear relationships characterized as "sadomasochistic," anger is far less essential than power as a constituent ingredient. Corruption of power is intrinsic to sadomasochistic relations.

Chapter 8

1. Mihaly Csikszentmihalyi, 1990, *Flow: The Psychology of Optimal Experience*. New York: Harper and Row, p. 40.

2. See Ellen Sarasohn Glazer, 2000, "My Money My Life: Cash in Time, Gone with the Wind," *New York Times*, 13 February, section 3, p. 12.

3. Ethel S. Person, 1995, *By Force of Fantasy: How We Make Our Lives*. New York: Basic Books, pp. 97, 114–121.

4. Daniel J. Levinson, with C. N. Darrow, E. B. Klein, M. H. Levinson, and B. McKee, 1978, *The Seasons of a Man's Life*. New York: Knopf, pp. 97–101.

5. Self-control encompasses skills in two areas. First, there is *self-regulation*—the child's ability to control sleep patterns, appetite, bowels, and other aspects of physicality. Second, there is *self-care*—the ability to maintain bodily cleanliness and health, to listen to the body instead of closing the mind against it. Eventually, self-control comes to include the rudiments of mastery in extended domains—children's sense of being able to manage their time, to do their chores and homework, and to order their lives in accordance with realistic external demands.

6. Frank Sulloway, 1996, *Born to Rebel*. New York: Pantheon.

7. Erna Furman, 1998, *Self-Control and Mastery in Early Childhood: Helping Young Children Grow*. Madison, Conn.: International Universities Press, p. 91.

8. The same process also applies to psychoanalysis, considered as a form of remediation for deficits in self-mastery. The goal is to become more autonomous, yet when things go well this is achieved by allowing oneself to depend on the person of the analyst and on the freedom and availability of the therapeutic relationship, so that one does not have to take new and perhaps long overdue steps toward autonomy utterly alone. It has been remarked, notably by the psychoanalytic theorist Hans Loewald, that in this way the analytic relationship is analogous to successful parenting.

9. Joseph Noshpitz, 1979, "Disturbances in Early Adolescent Development," in *The Course of Life*, vol. 2, ed. Stanley I. Greenspan and George H. Pollack. Maryland: U.S. Department of Health and Human Services, p. 329.

10. Viorst, op cit., p. 75.

11. Althea Horner, 1995 [1989], *The Wish for Power and the Fear of Having It*. Northvale, N.J.: Jason Aronson, p. 85.

12. Clinically, what we find is that the Oedipal stage becomes problematic only when the parents "heat it up" in words or deeds, making the child uncertain where imagination ends and real-

ity begins. For example, Little Hans, in Freud's first case study of the Oedipal triangle, had to deal with very real complications—his parents' marriage was troubled, and his mother took him into her bed to sleep at night. In the first Oedipus complex, the child reasons that if he could rid himself of his rival, he would have exclusive possession of the object of the competition (usually his mother). Therefore, on a preconscious level, the boy sometimes symbolizes his aggression as murderous violence with the aim of ridding himself of his competitor. If things do not go well at this stage of development, he may (consciously or unconsciously) remain truly angry at his father and fearful of retaliation, or he may have to suppress his feelings. For a girl and her mother, the competition may be ongoing and noisy, or subterranean and depressed. In many patients with an obsessional neurosis or a success phobia, there is a clear-cut history of a dramatic personality change in early or middle childhood, in which a very aggressive child metamorphosed into a model child, sometimes to the relief of the parents but at the cost of his or her own assertiveness and creativity.

13. Contrary to popular opinion, adolescence need not be a time of renewed strife between parents and children. But when strife does break out—or, worse, when the child settles comfortably into a pattern of collusion with one parent or the other—there can be lasting consequences for how the child will later deal with issues of autonomy. It is the child's healthy wish not to be compromised in this way that makes for stormy scenes when things do go awry.

14. Susanna Rodell, 1998, "Lives," *New York Times Magazine*, 10 May.

15. Nicholas Evans, 1995, *The Horse Whisperer*. New York: Bantam Doubleday, pp. 11, 14. The fascination many of us felt as we watched *Chimere*, the equestrian dance theater directed by Zingaro, who is part-guru, part-animal-trainer, part-choreographer, also has much to do with the intricacies of the power balance we strike with animals. Zingaro has an instinctive sense of how to play to the deep yearning we all have to both master and be one with another creature.

16. This is a force that D. W. Winnicott calls aggression and that others have described as a life force (*élan vital*). See Chapter 1.

17. Bruno Bettelheim, 1976, *The Uses of Enchantment: The Meaning and Importance of Fairy Tales*. New York: Knopf, p. 274.

18. Ruth La Ferla, 2000, "Like Magic, Witchcraft Charms Teenagers." *New York Times*, 13 February, section 9, pp. 1–2.

19. Quoted by La Ferla.

20. Ibid.

21. The witchcraft described here is different from that of the Goths and Satanists who came to public attention in the context of the shootings in Columbine.

22. Eric Klinger, 1990, *Daydreaming: Using Waking Fantasy and Imagery for Self-Knowledge and Creativity*. Los Angeles: Tarcher, p. 28.

23. Jerome Singer, 1979, *The Inner World of Daydreaming*. New York: Harper and Row, p. 159.

24. Sigmund Freud, "Creative Writers and Day-Dreaming," 1908 [1909], S.E., Vol. 9, p. 153.

25. I reported Mr. Kenney's use of literature in lieu of independently generated fantasies in my book *By Force of Fantasy*, op. cit.

26. Levinson discusses the mentor relationship in detail, op. cit., pp. 9–101.

27. This vignette and the next are cases of the late Lionel Ovesey, which we prepared for publication in a book about sexuality that we planned to write together. He died before we brought the project to fruition. To the best of my knowledge, these cases were not published in any of his papers.

28. These adaptations were first theorized in great detail by Lionel Ovesey. He suggested that there were two fantasies in which the penis could take on the function of a breast. In the first, the father's penis appears to be a feeding organ, similar to the mother's breast, and his semen is equated with milk. Then a patient may produce a dream image of sucking the penis. The second involves the female's incorporation of the father's penis by mouth or vagina, or the male's

incorporation of the penis by mouth or anus. In this way, the donor's masculine strength becomes available to the dependent subject. (Fantasies that make use of the penis for dependent gratification are not restricted to homosexual men but may also occur in heterosexual men—sometimes leading to panic about being homosexual.)

29. "Following Up: No More Dramas for a 'Dull' Mr. and Mrs." *New York Times* metropolitan section, 10 December 2000.
30. *Psychosomatic Medicine*, 1990, 52(3, May–June): 247–270.
31. "Time-Bomb Genes," *New York Magazine*, 8 February 1999, pp. 29ff, 89.

Chapter 9

1. Ethel S. Person, 1999, *The Sexual Century*, New Haven, Conn.: Yale University Press, pp. 341–343.
2. Molly Haskell, 2001, "Swaggering Sexuality before the Mandated Blush," *New York Times*, 13 May, p. MT 15.
3. Simone de Beauvoir, 1953, *The Second Sex*. New York: Knopf.
4. Natalie Angier, 1999, *Woman: An Intimate Geography*. Boston and New York: Peter Davidson/ Houghton-Mifflin, p. 308.
5. Adrienne Rich, 1979, *On Lies, Secrets, and Silence: Selected Prose 1966–1978*. New York: Norton, pp. 196–197.
6. Ibid., p. 271.
7. Ibid., p. 272. Here, she is quoting a line from her book *Of Woman Born*.
8. Juliet Mitchell, 1997, "Psychoanalysis and Feminism" in *Psychology of Society*, ed. Richard Sennett. New York: Vintage, p. 351.
9. Elaine Showalter, 1985, "The Death of Lady (Novelist): Wharton's "House of Mirth," *Representations* 9 (Winter): 133–149.
10. Laurie J. Flynn, 2001, "Survey on Women's Role in Silicon Valley," *New York Times*, 23 April, p. C3.
11. Ethel S. Person, 1982, "Women Working: Fears of Failure, Deviance, and Success," *Journal of the American Academy of Psychoanalysis* 10(1): 67–84.
12. See Ethel S. Person, 1986, "Working Mothers: Impact on the Self, the Couple, and the Children," in *The Psychology of Today's Woman: New Psychoanalytic Visions*, ed. D. Cantor and T. Bernay. Hillsdale, N.J.: Analytic Press.
13. Caroline Seebohm, 1997, *No Regrets: The Life of Marietta Tree*. New York: Simon and Schuster.
14. Dawn Steele, 1994, *They Can Kill You But They Can't Eat You: Lessons from the Front*. New York: Pocket Books. See also Bernard Weinraub, 1997, "Dawn Steele, Studio Chief and Producer, Dies at 51," *New York Times*, 22 December.
15. See, for example, J. M. Bardwick, 1979, *In Transition: How Feminism, Sexual Liberation, and the Search for Self-Fulfillment Have Altered Our Lives*. New York: Holt, Rinehart and Winston.
16. Donna McCrohan, 1978, *The Honeymooners' Companion: The Kramdens and the Nortons Revisited*. New York: Workman, p. 119.
17. Michael A. Messner, 1992, *Power at Play: Sports and the Problem of Masculinity*. Boston: Beacon.
18. E. A. Rotundt, quoted in Messner, p. 14.
19. Ibid., p. 15.
20. Elliot J. Gorm, 1986, *The Manly Art: Bare-Knuckle Prize Fighting in America*. Ithaca, N.Y.: Cornell University Press. Quoted in Messner, p. 15.
21. Ibid., p. 16.
22. Ibid., p. 18.

23. R. W. Connell, 1992, "Drumming Up the Wrong Tree: The Men's Movement," *Tikkun* 7(1): 31–36. Quoted passages are from pp. 32 and 33.
24. Ibid., quotes from pp. 32–33.
25. Lionel Tiger, 1999, *The Decline of Males*. New York: Golden Books. Also: "Who Needs Men? Addressing the Prospect of a Matriarchal Millennium" (conversation with Lionel Tiger and Barbara Ehrenreich, moderated by Colin Harris). *Harper's*, June 1999, pp. 34–46. Quotations here are from "Who Needs Men?" pp. 34, 35, 41–42.
26. The terms "open" and "closed" programs were coined by Ernst Mayr. See Konrad Lorenz, 1981, *The Foundations of Ethology*. New York: Springer.
27. R. L. Jacobs and D. C. McClelland, 1994 "Moving Up the Corporate Ladder: A Longitudinal Study of the Leadership Motive Pattern and Managerial Success in Men and Women," *Consulting Psychology Journal* (Winter): pp. 32–34. Quoted in Linda Austin, 2000, *What's Holding You Back*. New York: Basic Books.
28. Ibid., p. 182.
29. Ibid.
30. Ruth Jacobson and David McClelland, quoted in Austin, op. cit., p. 182.
31. Ibid., p. 190.
32. Ibid., p. 182.
33. Austin, *What's Holding You Back*, p. 187.
34. Roberta Siegel quoted in Austin, p. 185.
35. Ethel S. Person, 1995, *By Force of Fantasy: How We Make Our Lives*. New York: Basic Books, p. 197.

Chapter 10

1. W. W. Meissner, 1997, "The Self and the Principle of Work," in *Work and Its Inhibitions*, ed. C. W. Socarides and Selma Kramer. New York: International Universities Press, p. 35.
2. Daniel J. Levinson, 1978, *The Seasons of a Man's Life*, New York: Knopf, p. 1.
3. Mihaly Csikszentmihalyi, 1990, *Flow: The Psychology of Optimal Experience* New York. Harper, pp. 157–158
4. Ibid., p. 160. The subsequent quotations are also from p. 160.
5. John Kenneth Galbraith, 1983, *The Anatomy of Power*. Boston: Houghton Mifflin.
6. Herman Guttman and Ira Berlin. *Power and Culture: Essays on the American Working Class*. New York: Pantheon, 1987.
7. Michael Lewis, "The Artist in the Grey Flannel Pajamas: Who the New American Workers Think They Are," *New York Times Magazine*, 5 March 2000, section 6, pp. 45–48. Quotations are from p. 46.
8. For an engaging history of Hollywood entrepreneurs, see Otto Friedrich, 1987 [1986] *City of Nets: A Portrait of Hollywood in the 1940s*. New York: Harper.
9. Joseph Schumpeter, 1954, *Capitalism, Socialism, and Democracy*. New York: Harper and Row.
10. Quoted in M. Maccoby, 1976, *The Gamesman: The New Corporate Leaders*. New York: Simon and Schuster, p. 79.
11. Walter Benjamin, 1979, *Reflections: Essays, Aphorisms, Autobiographical Writings*, ed. and intro. Peter Demetz. New York: Harcourt Brace Jovanovich, p. 65.
12. Douglas McGregor, 1966, *Leadership and Motivation*. Cambridge, Mass · MIT Press, p. 67.
13. Abraham Zaleznick, 2001, "Power and Leadership in Complex Organizations," in *On Freud's Group Psychology and the Analysis of the Ego*, ed. Ethel S. Person, for the International Psychoanalytical Association. Hillsdale, N.J.: Analytic Press, pp. 95–96.
14. Michael Korda, 1975. *Power: How to Get It, How to Use it*. New York: Random House, chap. 4.

15. John O. Whitney and Tina Packer, 2000, *Power Plays.* New York: Simon and Schuster, p. 62. Much of this paragraph draws on Whitney.

16. Whitney and Packer, ibid., p. 62.

17. There are competing viewpoints—conveyed in a variety of studies and anecdotes, about the relative efficacy of strategies of cooperation and employee empowerment (bottom-up) versus those of control and command (top-down). Stephen Covey, author of *The Seven Habits of Highly Effective People* and an authority on leadership, grounds his business ethics in pragmatism. In discussing five different kinds of personal philosophies that can be applied to management—win/win, win/lose, lose/win, lose/lose, and win—Covey suggests that the most effective strategy varies, depending on one's goal. While Covey agrees that win/lose is the appropriate paradigm for a tennis game, he emphasizes the usefulness of flexibility in a business structure when the win/lose paradigm may undercut a company's profitability. If there is a negotiation rather than a game at stake, he argues that two win/lose people may put their egos in front of the outcome so that they will kill a negotiation, "blind to the fact that murder is suicide, that revenge is a two-edged sword" (Steven R. Covey, 1990, p. 210). One of Covey's major contributions is to identify how an overall win/lose bias may constitute an authoritarian approach ("I get my way and you don't get yours") and he identifies win/lose people as "prone to use position, power, credentials, possessions, or personality to get their way" (ibid., p. 207). Ego needs can override getting what you want in the deal.

    Covey proposes different models for negotiation. In deals between two separate entities, he favors the win/win strategy as ideal, insofar as it has the potential for promoting cooperation rather than competition. His strategies are particularly applicable for those who are in some kind of ongoing relationship with one another. Whether or not it is cooperation based on joint input that is meant to be taken into account or merely the appearance of valuing opinions from all levels of management is sometimes hard to say. In public companies, the CEO deals not just with his managers but with his board. At board meetings he may stimulate a discussion on policy but will have the votes he needs pinned down before the meeting ever begins. However, if he has not been doing well he may call the meeting only to discover that a coup to depose him has been organized. Steven R. Covey, 1990, *The Seven Habits of Highly Effective People: Powerful Lessons in Personal Change.* New York: Fireside/Simon and Schuster.

18. Hans Morgenthau, 1962, "Love and Power," *Politics in the 20th Century: The Restoration of American Politics.* Chicago: University of Chicago Press, pp. 7–14.

19. Erna Furman, "Child's Work: Developmental Aspect of the Capacity to Work and Enjoy It," in *Work and Its Inhibitions,* Eds. S.W. Socarides and Selma Kramer. New York: International Universities Press. p. 6.

Chapter 11

1. Rosamund Harding, as quoted in Anthony Storr, 1991 [1972], *Anatomy of Inspiration: The Dynamics of Creation.* New York: Penguin, p. 214.

2. Ibid.

3. Ibid., p. 50.

4. Arthur Koestler 1989 [1964], *The Act of Creation.* New York: Viking/Penguin, p. 181. The quotation from Goethe is on p. 151.

5. Joshua Widick is a dancer and choreographer who is also my assistant.

6. May Sarton, 1984, *At Seventy: A Journal.* New York: Norton, p. 10.

7. Sigmund Freud, 1908, "Creative Writers and Day-Dreaming," *S.E.* 9: 143–144.

8. Vivian Gussin Paley, 1990, *The Boy Who Would Be a Helicopter: The Uses of Storytelling in the Classroom.* Cambridge, Mass.: Harvard University Press.

9. Ethel S. Person, 1995, *By Force of Fantasy: How We Make Our Lives*. New York: Basic Books.
10. See Charles Kliegerman's report on Buddy Meyer's concept of the "secret sharer." Kliegerman, 1972, Panel Report on Creativity (Twenty-Seventh Annual International Psychoanalytic Congress, Vienna, 1971), *International Journal of Psycho-analysis* 54: 21–30.
11. Gardner presents an "anatomy of creativity seen through the lives" of Einstein, Picasso, Stravinsky, T. S. Eliot, Martha Graham, and Gandhi in addition to Freud.
12. Howard Gardner, 1993, *Creating Minds*. New York: Basic Books, pp. 43–44.
13. See also Leonard Shengold, 1993, *"The Boy Will Come to Nothing!" Freud's Ego Ideal and Freud as Ego Ideal*. New Haven: Yale University Press, chap. 6; and Stanley Coen, 1997, *Between Author and Reader: A Psychoanalytic Approach to Writing and Reading*, New York: Columbia University Press, chap. 4.
14. Thanks to my friend the psychoanalyst Dr. Barbara Rocah, for directing me to this source. S. Freud, 1960, *Letters of Sigmund Freud*, ed. E. L. Freud. New York: Basic Books, p. 4.
15. Gardner, op. cit., p. 57.
16. Josef Breuer and Sigmund Freud, 1900, *Studies on Hysteria*, S.E. 2:1–309.
17. Sigmund Freud, 1935, *An Autobiographical Study*. New York: Norton, p. 34.
18. Gardner, op. cit., pp. 60–61.
19. Albrecht Hirschmüller, 1989, *The Life and Work of Josef Breuer*. New York: New York University Press.
20. Gardner, op. cit., pp. 68–69.
21. Ibid., p. 139.
22. Sometimes, too, a creative person uses the consciousness of mortality as a spur—to transcend mortality by creating something enduring.
23. Edith Wharton, 1964 [1933], *A Backward Glance*. New York: Macmillan, p. 112.
24. Ibid., p. 113.
25. Ibid., p. 108.
26. Ibid., p. 115.
27. Ibid., pp. 112–113.
28. Olivia Coolidge, 1964, *Edith Wharton 1862–1937*. New York: Scribner, p. 131.
29. Ibid., p. 135.
30. Ibid., p. 201.
31. Ibid., p. 130.
32. Ibid., p. 137.
33. Ibid., p. 209,
34. Burroughs Mitchell, 1989, *The Education of an Editor*. Garden City, N.Y.: Doubleday, p. 25.
35. Maxwell Perkins, 1957, Introduction to Thomas Wolfe. *Look Homeward, Angel*. New York: Scribner, pp. viii–ix. The publisher received the Introduction— originally published separately in the *Harvard Library Bulletin* 1947 (3, Autumn)— from Perkins's secretary two days after the editor's death. Passages here are from pp. ix and xi.
36. A. Scott Berg, 1978, *Max Perkins: Editor of Genius*. New York: Thomas Congdon/Dutton, p. 315.
37. Lillian Ross, 1998, *Here but Not Here: My Life with William Shawn and The New Yorker*. New York: Random House.
38. Sigmund Freud, 1916, "Some Character Types Met with in Psychoanalytic Work," S.E., 14: pp. 316–331.
39. Elias Canetti, 1982 [1980], *The Torch in My Ear*. New York: Farrar Straus and Giroux. Passages cited are from pp. 122 and 245.
40. Elias Canetti, 1972 [1960], *Crowds and Power [Masse und Macht]*, New York: Continuum.
41. Freud, 1921, "Group Psychology and the Analysis of the Ego," S.E., p. 83.
42. Ethel S. Person, *By Force of Fantasy*. Op. cit.

Chapter 12

1. Elias Canetti, 1962 [1960], *Crowds and Power*, New York: Continuum, p. 397.
2. Claude Lévi-Strauss, 1987, quoted in Mihaly Csikszentmihalyi, 1993, *The Evolving Self: A Psychology for the Third Millennium*. New York: Harper Perennial.
3. Ibid., p. 221.
4. Max Beerbohm, 1919, *Seven Men*. London: William Heinemann, pp. 3–48.
5. Ibid., pp. 9–11
6. Ibid., p. 25.
7. Ibid., p. 26.
8. Ibid., p. 27.
9. Gretchen Kraft Rubin, 2000, *Power, Money, Fame, Sex: A User's Guide*. New York: Pocket Books, p. 158.
10. Michael Korda, 1999, *Another Life: A Memoir of Other People*. New York: Random House, pp. 245–325.
11. Ibid., pp. 246–247.
12. Ibid., p. 248.
13. Ibid., p. 253.
14. Ibid., pp. 253–254.
15. Louis Auchincloss, 1965, "The House of Mirth," in *Pioneers and Caretakers: A Study of Nine American Women Novelists*. New York: Dell, pp. 25–29.
16. Erica Goode, 1999, "For Good Health, It Helps to Be Rich and Important," *New York Times*, 1 June, science section, p. F1.
17. Dr. Clyde Hertzman of the University of British Columbia, quoted by Erica Goode.
18. Thorstein Veblen, 1912 [1899], *The Theory of the Leisure Class: An Economic Study of Institutions*. New York: Macmillan, p. 75.
19. Michael Cunningham, 1998, *The Hours*. New York: Farrar Straus and Giroux. The book plays with three stories about women: in 1923, Virginia Woolf wakes from a dream that leads her to Mrs. Dalloway; in the present, Clarissa Vaughan, in Greenwich Village, is planning a party for her closest friend, Richard, who is dying of AIDS; and in 1949 in Los Angeles, a third woman is planning a birthday party and reading Woolf.
20. Ibid., pp. 60–61.
21. Ibid., p. 19.
22. Ibid., p. 94.
23. Ibid., p. 203.
24. James Baldwin, 1993 [1961], "The Black Boy Looks at the White Boy," in *Nobody Knows My Name: More Notes of a Native Son*. New York: Dial Press, pp. 222–223.
25. Alex Williams, 1999, "To Have and Have More," *New York Magazine*, 14 June, p. 34.
26. Ralph Gardner, Jr., 1999, "Class Struggle on Park Avenue," *New York Magazine*, 14 June, p. 24.
27. Katherine Newman, 1993, *Declining Fortunes: The Withering of the American Dream*. New York: Basic Books, p. 3.
28. Elias Canetti, 1982 [1980] *The Torch in My Ear*. New York: Farrar, Straus and Giroux, p. 220.
29. Joe Wood, 1998, "Up from Brownsville/Alfred Kazin: Life and Work," *Dissent*, Fall, pp. 119–127. Quotations are from p. 125.
30. Robert Parker, 1993, *Double Deuce*. New York: Berkeley, p. 147.

Chapter 13

1. John Krakauer, 1996, *Into the Wild*. New York: Anchor/Doubleday, p. 134.
2. While many of us rely on one, two, or even all three of these strategies, there are a few among

us who come to terms with the limitations of our existence and larger numbers who narcotize themselves with one or another substance.

3. Erich Fromm, 1964, *The Heart of Man: Its Genius for Good and Evil*. New York: Knopf, pp. 6, 19–20.

4. Just as humankind envies the power of the Gods and Mafia members the power of figures like Don Corleone, so is envy endemic to any power hierarchy.

5. Mortals could claim divinity in Greek tragedy because Zeus "bestowed his seed upon mortal woman." Walter Kerr, 1967, *Tragedy and Comedy*. New York: Simon and Schuster, p. 93. Subsequent quotation are from pp. 107 and 122.

6. Quoted in Hans Morgenthau, 1946, *Scientific Man vs. Power Politics*. Chicago: University of Chicago Press, pp. 192–193.

7. André Malraux, 1969 [1934], *Man's Fate*. New York: Vintage, p. 228.

8. Morgenthau, op. cit., pp. 192–193.

9. The phrase is Walter Kerr's, op. cit., p. 97.

10. Thomas Merton, 1976, *The Seven Storey Mountain*. New York: Harcourt Brace Jovanovich, pp. 284–285. Copyright © 1976, by The Trustees of the Merton Legacy Trust.

11. Religious attachment may take the form of surrender to a superior power in another human being. The choice of the object can be highly idiosyncratic, to say the least. Bernice Perry, for instance, said she relied on Frank Sinatra's healing powers (*New York Times Magazine*, December 8, 1996, p. 44). She had an accident when she was in her forties and was unable to walk. She said at age seventy-two that she had prayed to God and to Frank Sinatra every day and that Sinatra gave her "the strength to get my feet off the bed." At the time of this story she paid "weekly tribute [to Sinatra] on her own public-TV show, 'Lady Bernice Perry Frankly Speaking in Sinatra Land.'" Apparently others shared her faith in Sinatra's power to help or heal them. Perry said: "He has been the inspiration and light of my life. . . . I will honor him as long as I'm alive." The story did not mention whether Perry ever met Sinatra. From a psychological rather than a religious perspective, identification with something greater than ourselves can mean someone or something far from holy and nonetheless can represent safety and transcendence.

12. Elizabeth Janeway, 1980, *Powers of the Weak*. New York: Knopf, p. 127.

13. Fyodor Dostoyevsky, 1993 [1980], "The Legend of the Grand Inquisitor," in *The Brothers Karamazov*. Trans. and intro. by David McDuff. London and New York: Penguin, chap. 5, book 5, pp. 283–304, p. 302.

14. Philip Rahv, 1966 [1949], *The Myth and the Powerhouse: Essays on Literature and Ideas*. New York: Noonday, p. 167.

15. Sigmund Freud, "Dostoyevsky and Parricide," *S.E.* 21:175–196, p. 177.

16. Op. cit., p. 287. In portraying the Cardinal, Dostoyevsky has drawn on the portrait of Tomás de Torquemada, the fifteenth-century cardinal, infamous for his role in the Inquisition.

17. Ibid., p. 293.

18. Ibid., p. 292.

19. Ibid.

20. Ibid., p. 296.

21. Dennis Dalton, 1998, "Dostoyevsky's Grand Inquisitor," in *Power Over People: Classical and Modern Political Theory*, Great Courses on Tape, Part II. Teaching Company.

22. Dostoyevsky, op. cit. p. 302.

23. Ibid.

24. Ibid.

25. Albert Camus, 1957, *The Fall*. New York: Knopf, p. 133.

26. Mario Puzo, 1997 [1964], *The Unfortunate Pilgrim*. New York: Ballantine, p. xi.

27. Mario Puzo, 1978 [1969], *The Godfather*. New York: Penguin, p. 14.

28. Ibid., p. 50.
29. Ibid., p. 25.
30. Ibid.
31. The Don also goes outside his organization to enlist political power through payoffs to police, judges, and even senators. At his daughter's wedding a United States Senator calls to apologize for not personally attending, but says he had no alternative since F.B.I. men were taking down the license numbers of those inside. Of course, it was a message of the Don, well-informed by his insiders at the F.B.I., who had made sure the Senator was warned not to come. Ibid., p. 41.
32. Ibid., p. 56.
33. Ibid., p. 69. This psychological power is akin to the kind of power displayed in the Inquisitor's act of burning heretics at the stake.
34. Drawing on Freud. Rieff argues that whereas Christianity proclaimed the ultimate authority to be the source of love, "Freud discovered the love of authority." Rieff, 1961, *Freud: The Mind of the Moralist*. New York: Doubleday, p. 168.
35. The same impulse can explain cults. Even people who are not tempted by religions, new or old, or by mass movements may be inclined to make gods and goddesses of their cultural icons.
36. Sigmund Freud, 1921, *Group Psychology and the Analysis of the Ego*, S.E. 18. p. 69.
37. Ibid., p. 127.
38. Ibid.
39. Ibid.
40. Ibid.
41. Ibid., p. 92.
42. Transference is understood literally as a transference of the patient's revived childhood feelings for his parents to the person of the analyst. The psychoanalyst is heir to the overvaluation accorded to his or her parents during childhood. Just as the child was dependent on the parents for protection and safety and experienced power vicariously through identification, so, too, in transference does the patient see the analyst as having the same kind of power. Psychoanalysts understand the propensity for self-subordination and surrender as a manifestation of this transference.
43. Some analysts—including Otto Rank, Jung, and some of the existential psychoanalysts, among them Erich Fromm and Rollo May—have emphasized existential anxiety as a major part of our psychic vulnerability.
44. Similarly, Dostoyevsky, in the Legend of the Grand Inquisitor, argues that the Cardinal exiled Christ and put Satan in his place.
45. Puzo, *The Godfather*, p. 324.
46. John G. Stoessinger, 1965 [1961], *The Might of Nations: World Politics in Our Time*. New York: Random House, p. 26.
47. In its failure to consider the individual's integration into the larger social world or, conversely, the impact of the social world on the individual psyche, psychoanalytic theory is in the tradition of several millennia of western thought, which has long cherished the belief that the psyche is fundamentally ahistorical. Sennett describes the ahistorical position succinctly: "The human being was a creature placed in the circumstances of history but not essentially a product of those circumstances." (Richard Sennett, 1980, *Authority*. New York: Knopf, p. 6.) That position was unchallenged until nineteenth-century social theorists, building on the earlier work of the Italian philosopher Giambattista Vico, upended the ahistorical viewpoint. Unfortunately, psychoanalytic interest has lagged behind. Only recently have psychoanalysts begun to acknowledge the broader historical perspective, in particular as regards the way social arrangements and beliefs affect sex and gender. Another intellectual task that psychoanalysts have only begun to take with any seriousness is to do the

reverse kind of analysis: to explain how certain psychological propensities that appear to be hardwired and thus immune to history may nonetheless turn out to be agents of history.

Chapter 14

1. Harriet Rubin, 1997, *The Princessa: Machiavelli for Women*. New York: Currency/Doubleday, p. 14.
2. Why these characteristic physical movements evolved is unclear, but research has found that after middle childhood they are relatively stable. Moreover, people's characteristic ways of organizing physical activity in space correspond to psychological attitudes. Frances La Barre, 2001, *On Moving and Being Moved: Nonverbal Behavior in Clinical Practice*. Hillsdale, N.J.: Analytic Press, pp. 35–38, 149–150.
3. My account of Roosevelt draws primarily on the following sources: Joseph Alsop, 1998 [1982], *FDR*. New York: Gramercy; Hugh Gregory Gallagher, 1985, *FDR's Splendid Deception*. New York: Dodd, Mead; Gary Wills, 1994, *Certain Trumpets: The Call of Leaders*. New York: Simon and Schuster. The quotation here is from Alsop, p. 73.
4. Geoffrey C. Ward, 1985, *Before the Trumpet: Young Franklin Roosevelt*. New York: Harper and Row, pp. 251, 253.
5. Alsop, op. cit., p. 73.
6. Teddy's daughter, Alice Roosevelt Longworth, is supposed to have "quipped that her father wanted to be the bride at every wedding, the corpse at every funeral." Bonnie Angelo, 2001 [2000], *First Mothers*. New York: Harper Perennial, pp. 1–39.
7. Ralph Waldo Emerson, 1926, "Self-Reliance," in *Emerson's Essays*, intro. Irwin Edman. New York: Harper Colophon, p. 35.
8. When Emerson was very young he was urged to make obeisance to some church doctrines. He declined, insisting that he wanted to live wholly from within. His adviser suggested that this impulse might come from below rather than from above. Emerson replied, "They do not seem to me to be such; but if I am the Devil's child I will live then from the Devil" (p. 36).
9. My account of Roosevelt's illness is based on Alsop and Gallagher.
10. Quoted in Gallagher, op. cit., p. 11.
11. Ibid., p. 18
12. Ibid., p. 20.
13. Ibid., p. 24.
14. Alsop, op. cit., p. 96.
15. Angelo, op. cit., p. 37.
16. Wills, op. cit., pp. 13–17.
17. Emerson, op cit., p. 41. Emerson also wrote: "Every true man is a cause, a country, and an age; requires infinite spaces and numbers and time fully to accomplish his thoughts;—and posterity seem to follow his steps as a procession. A man Caesar is born, and for ages after we have a Roman Empire. Christ is born, and millions of minds so grow and cleave to his genius that he is confounded with virtue and the possibility of man. An institution is the length and shadow of one man; as, the Reformation, of Luther; Quakerism, of Fox; Methodism, of Wesley; Abolition, of Clarkson. Scipio, Milton called 'the height of Rome'; 'And all history resolves itself very easily into the biography of a few stout and earnest persons'" (p. 44). The following quotations are from pp. 45 and 61.
18. Rainer Maria Rilke, 1954 [1934], *Letters to a Young Poet*, trans. M. D. Herter. New York: Norton, p. 69.
19. Sojourner Truth, 1991, *The Narrative of Sojourner Truth*, ed. Henry Louis Gates, Jr. New York: Schomberg Library of Nineteenth Century Black Women Writers, p. 116.
20. Quoted in Joya Karas, 1941–1946, *Music in Terezin*. New York: Beaufort, p. 196.

Epilogue

1. Even Otto Kernberg, one of the most brilliant of contemporary psychoanalytic commentator on groups, mentions power but does not theorize it. Kernberg, 1998 [1977], *Ideology, Conflict, and Leadership in Groups and Organizations*. New Haven: Yale University Press. In fact, there is no entry for power in his index.
2. Rollo May, 1972, *Power and Innocence*. New York: Norton, pp. 20–21.
3. Alfred North Whitehead, 1949, *Adventures of Ideas*. New York: Macmillan.
4. Richard Almond, 1997, "Omnipotence and Power," in *Omnipotent Fantasies and the Vulnerable Self*, ed. Carolyn Ellman and Joseph Reppen. Northvale, N.J.: Jason Aronson, pp. 1–37. Quotation, p. 2.
5. John Mack, 1994, "Power, Powerlessness, and Empowerment in Psychotherapy," *Psychiatry*, 57:179–199.
6. Sigmund Freud, 1900, "The Interpretation of Dreams," *S.E.* 4. Quotations are from pp. 196, 197.
7. Mack, op. cit., p. 187.
8. Gail Berry, 1995, "Freud's Family Romance: A Leitmotiv and Its Legacy." Unpublished paper. Presented to the American Academy of Psychoanalysis, 19 May in Miami.
9. Carl E. Schorske, 1980, "Politics and Patricide," in *Le Fin de Siècle*. Vienna and New York: Knopf. Quotations are from pp. 184–186, 200, 203.
10. Dennis Klein, 1981, *The Jewish Origins of the Psychoanalytic Movement*. Chicago: University of Chicago Press.
11. The passage continues: "These words from Virgil's *Aeneid* are spoken by Juno, divine defender of Semitic Dido against Aeneas, founder of Rome. Having failed to persuade Jupiter to let Aeneas marry Dido ('to bend the higher powers'), Juno summons from Hell a fury, Allecto, who unleashes seething passions of sex and military aggression in the camp of Aeneas' allies." Schorske, op. cit., p. 200. I am grateful to the psychoanalyst Paul Lippmann for pointing out Schorske's reference to this legend.
12. One of the first accounts is by Paul Roazen, 1971, *Freud and His Followers*, 1971, New York: New American Library, pp. 174–224. A large part of this section is based on Roazen.
13. *The Interpretation of Dreams, S.E.* 4:93.
14. Roazen, op. cit., p. 178.
15. Ibid., p. 182.
16. Ernest Jones, *The Life and Work of Sigmund Freud*. New York: Basic Books, Vol. II, pp. 69–70. Subsequent quotations are from p. 71.
17. Henri Ellenberger, 1970. *The Discovery of the Unconscious*. New York: Basic Books, p. 611.
18. Freud, "Analysis Terminable and Interminable," *S.E.* 23: 252–253.
19. The matter was actually somewhat more complicated. The reason why Freud felt free to subsume aggression under the libido was that he still held a belief, which was part of Fliess's legacy, that there were two kinds of libido—a masculine, active kind and a feminine, passive kind, each of which was present in both men and women. In an earlier discussion of Adler's ideas, Freud had retorted that Adler's "aggression" was nothing more than the assertive masculine stream of the libido. In response to this critique, Adler began reviewing the literature on contemporary theories of bisexuality including Fliess's, and presented his revised theory, the theory of masculine protest. It may be noted that Adler's revised theory was social and culturalist whereas Freud's theory was biological and "essentialist."
20. Roazen, op. cit., p. 185.
21. Max Graf, 1942, "Reminiscences of Professor Sigmund," *Psychoanalytic Quarterly*, 31(4):474–475.
22. Carl Jung, 1968, *Memories, Dreams, Reflections*. London: Routledge and Kegan Paul.
23. Jones, op. cit., p. 304.

24. Jung, 1968, op. cit.
25. Quoted in Jones, op. cit., Vol. III, p. 208.
26. Freud, 1921, "Group Psychology and the Analysis of the Ego," S.E. 18 80–81.
27. Thomas Szasz, 1963, "Freud as Leader," *Antioch Review*, p. 153.
28. Roazen, op. cit., p. 186. The quotation from Erikson is also from p. 186.
29. Rollo May, 1969, *Love and Will*. New York: Norton, p. 182. May observes: "If the complete determinism and theory for which Freud argued were truly practiced, no one could be cured in psychoanalysis" (p. 195).
30. Alan Wheelis, quoted in Rollo May, ibid., p. 289.
31. Richard Webster, 1995, *Why Freud Was Wrong: Sin, Science and Psychoanalysis*. New York: Basic Books, p. 390.
32. Freud to Jones, 1 August 1912. Quoted in Phyllis Grosskurth, 1991, *The Secret Ring: Freud's Inner Circle and the Politics of Psychoanalysis*. Reading, Mass.: Addison-Wesley, pp. 47–48.
33. François Roustang, 1986 [1976], "Dire Mastery: Discipleship from Freud to Lacan," trans. Ned Lukacher. Washington, D.C.: American Psychiatric Press, pp. 13, 21. The quotation from Freud is found in *On the History of the Psychoanalytic Movement*, S.E. 14:43.
34. Kernberg, op. cit., p. 235.
35. To make psychoanalysis a scientific discipline, we must relinquish the equation so often made between the meaning of clinical themes and developmental causality. Meaning can be separated from assumptions of continuity insofar as the latter imply a causal chain. Many analysts have criticized assumptions of continuity and causality routinely made in psychoanalysis, along with the other historical sciences such as history, evolution, and developmental psychology. However, it would be inaccurate to claim that psychoanalysis is simply a science of meaning and therefore does not belong to the natural sciences. Psychoanalysis is a natural science insofar as it deals with the composition of self-sustaining characteristics of current mental organization.
36. Arnold H. Modell, 1978, "Affects and the Complementarity of Biological and Historical Meaning," in *The Annual of Psychoanalysis*, vol. 6. New York: International Universities Press.
37. Gerald L. Klerman, 1982, "Testing Analytic Hypotheses: Are Personality Attributes Predisposed to Depression?" in *Psychoanalysis: Critical Explorations in Contemporary Theory and Practice*, ed. A. M. Jacobson and D. X. Parmalee. New York: Brunner/Mazel.
38. Stephen Marcus, 1982, "Culture and Psychoanalysis," *Partisan Review*: 224–252.
39. Freud, 1924, "The Economic Problem of Masochism," S.E. 19:163.
40. D. W. Winnicott, 1992 [1950–1955], "Aggression in Relation to Emotional Development," in *Collected Papers: Through Paediatrics to Psycho-Analysis*. New York: Brunner/Mazel pp. 204–218.
41. Freud, 1921, "Group Psychology and the Analysis of the Ego," S.E. 18: 69.

Bibliography

Aeschylus. *Prometheus Bound*. (estimated date, shortly before 458 B.C.). In *Great Books of the Western World*, vol. 5. Ed. Robert Maynard Hutchins. Translated into English verse by G. M. Lookson. Chicago: Encyclopedia Britannica, Inc., University of Chicago, 1952, pp. 40–51.

Alberoni, Francesco. *Falling in Love*. Trans. Lawrence Venuti. New York: Random House, 1983.

Almodovar, Pedro (Director). *All About My Mother* (Motion Picture). Culver City, Ca: Columbia TriStar Home Video, 1999.

Almond, Richard. "Omnipotence and Power." In *Omnipotent Fantasies and the Vulnerable Self*. Ed. Carolyn Ellman and Joseph Reppen. Northvale, N.J.: Jason Aronson, 1997, pp. 1–37.

Alsop, Joseph. *FDR*. New York: Gramercy, 1998.

Angelo, Bonnie. *First Mothers: The Women Who Shaped the Presidents*. New York: Harper Perennial, 2001.

Angier, Natalie. *Woman: An Intimate Geography*. Boston and New York: Peter Davidson/ Houghton-Mifflin, 1999.

Arendt, Hannah. *The Human Condition*. Chicago: University of Chicago Press, 1958.

Aristophanes. *Lysistrata*. Trans., Douglass Parker. Ann Arbor: University of Michigan Press, 1964.

Auchincloss, Louis. "The House of Mirth: In Old and New York." In *Pioneers and Caretakers: A Study of Nine American Women Novelists*. New York: Dell, 1965.

Auden, W. H. "In Memory of Ernst Toller." In *Collected Poems*. Ed. Edward Mendelson. New York: Random House, 1976.

Austin, Linda. *What's Holding You Back: 8 Critical Choices for Women's Success*. New York: Basic Books, 2000.

Bair, Deidre. *Simone de Beauvoir: A Biography*. New York: Summit, 1990.

Baker, Al. "Sex and Power vs. Law and Order: Abuse Charges Against Police Underscore a Historic Tension." *New York Times* (28 January 2001), section 1, p. 21.

Baldwin, James. "The Black Boy Looks at the White Boy." In *Nobody Knows My Name: More Notes of a Native Son*. New York: Dial Press, 1993 [1961].

Bardwick, Judith M. *In Transition: How Feminism, Sexual Liberation, and the Search for Self-Fulfillment Have Altered Our Lives*. New York: Holt, Rinehart and Winston, 1979.

Bataille, Georges. *Eroticism: Death and Sexuality*. Trans. by Mary Dalwood. San Francisco: City Lights, 1986.

Becker, Ernest. *The Denial of Death*. New York: Free Press, 1973.

Bedell, Geraldine. "Nothing's Weak about Women." *London Sunday Express* (14 March 1999), p. 34.

Beerbohm, Max. *Seven Men*. London: William Heinemann, 1919.

Benjamin, Jessica. *The Bonds of Love: Psychoanalysis, Feminism, and the Problem of Domination*. New York: Pantheon, 1988.

Benjamin, Walter. *Reflections: Essays, Aphorisms, Autobiographical Writings*. Ed. and intro. Peter Demetz. New York: First Harvest / HBJ Edition, 1979.

Berg, A. Scott. *Lindbergh*. New York: G.P. Putnam and Sons, 1998.

———. *Max Perkins: Editor of Genius*. New York: Thomas Congdon/Dutton, 1978.

Berle, Adolph. *Power*. New York: Harcourt, Brace, and World, Inc., 1969.

Berry, Gail. "Freud's Family Romance: A Leitmotiv and Its Legacy." Unpublished paper presented to the American Academy of Psychoanalysis, Miami, 19 May 1995.

Bettelheim, Bruno. *The Uses of Enchantment: The Meaning and Importance of Fairy Tales*. New York: Knopf, 1976.

Blake, William. *The Marriage of Heaven and Hell*. New York: Gramercy Books, 1993.

Blass, Thomas (ed.). *Obedience to Authority: Current Perspectives on the Milgram Paradigm*. Mahwah, New Jersey and London: Lawrence Erlbaum, 2000.

Bordo, Susan. *The Male Body: A New Look at Men in Public and in Private*. New York: Farrar Straus and Giroux, 2001.

Bowlby, John. *Attachment and Loss. Vol. 1: Attachment*, 1969, *Vol. 2 Separation, Anxiety, and Anger*, 1974. *Vol. 3: Loss, Sadness, and Depression*, 1980. New York: Basic Books.

Brame, Gloria G., William D. and Jon Jacobs. *Different Loving: The World of Sexual Dominance and Submission*. New York: Villard/Random House, 1996.

Brantley, Ben. "Grim Waltz of Desire." *New York Times* (26 March 1999), p. E1.

Brenner, Marie. *Great Dames: What I Learned from Older Women*. New York: Random House, 2000.

Breuer, Josef, and Sigmund Freud. *Studies on Hysteria. Standard Edition of the Complete Psychological Works of Sigmund Freud (S.E.)*, 24 vols. Ed. J. Strachey, vol. 2 (1900). London: Hogarth, 1953–1974, pp. 1–309.

Browning, Frank. *The Culture of Desire: Paradox and Perversity in Gay Lives Today*. New York: Modern Library, 1994.

Brownmiller, Susan. *Against Our Will: Men, Women, and Rape*. New York: Bantam, 1976.

Brzezinski, Zbigniew K. *The Soviet Bloc: Unity and Conflict*. Cambridge, Mass.: Harvard University Press, 1960.

Bunuel, Luis (Director) *Belle du Jour*. (Motion Picture). London: Warner Home Video, 2000 [1967].

Camus, Albert. *The Fall*. New York: Knopf, 1957.

Canetti, Elias. *Crowds and Power [Masse und Macht]*. New York: Continuum, 1972 [1960].

———. *The Torch in My Ear*. New York: Farrar Straus and Giroux, 1982 [1980].

Caruso, Fred (Producer) and David Lynch (Director). *Blue Velvet* (Motion Picture). Santa Monica, Ca.: De Laurentiis Entertainment Group, 1986.

Chasseuet-Smirgel, Janine. *Creativity and Perversion*. New York: Norton Books, 1984.

Cheever, John. "Journals." *New Yorker* (21 January 1991) 66:28–40.

Chodorow, Nancy. *Femininities, Masculinities, Sexualities: Freud and Beyond*. Lexington: University of Kentucky Press, 1994.

Coen, Stanley J. *Between Author and Reader: A Psychoanalytic Approach to Writing and Reading*. New York: Columbia University Press, 1994.

Connell, R. W. "Drumming Up the Wrong Tree: Men's Movement," *Tikkun* (January-February 1992) 7:31–36.

Coolidge, Olivia. *Edith Wharton 1862–1937*. New York: Scribner, 1964.

Covey, Steven, R. *The Seven Habits of Highly Effective People: Powerful Lessons in Personal Change*. New York: Fireside/Simon and Schuster, 1990.

Csikszentmihalyi, Mihaly. *The Evolving Self: A Psychology for the Third Millenium*. New York: Harper Perennial, 1993.

———. *Flow: The Psychology of Optimal Experience*. New York: HarperCollins, 1990.

Cunningham, Michael. *The Hours*. New York: Farrar Straus and Giroux, 1998.

Daldry, Stephen (Director) and Lee Hall (Writer). *Billy Elliot* (Motion Picture). Universal City, Ca.: Universal Studios, 2000.

Dalton, Dennis. "Dostoevsky's Grand Inquisitor." In *Power Over People: Classical and Modern Political Theory*, Great Courses on Tape, Part II. Teaching Company, 1998.

De Beauvoir, Simone. *The Second Sex*. New York: Knopf, 1953.

De St. Jorre, John. "The Unmasking of O." *New Yorker* (1 August 1994) 70:42–50.

Diamond, M., and Sigmundson, H. K. "Sex Reassignment at Birth: Long-Term Review and Clinical Implications." *Archives of Pediatric and Adolescent Medicine* (1997) 151:298–304.

Doonan, Simon. " 'Girl' Just Wants to have Fun." *New York Times*, Dec. 28, 1997.

Dostoyevsky, Fyodor. "The Legend of the Grand Inquisitor." In *The Brothers Karamazov*. Trans. and intro. David McDuff. London and New York: Penguin [1880], 1993, chap. 5, book 5, pp. 283–304.

Eissler, Kurt. "Notes on Problems of Technique in the Psychoanalytic Treatment of Adolescents: With Some Remarks on the Perversions." In *Psychoanalytic Study of the Child* (1958) 13:223–254.

Ellenberger, Henri. *The Discovery of the Unconscious*. New York: Basic Books, 1970.

Elroy, James. *My Dark Places: An L.A. Crime Memoir*. New York: Vintage/Random House, 1997 [1996].

Emde, Robert. "Fantasy and Beyond: A Current Development Perspective on Freud's 'Creative Writers and Day-Dreaming,' " *On Freud's "Creative Writers and Day-Dreaming,"* ed. Ethel S. Person, Peter Fonagy, and Servulo Figueira. New Haven, Conn.: Yale University Press, 1995, pp. 133–163.

Emerson, Ralph Waldo. "Self Reliance." In *Emerson's Essays*. Intro. Irwin Edman. New York: Harper Collophon, 1926.

Epstein, Cynthia. "The Major Myth of the Woman's Movement." *Dissent* (Fall 1999), p. 85.

Evans, Nicholas. *The Horse Whisperer*. New York: Bantam, 1995.

Faderman, Lillian. *Odd Girls and Twilight Lovers: A History of Lesbian Life in Twentieth Century America*. New York: Columbia University Press, 1991.

Fairbairn, W. R. D. *An Object-Relations Theory of Personality*. New York: Basic Books, 1952.

Faludi, Susan. *Stiffed: The Betrayal of the American Man*. New York: Morrow, 2000.

Farmer, Richard, as told to Rebecca Gooch, "Atlas Drugged," in *Maxim for Men*, June 1999, pp. 95–98.

Fiedler, Leslie. *Love and Death in the American Novel*. Rev. ed. New York: Stein and Day, 1986 [1960].

Fitzgerald, F. Scott. *Tender Is the Night*. New York: Scribner, 1934.

Flaubert, Gustave. *The Letters of Gustave Flaubert 1830–1857*. Selected, ed., and trans. by Francis Steegmuller. Cambridge, Mass.: Belknap Press of Harvard University Press, 1980 [1977].

Flynn, Laurie J. "Survey on Women's Role in Silicon Valley." *New York Times* (23 April 2001).

Foucault, Michael. *The History of Sexuality*, Vol. 1. New York: Random House, 1978.

Foushee, H. Clayton, and Robert L. Helmreich. "Group Interaction and Flight Crew Performance." In *Human Factors in Aviation*. Ed. E. L. Wiener and D. C. Nagel. New York: Academic Press, pp. 189–227.

French, Marilyn. *Beyond Power: On Women, Men, and Morals*. New York: Ballantine, 1985.

Freud, Anna. "Beating Fantasies and Daydreams" in *The Writings of Anna Freud*, Vol. 1 (1922–1935). Madison, Conn.: International Universities Press, 1974.

Freud, Sigmund. *Letters of Sigmund Freud*. Selected and ed. by Ernst L. Freud. New York: Basic Books, 1960.

———. *An Autobiographical Study*. New York: W. W. Norton, 1935.

———. *The Standard Edition of the Complete Psychological Works of Sigmund Freud* (S.E.), 24 vols. Ed. and trans. J. Strachey. London: Hogarth Press, [1924, 1925] 1974 20:1–73.

———. "Analysis Terminable and Interminable." S.E. (1937) 23:252–253.

———. "Beyond the Pleasure Principle." S.E. 1 (1920) 18:1–64.

———. "Creative Writers and Day-Dreaming." S.E. ([1907], 1908) 9:141–154.

———. "Dostoyevsky and Parricide." S.E. (1928 [1927]) 21:168–196.

———. "The Economic Problem of Masochism." S.E. (1924) 19:155–170.

———. "Femininity." S.E. (1922) 22:112–135.

———. "The Future of an Illusion." S.E. (1927) 21:3–56.

———. "Group Psychology and the Analysis of the Ego." S.E. (1921) 18:67–143.

———. "Inhibitions, Symptoms, and Anxiety." S.E. (1926) 20:75–175.

———. "The Interpretation of Dreams." S.E. (1900) 4:1–338 and 5:339–627.

———. "Observations on Transference Love." S.E. (1915) 12:149–157.

———. "Some Psychical Consequences of the Anatomical Distinction between the Sexes." S.E. (1925) 19:241–258.

Fried, Joseph. "Following Up: No More Dramas for a 'Dull' Mr. and Mrs.," *New York Times* (10 December 2000), section 1, p. 57.

Friedman, Richard and Jennifer Downey. "Biology and the Oedipus Complex." *Psychoanalytic Quarterly* (1995) 64:234–264.

Friedrich, Otto. *City of Nets: A Portrait of Hollywood in the 1940s*. New York: Harper and Row, [1986], 1987.

Fromm, Erich. *The Heart of Man: Its Genius for Good and Evil*. New York, Evanston, and London: Knopf, 1964.

Furman, Erna. *Self-Control and Mastery in Early Childhood: Helping Young Children Grow*. Madison, Conn.: International Universities Press, 1998.

———. "Child's Work: Developmental Aspects of the Capacity to Work and Enjoy It." In *Work and Its Inhibitions: Psychoanalytic Essays*. New York: International Universities Press, 1997, pp. 3–18.

Gabler, Neal. "Male Bonding: Why Is James Bond So Popular? He's a Baby Boomer Writ Large." *Modern Maturity* (January-February 2000), pp. 52ff.

Gagnon, John, and William Simon. *Sexual Conduct: The Social Sources of Human Sexuality*. Chicago: Aldine, 1973.

Galbraith, John Kenneth. *The Anatomy of Power*. Boston: Houghton Mifflin, 1983.

Gallagher, Hugh Gregory. *FDR's Splendid Deception*. New York: Dodd, Mead, 1985.

Gardner, Howard. *Creating Minds*. New York: Basic Books, 1993.

Gardner, Ralph Jr. "Class Struggle on Park Avenue." *New York Magazine* (14 June 1999) 32:22ff.

Gaylin, Willard. *Feelings: Our Vital Signs*. New York: Harper and Row, 1979.

Ginsberg, George, William Frosch, and Theodore Shapiro. "The New Impotence." In *Archives of General Psychiatry* (1972) 26:218–220.

Glazer, Ellen Sarasohn. "My Money My Life: Cash in Time, Gone with the Wind." *New York Times* (13 February 2000), 3, section 3, p. 12.

Goetz, Ruth Goodman and Augustus Goetz. *The Heiress* (typescript). Dramatists' Play Service, 1975 [1946].

Goode, Erica. "For Good Health, It Helps to Be Rich and Important." *New York Times* (1 June 1999), p. F1.

Gorm, Elliott J. *The Manly Art: Bare-Knuckle Prize Fighting in America.* Ithaca, N.Y.: Cornell University Press, 1986.

Gornick, Vivian. "*The Second Sex* at Fifty," *Dissent* (Fall 1999), pp. 69–72.

Gosse, Edmund. "The Mayor-elect of Rye." In *Henry James: Interviews and Recollections.* Ed. Norman Page. New York: St. Martin's Press, 1984 [1940].

Graf, Max. "Reminiscences of Professor Sigmund." *Psychoanalytic Quarterly* (1942):31(4) 474–475.

Graham, Katharine. *Personal History.* New York: Knopf, 1997.

Grosskurth, Phyllis. *The Secret Ring: Freud's Inner Circle and the Politics of Psychoanalysis.* Reading, Mass.: Addison-Wesley, 1991.

Gussow, Max. "Mario Puzo, Author Who Made 'The Godfather' a World Addiction, Is Dead at 78." *New York Times* (3 July 1999), p. B7.

Guttman, Herbert G., and Ira Berlin. *Power and Culture: Essays on the American Working Class.* New York: Pantheon, 1987.

Hardwick, Elizabeth. *Seduction and Betrayal: Women and Literature.* New York: Vintage, 1974.

Harris, Colin, moderator. "Who Needs Men? Addressing the Prospect of a Matriarchal Millennium." *Harper's Magazine* (June 1999) 298:33–42.

Haskell, Molly. *Holding My Own in No Man's Land: Women and Men and Film and Feminists.* New York: Oxford University Press, 1977.

———. "Swaggering Sexuality before the Mandated Blush." *New York Times* (13 May 2001) sec. 2A, p. 15.

Helmreich, R. L., J. A. Wilhelm, S. E. Gregorich, and T. R. Chivster. "Preliminary Results from Evaluation of Cockpit Resource Management Training: Performance Ratings of Flight Crews." *Aviation, Space, and Environmental Medicine,* 1990, 61:576–579.

Hillman, James. *Kinds of Power: A Guide to Its Intelligent Uses.* New York: Currency/Doubleday, 1995.

Hirigoyen, Marie-France. *Stalking the Soul: Emotional Abuse and the Erosion of Identity.* Canada: Helen Marks Books. Paris: Éditions La Découverte et Syros, 2000 [1998].

Hirschmüller, Albrecht. *The Life and Work of Josef Breuer: Physiology and Psychoanalysis.* New York: New York University Press, 1989.

Holy Bible: Containing the Old and New Testaments. New Revised Standard Version. New York: Oxford University Press, 1989.

Horner, Althea. *The Wish for Power and the Fear of Having It.* Northvale, N.J.: Jason Aronson, 1995 [1989].

Horney, Karen. "The Denial of the Vagina: A Contribution to the Problem of the Genital Anxieties Specific to Women." *International Journal of Psycho-Analysis* (1933) 14:57–70.

———. "The Dread of Women: Observations on a Specific Difference in the Dread Felt by Men and by Women Respectively for the Opposite Sex." *International Journal of Psycho-Analysis* (1932) 13:348–360.

———. "The Flight from Womanhood: The Masculinity Complex in Women, as Viewed by Men and by Women." *International Journal of Psycho-Analysis* (1932) 7:324–339.

———. "On the Genesis of the Castration Complex in Women." *International Journal of Psychoanalysis* (1924) 5:50–65.

Horowitz, Craig. "Time-Bomb Genes." *New York Magazine* (8 February 1999) 32 (5):28ff.

Huxley, Aldous. *The Devils of Loudun,* paperback edition. New York: Carroll and Graf, 1986 [1952].

Ibsen, Henrik. *A Doll's House.* New York: Appleton, 1889.

Ironson, G., A. LaPerriere, M. Antoni, P. Ohearn, N. Schneiderman, N. Klimas, and M. A. Fletcher. "Changes in Immune and Psychological Measures as a Function of Anticipation and Reaction to News of HIV-1 Antibody Status." *Psychosomatic Medicine* (1990) 52(3):247–70.

Isaacs, Susan. *Long Time No See*. New York: HarperCollins, 2001.

Jacobs, R. L. and D. C. McClelland. "Moving Up the Corporate Ladder: A Longitudinal Study of the Leadership Motive Pattern and Managerial Success in Men and Women." *Consulting Psychology Journal* (Winter 1994), pp. 32–34.

James, Henry. "The Beast in the Jungle." In *The Altar of the Dead: The Beast in the Jungle, The Birthplace, and Other Tales*. New York: Scribner, 1909.

————. *Interviews and Recollections*. Ed. Norman Page. New York: St. Martin's Press, 1984 [1940].

James, William. *The Varieties of Religious Experience: A Study in Human Nature*. New York: New American Library, a Mentor Book, 1958, [1902].

Janeway, Elizabeth. *The Powers of the Weak*. New York: Knopf, 1980.

Jones, Ernest. "The Early Development of Female Sexuality." *International Journal of Psychoanalysis* (1927) 8:459–472.

————. "Early female sexuality." *International Journal of Psychoanalysis* (1935) 16:263–275.

————. *The Life and Work of Sigmund Freud*, 3 vols. New York: Basic Books, 1957.

————. "The Phallic Phase." *International Journal of Psychoanalysis* (1933) 14: 1–33.

Jung, Carl. *Memories, Dreams, Reflections*. London: Routledge and Kegan Paul, 1963.

Kagan, Jerome. *The Nature of the Child*. New York: Basic Books, 1984.

Karas, Joya. *Music in Terezin*. New York: Beaufort Books, 1941–46.

Kasander, Kees (Producer) and Peter Greenaway (Director and Writer). *The Cook, The Thief, His Wife and Her Lover* (Motion Picture). Troy, MI: Allarts Cook, Erato Films and Film Inc., 1989.

Kennedy, Paul. *The Rise and Fall of the Great Powers*. New York: Vintage, 1987.

Kernberg, Otto F. *Aggression in Personality Disorders and Perversion*. New Haven: Yale University Press, 1992.

————. *Ideology, Conflict, and Leadership in Groups and Organizations*. New Haven: Yale University Press, 1998.

————. *Internal World and External Reality*. New York: Jason Aronson, 1985.

Kerr, Walter. *Tragedy and Comedy*. New York: Simon and Schuster, 1967.

Klein, Dennis. *The Jewish Origins of the Psychoanalytic Movement*. Chicago: University of Chicago Press, 1985.

Klerman, Gerald L. "Testing Analytic Hypotheses: Are Personality Attributes Predisposed to Depression?" In *Psychoanalysis: Critical Explorations in Contemporary Theory and Practice*. Ed. A. M. Jacobson and D. X. Parmalee. New York: Brunner/Mazel, 1982.

Kliegerman, Charles. "Panel Report on 'Creativity'" (Twenty-seventh Annual Psychoanalytic Congress, Vienna). *International Journal of Psychoanalysis* (1971) 54:21–30.

Klinger, Eric. *Daydreaming: Using Waking Fantasy and Imagery for Self-Knowledge and Creativity*. Los Angeles: Tarcher, 1990.

Koestler, Arthur. *The Act of Creation*. New York: Viking Penguin, 1989 [1964].

Kohn, Alfie. "In Pursuit of Affluence at a High Price." *New York Times* (2 February 1999), p. F7.

Korda, Michael. *Another Life: A Memoir of Other People*. New York: Random House, 1999.

————. *Power: How to Get It, How to Use It*. New York: Random House, 1975.

Krakauer, Jon. *Into the Wild*. New York: Anchor, 1996.

Kuczynski, Alex. "Oprah, Coast to Coast: A Phenomenon Struts Her Stuff on the Newsstands," *New York Times* (2 October 2000), p. C1.

La Barre, Frances. *On Moving and Being Moved: Nonverbal Behavior in Clinical Practice*. Hillsdale, N.J.: The Analytic Press, 2001.

La Ferla, Ruth. "Like Magic, Witchcraft Charms Teenagers." *New York Times* (13 February 2000), section 9, pp. 1–2.

Lahr, John. "Making Willie Loman: A. Miller's Death of a Salesman Notebooks." *New Yorker* (25 January 1999) 74:42–49.

———. "The Whirlwind: How Kenneth Tynan Reinvented Theatre Criticism—and Himself." *New Yorker* (7 August 2000) 76: 42–47.

Lasch, Christopher. *The Culture of Narcissism*. New York: Norton, 1978.

Lawner, Peter. "Trust and Trusting in Love Relations." In *Love: Psychoanalytic Perspectives*. Ed. Judith Lasky and Helen Silverman. New York: New York University Press, 1988, pp. 133–146.

Lear, Jonathan. *Open Minded: Working Out the Logic of the Soul*. Cambridge, Mass.: Harvard University Press, 1999.

Lee, Felicia R. "Coping: Looking for Mr. Goodbucks." *New York Times* (6 March 2000), section 14, p. 1.

———. "A Feminist Survivor with the Eyes of a Child." *New York Times* (4 July 2000), p. E1.

Leo, John. "The 'Modern Primitives.'" *U.S. News and World Report* (31 July 1995) 119: 16.

Levinson, Daniel J. *The Seasons of a Man's Life*, with C. N. Darrow, F. B. Klein, M. II. Levinson, and B. McKee. New York: Knopf, 1978.

Lewis, Michael. "The Artist in the Gray Flannel Pajamas: Who the New American Workers Think They Are." *New York Times Magazine* (5 March 2000) 6:45–48.

Lichtenstein, Heinz. "Identity and Sexuality: A Study of their Interrelationship in Man." *Journal of the American Psychoanalytic Association* (1961) 9: 179–260.

Lindholm, Charles. *Charisma*. Cambridge, Mass.: Basil Blackwell, 1990.

Lorenz, Konrad. *The Foundations of Ethology*. New York: Springer, 1981.

Loughery, John. *The Other Side of Silence. Men's Lives and Gay Identities—A Twentieth-Century History*. New York: Holt/John Macrae, 1999.

Maccoby, Michael. *The Gamesman: The New Corporate Leaders*. New York: Simon and Schuster, 1976.

MacInnes, John. *The End of Masculinity: The Confusion of Sexual Genesis and Sexual Difference in Modern Society*. Buckingham and Philadelphia: Open University Press, 1998.

Mack, John. "Power, Powerlessness, and Empowerment in Psychotherapy." *Psychiatry* (1994) 57: 179–199.

Malcolm X and Alex Haley. *The Autobiography of Malcolm X*. New York: Ballantine 1999 [1965].

Malraux, Andre. *Man's Fate*. New York: Vintage Books 1969, [1934].

Marcus, Stephen. "Culture and Psychoanalysis." *Partisan Review* (1982), pp. 224–252.

Marshall, Alan (Producer) and Paul Verhoeven (Director). *Basic Instinct* (Motion Picture). Santa Monica, Ca.: Artisan Home Entertainment. 1998. [1992].

Maslow, Abraham H. "The Need to Know and the Fear of Knowing." *Journal of General Psychology* (1963) 68: 111–125.

Masson, Jeffrey M. (trans. and ed.). *The Complete Letters of Sigmund Freud, to Wilhelm Fliess, 1887–1904*. Cambridge, Mass.: Belknap Press of Harvard University Press, 1985.

May, Rollo. *Love and Will*. New York: Norton, 1969.

———. *Power and Innocence: A Search for the Sources of Violence*. New York: W. W. Norton & Company, 1998 [1972].

McAdams, Dan P. *Intimacy: The Need to Be Close*. New York: Doubleday, 1989.

McCrohan, Donna. *The Honeymooners' Companion: The Kramdens and the Nortons Revisited*. New York: Workman, 1978.

McDougall, Joyce. *Plea for a Measure of Abnormality*. New York: International Universities Press, 1980.

McGregor, Douglas. *Leadership and Motivation*. Cambridge, Mass.: MIT Press, 1966.

Meissner, W. W. "The Self and the Principle of Work." In *Work and Its Inhibitions*. Ed. C. W. Socarides and Selma Kramer. New York: International Universities Press, 1997, pp. 35–60.

Merkin, Daphne. "The Black Season: Reflections of Life in an Institution." *New Yorker* (8 January 2001) 76: 32–39.

———. "Dreaming of Hitler." In *Dreaming of Hitler*. San Diego: Harvest/Harcourt Brace, 1997, pp. 346–363.

———. "Spanking: A Romance." In *Dreaming of Hitler*. San Diego: Harvest/Harcourt Brace, 1997, pp. 59–65.

Merton, Thomas. *The Seven Storey Mountain*. New York: Harcourt Brace Jovanovich/Trustees of the Merton Legacy Trust, 1976.

Messner, Michael A. *Power at Play: Sports and the Problem of Masculinity*. Boston: Beacon, 1992.

Milgram, Stanley. *Obedience to Authority*. New York: Harper and Row, 1974.

Millet, Kate. *Sexual Politics*. Garden City, N.Y.: Doubleday, 1970.

Mitchell, Burroughs. *The Education of an Editor*. Garden City, N.Y.: Doubleday, 1980.

Mitchell, Juliet. "Psychoanalysis and Feminism." In *Psychology of Society*. Ed. Richard Sennett. New York: Vintage, 1997, p. 364.

Modell, Arnold H. "Affects and the Complementarity of Biological and Historical Meaning." In *The Annual of Psychoanalysis*, vol. 6. New York: International Universities Press, 1978, pp. 167–180.

Money J., F. Schwartz, and V. C. Davis. "Adult Erotosexual Status and Fetal Hormonal Masculinization and De-Masculinization: 46 XX Congenital Virilizing Adrenal Hyperplasia and 46 XY Androgen-Insensitivity Syndrome Compared." *Psychoneuroendocrinology* (1984) 9: 405–515.

Moore, Susanna. *In the Cut*. New York: Plume, 1999 [1995].

Moore, Thomas. Afterword to Marie-France Hirigoyen, *Stalking the Soul: Emotional Abuse and the Erosion of Identity*. Canada: Helen Marks and Paris: Éditions La Découverte et Syros, 2000, [1998].

Morgenthau, Hans. "The Demands of Prudence." In *Politics and the Twentieth Century: Volume 3, The Restoration of American Politics*. Chicago: University of Chicago Press, 1962.

———. "Love and Power." In *Politics in the Twentieth Century: The Restoration of American Politics*, Vol. 3. Chicago: University of Chicago Press, 1962.

———. *Truth and Power: Essays of a Decade, 1960–1970*. New York: Praeger, 1970.

———. *Scientific Man versus Power Politics*. Chicago: University of Chicago Press, 1946.

Morgenthau, Hans, and Ethel S. Person. "The Roots of Narcissism," *Partisan Review* (1978) 45(3):337–347.

Morrison, Toni. *The Bluest Eye*. New York: Penguin, 1970.

Newman, Katherine S. *Declining Fortunes: The Withering of the American Dream*. New York: Basic Books, 1993.

Noshpitz, Joseph. "Disturbances in Early Adolescent Development." In *The Course of Life*, Vol. 2. Ed. Stanley I. Greenspan and George H. Pollack. Maryland: U.S. Department of Health and Human Services, 1979, pp. 309–356.

O'Donnell, Damian (Director) and Khan-Din, Ayub (Writer). *East is East* (Motion Picture). Los Angeles: Miramax Films, 2000.

O'Donnell, Lynn (Producer) and Terry Zwigoff (Producer and Director). *Crumb*. (Motion Picture). Culver City, Ca.: Columbia TriStar Home Video, 1994.

O'Neill, Eugene. "The Iceman Cometh." In *Best American Plays: Third Series, 1945–1951*. Ed. John Gassner. New York: Crown, 1963, pp. 164–165.

Olds, Sharon. "The Takers."

Ornstein, Anna. "The Dread to Repeat: Comments on the Working-through Process in Psychoanalysis." *Journal of the American Psychoanalytic Association* (1991) 39 (2): 377–398.

Pace, Eric. "Anne Morrow Lindbergh. Dead at 94: Champion of Flight and Woman's Concerns." *New York Times* (8 February 2001), p. A29.

Paglia, Camille. "At Home with Mario Puzo: It All Comes Back to Family." *New York Times* (8 May 1997), p. C1.

Paley, Vivian Gussin. *The Boy Who Would Be a Helicopter: The Uses of Storytelling in the Classroom*. Cambridge, Mass.: Harvard University Press, 1990.

Parker, Robert. *Double Deuce*. New York: Berkeley, 1993.

Pascal, Blaise. *Pensées*. Intro. by T. S. Eliot. New York: Dutton, 1958.

Perkins, Maxwell. Intro. in Thomas Wolfe, *Look Homeward, Angel*. New York: Scribner/Simon and Schuster, 1957.

Perry, Bernice. *New York Times Magazine* (8 December 1996), p. 44.

Perry, Samuel, Lawrence Jacobsberg, and C. Card. "Severity of Psychiatric Symptoms After HIV Testing." *American Journal of Psychiatry* (May 1993) 150:775–779.

Person, Ethel S. *By Force of Fantasy: How We Make Our Lives*. New York: Basic Books, 1995.

———. "Change Moments in Therapy." In *Changing Ideas in a Changing World: The Revolution in Psychoanalysis—Essays in Honor of Arnold Cooper*. Ed. Peter Fonagy and Robert Michels. London and New York: Karnac, 2000.

———. *Dreams of Love and Fateful Encounters: The Power of Romantic Passion*. New York: Norton, 1988.

———. "The Influence of Values in Psychoanalysis: The Case of Female Psychology." In *Psychiatric Update: The American Psychiatric Association Annual Review*, vol. 2. Ed. Lester Grinspoon. Washington D.C.: American Psychiatric Press, 1983, pp. 36–50.

———. "Male Sexuality and Power." *Psychoanalytic Inquiry* (1986) 6:3–25. Reprinted in *The Sexual Century*. New Haven: Yale University Press, 1999.

———. "The Omni-Available Woman and Lesbian Sex: Two Fantasy Themes and Their Relationships to the Male Development Experience." In *The Psychology of Men*. Ed. Gerald Fogel, Frederick Lane, and Robert S. Liebert. New York: Basic Books, 1986, pp. 236–259.

———. "The Powers of the Strong and the Powers of the Weak." In *At the Threshold of the Millennium: A Selection of the Proceedings of the Conference*, Vol. III. Ed. Maria Rosa Fdort Brescia and Moises Lemlij. Lima, Peru: SIDEA, 1999.

———. *The Sexual Century*. New Haven: Yale University Press, 1999.

———. "Women Working: Fears of Failure, Deviance, and Success." *Journal of the American Academy of Psychoanalysis* (1982) 10:67–84.

———. "Working Mothers: Impact on the Self, the Couple, and the Children." In *The Psychology of Today's Woman: New Psychoanalytic Visions*. Ed. D. Cantor and T. Bernay. New Jersey: The Analytic Press, 1986.

Pommer, Erich (Producer) and von Sternberg, Josef (Director). *The Blue Angel* (Motion Picture). Germany: Pacific Film Archive, 1930.

Porter, Katherine Anne. "Orpheus in Purgatory." In *The Collected Essays*. New York: Dell, 1973, pp. 53–57.

Priestley, J. B. *Literature and Western Man*. New York: Harper, 1960.

Puzo, Mario. *The Fortunate Pilgrim*. New York: Random House/Ballantine, 1997.

———. *The Godfather*. New York: Penguin, 1978 [1969].

Quinn, Sally. Quoted in "Life of the Party: Journalist/Hostess/Washington Insider Sally Quinn Issues a Manners Manual." In *W* (November 1997), pp. 62–64.

Quindlen, Anna. *Black and Blue*. London: Arrow, 1999.

Rahv, Philip. *The Myth and the Powerhouse: Essays on Literature and Ideas*. New York: Noonday, 1966 [1949].

Ricapito, Maria. " 'Girl' Just Wants to Have Fun." *New York Times* (28 December 1997), section 9, p. 2.

Rich, Adrienne. *On Lies, Secrets, and Silence: Selected Prose 1966–1978*. New York: Norton, 1979.

Rieff, Philip. *Freud: The Mind of the Moralist*. New York: Doubleday/Anchor, 1961.

Rilke, Rainer Maria. *Letters to a Young Poet*. Trans. M. D. Herter. New York: Norton, 1954.

Roazen, Paul. *Freud and His Followers*. New York: New American Library, 1971.

Robin et al., as told to Jennie L. Frankel, Terry Maxine Frankel, and Joanne Parrent. *You'll Never Make Love in This Town Again.* Beverly Hills, Ca.: Dove, 1995.

Robinson, Paul. *The Modernization of Sex.* New York: Harper and Row, 1976.

Rodell, Susanna. "Lives; Why I Really Learned to Ride." *The New York Times* (10 May 1998), section 6, p. 66.

Roiphe, Anne. *Lovingkindess.* New York: Summit, 1987.

Rosenthal, A. M. *Thirty-Eight Witnesses: The Kitty Genovese Case.* Los Angeles: University of California Press, 1999.

Ross, Lillian. *Here but not Here: My Life with William Shawn and The New Yorker.* New York: Random House, 1998.

Ross, Nathan. "The Primacy of Genitality in the Light of Ego Psychology." *Journal of the American Psychoanalytic Association* (1970) 18:267–280.

Rousseau, Jean-Jacques. *The Confessions of Jean-Jacques Rousseau.* New York: Modern Library, 1945.

Roustang, François. "Dire Mastery: Discipleship from Freud to Lacan." Trans. Ned Lukacher. Washington, D.C.: American Psychiatric Press, 1986 [1976].

Rowling, J. K. *Harry Potter and the Sorcerer's Stone.* New York: Levine, 1997.

Rubin, Gretchen Kraft. *Power, Money, Fame, Sex: A User's Guide.* New York: Pocket Books, 2000.

Rubin, Harriet. *The Princessa: Machiavelli for Women.* New York: Currency/Doubleday, 1997.

Rubinfine, David. "Problems of Identity." *Journal of the American Psychoanalytic Association* (1958) 6:131–142.

Russell, Bertrand. *Power: A New Social Analysis.* New York: Norton, 1938.

Sarton, May. *At Seventy: A Journal.* New York: Norton, 1984.

Schulman, Michael. "On the Problem of the Id in Psychoanalytic Theory." *International Journal of Psychoanalysis* (1987) 68:161–174.

Schorske, Carl E. "Politics and Patricide." In *Le Fin de Siècle.* Vienna and New York: Knopf, 1980.

Schumpeter, Joseph. *Capitalism, Socialism, and Democracy.* New York: Harper and Row, 1954.

Seebohm, Caroline. *No Regrets: The Life of Marietta Tree.* New York: Simon and Schuster, 1997.

Sennett, Richard. *Authority.* New York: Knopf, 1980.

Sexton J. B., E. J. Thomas, and R. L. Helmreich. "Error, Stress, and Teamwork in Medicine and Aviation: Cross-Sectional Surveys." *British Medical Journal* (2000) Vol. 320 (7237): 745–749.

Shaw, George Bernard. *The Quintessence of Ibsenism.* New York: Hill and Wang, 1922.

Shengold, Leonard. *"The Boy Will Come to Nothing!" Freud's Ego Ideal and Freud as Ego Ideal.* New Haven: Yale University Press, 1993.

Showalter, Elaine. "The Death of Lady (Novelist): Wharton's House of Mirth." In *Representations* (Winter 1985) 9:133–149. Also reprinted in *House of Mirth, Edith Wharton.* Ed. Elizabeth Ammons. New York: Norton, 1999, pp. 357–372.

Shulevitz, Judith. "The Fall of Man." (Review of *Stiffed*). *New York Times Book Review* (8 October 1999) 104: 8–9.

Simon, Bennett. "The Power of the Wish and the Wish for Power: A Discussion of Power and Psychoanalysis." *Psychoanalytic Inquiry* (1986) 6: 119–131.

Singer, Jerome. *The Inner World of Daydreaming.* New York: Harper and Row, 1979.

Sontag, Susan. "Fascinating Fascism." In *Under the Sign of Saturn.* New York: Anchor/Doubleday, 1980.

Spitz, René. *No and Yes: On the Genesis of Human Communication.* Madison, Conn.: International Universities Press, 1957.

Steegmuller, Francis (ed. and trans.). *The Letters of Gustave Flaubert 1830–1857.* Cambridge, Mass.: T. B. Belknap Press of Harvard University Press and London, England, 1980, [1977].

Steele, Dawn. *They Can Kill You But They Can't Eat You: Lessons From the Front.* New York: Pocket Books, 1994.

Stern, Dan. *The Interpersonal World of the Infant: A View from Psychoanalysis and Developmental Psychology*. New York: Basic Books, 1984.

Stoessinger, John G. *Might of Nations: World Politics in Our Time*. New York: Random House, 1965 [1961].

Storr, Anthony. *The Dynamics of Creation*. New York: Penguin, 1991 [1972].

———. "Psychoanalysis and Creativity." In *Churchill's Black Dog, Kakfka's Mice, and Other Phenomena of the Human Mind*. New York: Grove, 1988.

———. *Solitude: A Return to the Self*. New York: The Free Press, 1988.

Stratton-Porter, Gene. *A Girl of the Limberlost*. New York: Doubleday, 1910.

Sulloway, Frank. *Born to Rebel: Birth Order, Family Dynamics, and Creative Lives*. New York: Pantheon, 1996.

Szasz, Thomas. "Freud as Leader." *Antioch Review*, 1963.

Talbot, Toby. *Gone*. (Unpublished novel).

Tannen, Deborah. *You Just Don't Understand: Women and Men in Conversation*. New York: Ballantine, 1989.

Tarnow, Eugene. "Self-Destructive Obedience in the Airplane Cockpit and the Concept of Obedience Optimization." In *Obedience to Authority: Current Perspectives on the Milgram Paradigm*. Ed. T. Blass. Hillsdale, N.J.: Lawrence Erlbaum, 2000, pp. 111–123.

Thomas, Alexander and Stella Chess. *Temperament and Development*. New York: Brunner/Mazel, 1977.

Thomas, Charles H. "Zimmerman's Bookstore." In *First History/The Old Thompson Block: A Torch of Bohemia*. *Filson Club History Quarterly* (October 1997), pp. 415–421.

Thompson, Clara. "Some Effects of the Derogatory Attitude Towards Female Sexuality." *Psychiatry* (1950) 13:249–354.

Tiger, Lionel. *The Decline of the Male*. New York: Golden Books, 1999.

Timberg, Robert. *The Nightingale's Song*. New York: Touchstone, 1996.

Time Out New York (4–11 February 1999), p. 14.

Trevathan, Wenda. *Human Birth: An Evolutionary Perspective*. New York: De Gruyter, 1987.

Truth, Sojourner. *The Narrative of Sojourner Truth*. Ed. Henry Louis Gates, Jr. New York: Schomberg Library of Nineteenth Century Black Women Writers, 1991.

Udwin, Leslie (Producer) and Damian O'Donnell (Director). *East is East* (Motion Picture). Based on the play by Ayub Khan-din. Burbank, Ca.: Miramax Home Entertainment, 2000.

Veblen, Thorstein. *The Theory of the Leisure Class: An Economic Study of Institutes*. New York: Macmillan, 1899.

Vidal, Gore. *Palimpsest: A Memoir*. New York: Penguin, 1995.

Viorst, Judith. *Imperfect Control: Our Lifelong Struggle with Power and Surrender*. New York: Simon and Schuster, 1998.

Walpole, Hugh. "James's Friendships." In *Henry James, Interviews and Recollections*. Ed. Norman Page. New York: St. Martin's Press, 1984 [1940].

Ward, Geoffrey C. *Before the Trumpet: Young Franklin Roosevelt*. New York: Harper and Row, 1985.

Webster, Richard. *Why Freud Was Wrong: Sin, Science, and Psychoanalysis*. New York: Basic Books, 1995.

Webster, Noah. *New International Dictionary of the English Language, 2nd edition*. Springfield, Mass.: G&C Merriam, 1951.

Weeks, Jeffrey. "Movements of Affirmation: Sexual Meanings and Homosexual Identities." *Radical History Review* (1970) 20: 164–179.

———. *Sexuality*. New York: Routledge, 1986.

Weinraub, Bernard. "Dawn Steele, Studio Chief and Producer, Dies at 51." *New York Times* (22 December 1997), p. B6.

Wertmuller, Lina. (Director) *Swept Away* (Motion Picture). New York: Axon Video, 1989 [1975].

Wharton, Edith. *A Backward Glance*. New York: Macmillan, 1964, [1933].

White, Robert W. "Motivation Reconsidered: The Concept of Competence." *Psychological Review* (1959): 66(5).

Whitehead, Alfred North. *Adventures of Ideas*. New York: Macmillan, 1949.

Whitney, John O. and Tina Packer. *Power Plays: Shakespeare's Lessons in Leadership and Management*. New York: Simon and Schuster, 2000.

Williams, Alex. "To Have and Have More." *New York Magazine* (14 June 1999) 32, pp. 32–35.

Wills, Gary. "A Guy I Like." *New York Review of Books* (20 July 1978), p. xxv.

———. *Certain Trumpets: The Call of Leaders*. New York: Simon and Schuster, 1994.

Winnicott, D. W. "Aggression and Its Roots." In *Deprivation and Delinquency*. Ed. Clare Winnicott, Kay Soers, and Madeline Davis. London and New York: Tavistock, 1984, pp. 84–99.

———. "Aggression in Relation to Emotional Development." In *Collected Papers: Through Paediatrics to Psychoanalysis*. New York: Brunner/Maze [1950–1955], 1984, pp. 204–218.

———. "The Capacity to Be Alone." In *The Maturational Process and the Facilitating Environment*. New York: International Universities Press, 1965 [1958].

Wolfe, Thomas. *Look Homeward, Angel*. New York: Scribner, 1957.

Wood, Joe. "Up from Brownsville: Alfred Kazin/Life and Work." *Dissent* (Fall 1998), pp. 119–127.

Yalom, Irvin. "Mama and the Meaning of Life." *Tales of Psychotherapy*. New York: Basic Books, 1999.

Zaleznick, Abraham. "Power and Leadership in Complex Organizations." In *On Freud's Psychology and Analysis of the Ego*. Ed. Ethel Person. Hillsdale, N.J.: The Analytic Press, 2001.

Zilbergeld, Bernard. *Male Sexuality*. New York: Bantam Books, 1978.

Index